MONROEVILLE PUBLIC LIBRARY
4000 GATEWAY CAMPUS BLVD
MONROEVILLE, PA 15146

# skeletons in the closet

tobin t. buhk and
stephen d. cohle, md

# skeletons in the closet

## stories from the county morgue

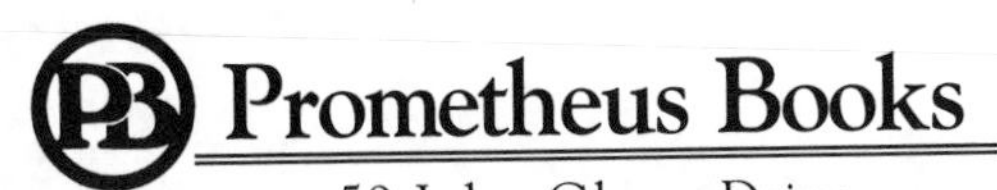

Prometheus Books
59 John Glenn Drive
Amherst, New York 14228-2119

MONROEVILLE
PUBLIC LIBRARY
APR 24 '08

Published 2008 by Prometheus Books

*Skeletons in the Closet: Stories from the County Morgue.* Copyright © 2008 by Tobin T. Buhk and Stephen D. Cohle. All rights reserved. No part of this publication may be reproduced, stored in a retrieval system, or transmitted in any form or by any means, digital, electronic, mechanical, photocopying, recording, or otherwise, or conveyed via the Internet or a Web site without prior written permission of the publisher, except in the case of brief quotations embodied in critical articles and reviews.

Inquiries should be addressed to
Prometheus Books
59 John Glenn Drive
Amherst, New York 14228–2119
VOICE: 716–691–0133, ext. 210
FAX: 716–691–0137
WWW.PROMETHEUSBOOKS.COM

12 11 10 09 08     5 4 3 2 1

Library of Congress Cataloging-in-Publication Data

Buhk, Tobin T.
Skeletons in the closet : stories from the county morgue / by Tobin T. Buhk and Stephen D. Cohle.
p. cm.
Includes bibliographical references and index.
ISBN 978–1–59102–603–7
1. Forensic pathology. 2. Death—Causes. I. Cohle, Stephen D. II. Title.

RA1063.4.B85 2008
614'.1—dc22
2007051812

Printed in the United States on acid-free paper

# Contents

# *note on the text*

An asterisk denotes the first use of a pseudonym. In cases that did not lead to significant court action, or in cases that have not yet been completely adjudicated, or in cases where anonymity is in the interest of good taste, the authors created pseudonyms and in some instances altered nonessential details to preserve the anonymity of the victims. The forensic science, however, is unaltered.

# "moonlighting"

Kent County Morgue
Spectrum Hospital's Blodgett Campus
Early Winter 2006

The moonlight lights up the forest like lighting on a movie set and illuminates the snow carpet that covers the forest floor, bathing everything in hues of blue. Despite the hour (midnight), one can read a book outside. A good night to enjoy the snow, for soon, if one believes the forecast, the foot of snow on the ground will disappear, melted by the barrage of rain that will accompany temperatures in the forties. Tonight, though, the frigid temperatures and the slight wind chill the body and soul, like the touch of a very cold, cruel mistress.

A few shots of spirits or a few glasses of beer provide an added insulation against Mother Nature's cold caress. Liquid insulation and then speed: for many, particularly in Michigan's less populated northern counties, a typical mid-December Friday night.

It was for one young snowmobile rider.

A warm sensation, like a warm water bottle, filled his stomach and chest. The snowmobile's light bounced off the snow as he sped along the trail. He felt invincible on this mechanical Cyclops. Fifty miles per hour. More speed. Sixty. Faster. Sixty-five. More speed. Seventy. Faster. The light danced faster and faster—a wild, almost uncontrollable dance.

The crunching steel could be heard from a distance, *if* anyone was listening. And then the dancing light disappeared.

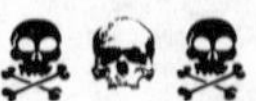

The sun has begun to rise and with it will come an unseasonably warm day in the forties—a warm contrast with the low twenties and endless volleys of freezing rain, sleet, and snow that has bombarded the area for days. Residents of West Michigan today will enjoy their first glimpse of the sun in weeks, and perhaps, with months of winter ahead, the last for some time.

It is a time when all things end and everything appears old. The deciduous trees have shed their leaves, and from the lobby of the hospital, the scene looks like the earth has flipped over and exposed the tree roots. The verdant grass has disappeared under a scalp of ice as if the earth's hair has turned white.

I waited in the lobby, anticipation rolling around my stomach like a stone. For eighteen months, I moonlighted as a high school teacher by week and a forensic pathology volunteer by weekend. Years of watching *Law & Order* and *CSI* motivated a potential career change and a fascination with forensics, which led me to the underworld of the Kent County Morgue. This morning, I would continue my education and reenter the morgue, motivated by a strange attraction pulling me back to this place. Like Persephone, I've eaten pomegranate in the underworld, and my time to return has come (my wife thinks I have a dark side). And like the Persephone of Greek myth, my foray into the underworld coincides with the onset of winter.

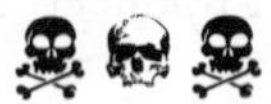

Dr. Stephen D. Cohle walks through the hospital lobby at about nine in the morning. In pale blue surgical scrubs and a blue T-shirt advertising "Yesterdog"—a local restaurant famous for its hotdogs—he looks like he's ready to begin prepping for surgery on the patient who waits for him a floor below.

Yet Dr. Cohle, known as "Doc" to his friends, cannot help this patient. It is not his job to discover what's wrong with this man's ticker or even to fix it. As Kent County's chief medical examiner, his job is to determine what caused the man's ticker to stop.

Dr. Cohle and I walk past the floral-patterned couches and easy chairs—the living room atmosphere of the lobby is complete with a Christmas tree decorated with small white bows—to a staircase and descend a few flights to the basement. Dr. Cohle moves through a cinder block–lined corridor to a security door labeled "Morgue." He punches in the key code required to enter the suite of rooms beyond this gray steel door, where he will meet this morning's patient.

Joel Talsma, the twenty-something autopsy assistant who will aid in the autopsy procedure this morning, sits munching on a bagel sandwich in the conference room alongside a deputy sheriff from Antrim County when Dr. Cohle arrives. Dr. Cohle serves as Kent County's chief medical examiner and forensic pathologist, but he also conducts autopsies for other counties, such as Antrim, that do not employ a forensic pathologist. Since Dr. Cohle's résumé contains over two decades of experience cracking some of the state's most vexing forensic mysteries, counties can rest assured that no matter how complex and convoluted the forensics of a particular case, its mysteries will likely be revealed under the bright fluorescent lights of the Kent County Morgue.

Antrim County to the north of Kent County consists of miles and miles of wooded, unpopulated acres—a playground for outdoor enthusiasts, such as hunters in the fall, snowmobile riders in the winter, and hikers and boaters in the spring and summer. Antrim County deputies, consequently, see several victims of snowmobile accidents each year, most from drunk or reckless driving.

The previous night would produce Antrim County's first snowmobile accident victim of the year, a bit belated. Usually, the deputy explains, the first victim falls after the first snowfall. Andrew McBride* and his brother Bryan,* after a few hours at a local bar, decided to go riding. Sometime during their outing—at about midnight—the brothers became separated. Andrew returned to the truck and waited.

Tired of waiting after twenty minutes, he drove his sled onto the trailer and left for home, where he assumed his brother would appear later (they lived together)—a strange, almost incomprehensible act of apparent carelessness for his brother's well-being, the deputy notes. Three hours later, other snowmobile riders discovered Bryan, the apparent victim of a crash. He died within the hour at a local hospital.

The deputy hands Dr. Cohle a stack of digital photographs. The pictures detail the damage done to McBride's snowmobile last night when its rider, who's lying on a table in the adjacent autopsy room, collided with a pine tree. The collision occurred just beyond a turn, so the deputy explained his theory that the victim didn't make the turn and lost control of the snowmobile. Unlike the scene of a car crash, the deputy notes, the snow does not capture skid marks that would indicate the driver's speed at the time of the accident. Andrew McBride, though, confirmed that he and Bryan liked to drive their snowmobiles fast. Very fast.

The head-on collision reduced the machine to a twisted, contorted pile of metal and threw the rider onto the ground next to it. A few hours later, at approximately three in the morning, a pair of snowmobile riders found McBride, breathing but unconscious. They attempted to resuscitate him, but despite their efforts, which were repeated within an hour by hospital personnel, Bryan McBride died—apparently the victim of a blunt force injury to the head when he hit the tree.

---

*An asterisk denotes the first use of a pseudonym. In cases that did not lead to significant court action, or in cases that have not yet been completely adjudicated, or in cases where anonymity is in the interest of good taste, the authors created pseudonyms and in some instances altered nonessential details to preserve the anonymity of the victims. The forensic science, however is unaltered.

An open-and-shut case, it appears. So why conduct an autopsy? Michigan law does not require an autopsy for any death, leaving the decision to the medical examiner. This man died when he struck the tree, so an autopsy becomes a superfluous exercise in anatomy, right?

Wrong.

Dr. Cohle has seen many of these "open-and-shut" cases over the years: the victim of a house fire on whose badly charred remains appeared three bullet wounds; a suicide victim who somehow managed to shoot herself in the head twice.

In the world of sports, sometimes a David will beat a Goliath because, to use a sports cliché, any team can win on any given Sunday; this possibility, to use another cliché, is why they play the games. In the morgue, any cause of death can appear on any given day, which is why they conduct autopsies. McBride's death and subsequent autopsy could reveal any number of ugly surprises.

In this case, anything *other* than a head injury could have occurred. The presence of a heavy metal, strychnine, or arsenic in his blood would indicate that someone poisoned him. HOMICIDE.

The presence of multiple depressed skull fractures, rather than the linear skull cracks one would expect from such an accident, would indicate that someone struck him over the head with something like a claw hammer. HOMICIDE.

Petechial or pinpoint hemorrhages—hundreds of tiny red dots that represent broken blood vessels—in the victim's eyes and face, coupled with abrasions on his neck, could indicate that someone throttled him. HOMICIDE.

"This is the victim." The deputy presents another photograph showing two brothers.

"Which one?" Dr. Cohle chuckles. Andrew and Bryan McBride were twins and almost indistinguishable from each other. This fact complicates the case, as it raises the question, which twin died in the accident? They believe Bryan McBride perished, but Dr. Cohle posits a scenario in which one twin, for whatever reason, switched identities with his dead brother. He entered the woods as Bryan McBride and after a tragic accident, exited the forest as Andrew McBride. Or an even more sinister possibility—he caused the accident.

"I hope you have fingerprints on file," Dr. Cohle notes. He knows that DNA offers no help in distinguishing one twin from the other. The DNA of identical twins is identical. They *can* use fingerprints, however, to identify the victim, *if* someone has a set of fingerprints on file for comparison. If not, well . . .

Bryan McBride, the apparent victim, has an extensive criminal history, the deputy notes, and fingerprints are on file. The brothers were like Cain and Abel—one a good boy, the other a troublemaker with a criminal jacket as thick as a dictionary. Neither was married, although Andrew McBride, if indeed he was the one who walked out of the forest last night, does have a steady girlfriend. This raises an interesting question. Did one brother erase his criminal past and acquire a girlfriend with one tragic accident?

As odd as it sounds, one twin could have engineered the accident to switch identities with his brother to shed the criminal record, to obtain a spouse or lover, or for some other motive. Now, the story that he left his brother in the woods to fend for himself takes on an insidious, Machiavellian connotation. Stranger things have happened; anyone who spends any amount of time around this underworld will realize that in forensic pathology, no fiction is stranger than the truth.

Therefore, in this case, the deputy acknowledges, fingerprints taken in the morgue this morning will prove vital in determining which brother died in the accident. And if necessary, Dr. Cohle can enlist the aid of a forensic dentist (see "The Sea Shall Give Up Her Dead"), who would examine the victim's teeth and compare them to antemortem dental records. While the brothers may have identical teeth, it is unlikely they have an identical dental history.

Dr. Cohle leads the motley procession of deputy, autopsy assistant, and teacher-cum-morgue volunteer into the autopsy room. The first thing a person sees when entering this room is a plaster-cast anatomical skeleton dangling from a post next to a support pillar. Its white bones indicate that it is a copy and not real. Real bones age and turn to a tea color. This morning, the skull is backward and its skeletal visage seems to be smiling.

Beyond the skeleton, the beige-tiled room, about the size of a two-stall garage, is where Dr. Cohle and his colleagues solve the most complex mysteries posed by the dead. The autopsy room has a very distinctive smell: a faint yet strong mixture of disinfectant and wintergreen, from the LorAnn Oil used to mask the smell of advanced decomposition that quickly floods the room when a body—a "stinker"—enters the room. After my eighteen-month "tour of duty," I acquired an aversion to anything wintergreen.

Along the south wall, two large workstations, with a scale for weighing organs dangling from the ceiling between them, dominate one side of the room. The opposite wall contains a large, stainless steel door—the refrigerator. Unlike its television counterparts of glistening stainless steel drawers, this refrigerator is rather small, about the size of a bathroom in a master suite. Bodies of victims lie cocooned in white sheets and black body bags on shelves line the walls.

The glass windows on either side of the refrigerator door are used as bulletin boards; taped onto one are various medical charts and scales, such as the Glasgow Coma Index, that provide essential reference materials to pathology personnel. The other glass window sports a collection of cartoons, including several *Far Side* comics, which indicate that even here, amid the human detritus left in the wake of tragedy, humor exists.

A scan of the cartoons indicates the kind of humor—wry, sardonic, sometimes cynical—morgue personnel enjoy or find relevant. One *Far Side* cartoon, for example, shows a man and a woman at a table in the middle of a desert, alone. A second table sits empty, but another couple is crawling toward it. The caption: "Well, it *was* a private table."

In another comic, one police officer reprimands another for drawing thought bubbles onto a chalk outline used to indicate placement of a body at a crime scene. Another shows two cows contemplating an anatomical drawing of a human, whose various body parts are labeled "Prime Rib," "Tenderloin," and other cuts of meat. Indeed, the comics represent the dark humor present in most professions, but here, the humor is a way to cut the sting of the tragedy.

The west wall contains a massive scale set into the floor used to weigh bodies and a table on which various items, such as a victim's clothes or possessions, are collected and packaged. From the morgue, the disposition of these items depends on the type of death: for homicides, these items will go to a police evidence technician, for other types of deaths, they may be returned to the victim's family. This morning, the snowsuit and boots the victim wore the night before lie on the floor.

The morgue's stereo also sits along the west wall next to a door that opens to another room, which contains various items used in daily business. It is also used as a temporary storage facility for evidence.

I duck into the room and pluck a pair of pale blue "booties," which keep a person from walking out of the morgue wearing shoes speckled with dots of blood from the morning autopsy. These spots may seem harmless, but each one could carry a virulent bloodborne pathogen. In fact, morgue personnel run the highest risk of contracting bloodborne illness; victims who enter the morgue often have a history of intravenous drug use, and their bodies host any number of diseases, including HIV and hepatitis. And the morgue personnel work around a number of sharp obstacles, such as sharp knife blades or edges of fractured bones, any of which could lead to an accidental cut.

On one of the tables in this room—the evidence room—I notice a cardboard box inside of which is a Styrofoam container. It looks like a package anyone might find sitting on the front porch, but the layperson would get quite a shock when he opens this box. It contains the heart of a high school student who, after finishing her event at a swim meet, collapsed and died. Dr. Cohle is a recognized authority in the subspecialty of cardiovascular pathology; in other words, he specializes in the heart. When pathologists need expert consultation on a case involving a heart, they send it or portions of it to Dr. Cohle, packaged in a bowling ball–sized box via FedEx. Dr. Cohle received portions of Terry Schiavo's heart this way, as well as others. As he did in the Schiavo case, Dr. Cohle will conduct a systematic study of the swimmer's heart to find out what made it stop.

The east wall of the autopsy room contains two light boxes used to illuminate x-rays and a door leading to a photography studio housing thousands of slides taken during autopsies in the years before digital photography. The slides represent a visual compendium of the dissections that occurred in the adjacent autopsy room.

In the center of the autopsy room sit the pieces of morgue furniture that stitch the place together: two large stainless steel autopsy tables, each with a sink at one end.

My gaze falls onto the person occupying one of the tables. Victims enter the morgue directly from the death scene or from the hospital where they were pronounced dead. The name John Doe will be replaced with either "Bryan McBride" or "Andrew McBride" after the fingerprints establish who died last night. The man is lying naked on the autopsy table. The last clothes he wore—a black snowsuit and boots—lie in a pile on the scale in a corner of the room.

"What are you doing?" I ask as I watch Joel run his hands over McBride's head and under the back of his neck. If the victim broke his neck or sustained a massive skull fracture, in most cases the autopsy assistant would be able to feel it.

He shakes his head. No neck fractures. No massive skull fractures.

I ask, "What's the most interesting case you've seen?" It's a natural question to ask. He pauses to think about the many cases, victims, and skeletons he's watched go into the ME's closet during his tenure assisting in autopsies.

"The lady in the lake," he responds. A husband and wife, while yachting in Lake Huron, disappeared without a trace. Authorities found the yacht floating in the middle of the lake, its occupants gone. Days later, the wife's body washed ashore. A toxicology analysis revealed the presence of carbon monoxide in her system, and police speculate that she and possibly her husband may have been swimming behind the yacht with the engine running, and that they inhaled exhaust, passed out, and drowned. The husband's body has never been found. Perhaps he didn't die. Perhaps he engineered his wife's accident and escaped to Canada where he lives under an assumed name. Anything is possible.

"What do you think happened?" I ask.

"Who knows?" Joel shrugs.

He produces a large syringe that would give even the most stout-hearted a pathological fear of needles and inserts it into the victim's eye. He pulls its plunger and it fills with clear fluid—vitreous humor. He fills a plastic beaker with the fluid that will go to the toxicology lab for testing. He has also placed four dots of blood on a DNA card—autopsy protocol includes completing a DNA card—which, as previously noted, will provide help in establishing identity, although not for this victim, since he was an identical twin.

Throughout the autopsy, Joel will take various fluid samples: blood from the femoral artery, gastric contents from the stomach, urine from the bladder. These samples may contain substances such as alcohol, drugs, or poisons. The presence of such a substance in the victim's body could help explain last night's accident. If it *was* an accident.

Dr. Cohle hands me a clipboard containing diagrams of a head: frontal, lateral, and top, or bird's-eye views. My job as volunteer this morning will partly consist of sketching any wounds.

He was a large man at six feet four and two hundred and forty pounds. He is bald except for a half-moon wedge of burnt-orange hair running across the back of his head from ear to ear. Unlike the majority of victims who enter the morgue, his eyes are open, revealing light blue irises that sharply contrast with his deep auburn hair and eyebrows. The left side of his body contains the evidence of the hospital personnel's vain struggle to revive him: EKG pads—white squares with shiny metal contact dots in their centers.

I begin to sketch the wounds, which doesn't take long: a bruise about the circumference of a baseball on the top of his head, likely caused by the helmet when he struck the pine tree; a line of pinpoint or petechial hemorrhages running across his eyebrow, likely caused by the pressure of the helmet; and pinpoint hemorrhages in his eyes. Most people imagine a mangled corpse when they think about an accident victim, but this victim's body looks about the same as a man who suffered a massive heart attack or a drug overdose.

His cause of death, Dr. Cohle notes, likely resides inside the skull.

Dr. Cohle and Joel roll the body to examine the back, which contains large purple blotches. The lack of blood pressure created by a beating heart causes blood to settle because of gravity. The skin becomes saturated with blood and appears purple or bruised. This *lividity* allows the medical examiner to determine the position of the victim when she or he died, as long as the body has not been moved for several hours after death. In this case, the victim's heart stopped while he lay on his back on a hospital gurney, so his back is purple.

Dr. Cohle dresses in a blue smock, and I pull surgical scrubs over my blue jeans and button-down shirt. Once the cutting begins, everyone in the autopsy room must wear a protective facemask with elastic strings that loop over the ears. The mask protects a person from inhaling air that might contain pathogens. When the medical examiner opens a lung infected with pneumonia or tuberculosis, the microorganisms could become airborne. In this way, a healthy person could catch a life-threatening illness from a corpse.

The mask contains a plastic visor and protects the eyes from any airborne human debris that could lead to an infection. If a drop of blood contaminated with hepatitis B struck a person in the eye, for example, that person would run the risk of acquiring the bloodborne infection.

Everyone is dressed for the morning's work. Joel draws his scalpel across McBride's chest, first from a point over the left shoulder to a point over the sternum, then from the right shoulder to the same point over the sternum, forming a V. From the base of the V, he cuts a line to a spot just above the navel to finish the Y-incision. The incision reveals the layers of skin and bright yellow fat (about an inch and a half thick in this victim) that sit like a blanket over the crimson muscle underneath. He places the flap of skin that he's cut (the top of the V) over McBride's face. He works his scalpel in a carving and sawing motion to separate the layers of skin and fat from the rib cage and sternum. Deep red, almost black lines of blood run down to the ends of the Y and spill onto the table, surrounding the victim's upper torso in a widening ring.

With the sternum now exposed, Joel snaps through the ribs with a long-handled instrument that looks like a tool used to prune tree branches. It is an apt analogy; the ribs break with the unsettling sound of wet branches snapping. Joel severs the ribs around the sternum to expose the underlying chest organs. With a tug and a sucking sound, the breastplate is removed to reveal the organs underneath. The intestines distend, looking like a pile of yellow-brown, translucent sausages.

Beginning with the heart and lungs, which he removes as one deep purple and red mass laced with lines of bright yellow fat, Joel will systematically remove all of the organs in the body cavity and place them in the large steel bowl resting between the victim's legs. When the bowl is filled, he will carry it to the workstation where Dr. Cohle will dissect each organ to determine what brought a premature end to this thirty-eight-year-old victim's life.

In a death apparently caused by a head injury, one wonders why the ME does not just open the victim's skull. While the details of this case suggest that McBride died of a head injury and that the key to his death lies inside his skull, some causes of death leave no conclusive forensic evidence. Drowning, for example, leaves no conclusive, telltale clues that prove the victim aspirated water. In such a case, the autopsy becomes an autopsy "of exclusion," during which the medical examiner rules out any other possible cause of death. To exclude all other possibilities, a complete autopsy—a dissection of the organs—must occur.

Besides, sometimes a victim's body contains ugly little surprises and hidden forensic clues that can turn an apparent accidental death into a murder investigation.

For example, the discovery of a fractured hyoid bone—the horseshoe-shaped bone in the throat structures—could possibly indicate someone strangled McBride, a finding that would force police to reevaluate the accident scenario. The totaled snowmobile would likely result from a staged accident if the victim *was* strangled—unless he caught his neck on something like a wire fence or a clothesline.

On the other hand, if Dr. Cohle finds severely occluded or blocked coronary arteries—a rare but not unheard of finding in a thirty-eight-year-old victim—he can conclude that he died of heart disease or a heart event such as a ventricular fibrillation (in the absence of fatal injury). In such a case, a cardiac arrhythmia could have led to a loss of consciousness, which caused him to lose control and hit a tree.

Without a complete autopsy, vital forensic evidence could go unseen. Murderers or the criminally negligent could go free, or innocent people could face charges for crimes they didn't commit. Sometimes the lack of a complete autopsy can even create reasonable doubt for a jury.

Thus, not studying each organ can lead to disastrous consequences, as it did in the case of a horrific car accident described by Dr. Cohle.

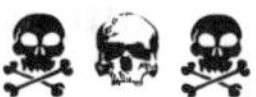

"You have to indulge me in this," Dr. Cohle states to the deputy as he draws a diagram of four vehicles—two (a pickup truck and an SUV) in front of a motorcycle and a third (another pickup truck) behind—on the whiteboard next to the workstation. "Here is an interesting case in which alcohol impaired a driver's judgment."

This case also illustrates the need for a complete, thorough autopsy and why the forensic pathologist can leave no anatomical stone unturned. In this case, the pathologist who conducted the autopsy did not open the victim's skull—an omission that in part created reasonable doubt. Dr. Cohle testified as an expert witness for the defense.

The first pickup truck stopped abruptly. The driver of the SUV managed to stop without colliding with the pickup, but the cyclist did not stop in time and ran into the back of the SUV. The driver of the second pickup truck, who was drunk, did not manage to stop in time and rear-ended the SUV, running over the cyclist in the process and crushing him.

But *what* killed the cyclist: a head injury caused by running into the SUV or injuries sustained when the second pickup truck ran over him? A long prison sentence awaited the intoxicated driver if the jury believed the latter possibility. Although eyewitnesses stated that the cyclist had slowed to ten to fifteen miles per hour when he hit the SUV, the rear of the SUV received significant damage, indicating that the cyclist could have sustained a lethal head injury when he struck it.

In other words, the collision with the SUV may have resulted in the injury that killed the cyclist, making the second pickup truck driver guilty of driving under the influence but not of vehicular homicide. At the least, the damage to the back of the SUV presented a reasonable doubt. The jury agreed and found that the intoxicated driver did not cause the cyclist's death.

While the cyclist may have survived even a serious head injury from the collision, the second pickup truck driver's actions eliminated that possibility. Yet the lack of a complete autopsy left unanswered the question of which injury killed the man and therefore created even more reasonable doubt. Of course, if that driver was sober, there would have been no controversy or court case.

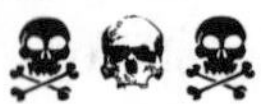

Back to McBride. In approximately twenty-five minutes, Joel has removed all of the internal organs, filling the bowl resting between McBride's feet on the stainless steel autopsy table. The torso now looks like an empty shell. One can see the inside of the spinal vertebrae, which appear off-white and curved, running the length of the torso.

"Big spleen," Doc notes, as he glances into the bowl containing the organs. Dr. Cohle takes each organ out and weighs it. He calls out the weights, and, using a blue marker, I note them on the dry erase board. These will become part of the official report produced from Dr. Cohle's verbal notes, which are dictated into a microphone attached to the workstation. The microphone is activated and deactivated with pedals at its base that look and work like piano pedals.

After a few minutes of examining the victim's throat structures, Doc has found some hemorrhaging, though not enough damage to indicate that the victim had been throttled, garroted, or strangled. This damage likely occurred during resuscitation attempts.

"That's an interesting x-ray," I note as Dr. Cohle cross-sections, or "bread loafs" the victim's heart. I noticed the x-ray of another morgue customer earlier and detected several anomalous objects apparently inside the torso. Objects that didn't belong there. In the black-and-white image, one can clearly make out several screws, nails, and staples.

"Did this victim swallow nails?" I ask.

Doc chuckles. "That's from a fire that destroyed a three-story apartment building," he explains.

Police believe a cigarette may have begun the conflagration. The x-ray is of one of the fire's victims. Appearances can deceive; he didn't swallow screws, nails, and staples. In a house fire case, when authorities remove the badly charred remains of a victim's body, they often unwittingly scoop up with the body debris from the fire. The metal debris sticks out in an x-ray like pegs in a Lite-Brite toy.

While Dr. Cohle examines each organ, Joel takes fingerprints of the victim. He daubs graphite on each of the fingers, painting each fingertip black. He sticks a white sticker on the right thumb. The graphite adheres to the sticker, and a fingerprint is produced. He places the sticker on a clear vellum sheet titled "OFFICE OF THE MEDICAL EXAMINER" in the box titled "RIGHT THUMB." A complete set of fingerprints—ten (unless the victim is missing a finger)—is taken.

One by one, Dr. Cohle dissects the victim's organs and stores small tissue samples from each in a "stock jar"—a Ball jar filled with formaldehyde. Should a need arise in the next three years to examine additional tissue from the case, he could obtain the tissue samples from the jar stored in an evidence room.

"The liver contains no fatty change," Dr. Cohle notes. "Fatty change" sometimes appears in alcoholics. Consumption of alcohol damages liver cells that subsequently acquire intracellular fat, and the organ's appearance changes from a brown to a light golden color.

"So he wasn't an alcoholic?" the deputy asks.

Doc shakes his head. "Not necessarily." The absence of fatty change, he explains to the deputy standing next to him, does not mean that the deceased didn't drink heavily or even compulsively. Not every heavy drinker's liver undergoes fatty change.

Therefore, the absence of fatty change does not necessarily rule out alcohol as a possible cause of the snowmobile accident. Perhaps one too many cocktails before his midnight ride led to McBride's collision with the pine tree. Many of the morgue's visitors come in feet-first as a result of alcohol-induced accidents.

"How fast was he traveling?" I ask the deputy.

The deputy shrugs. "No skid marks on snow. Unless we begin crashing sleds, we can't know. Some of these kids travel as fast as two hundred miles per hour."

"On snowmobiles?" I ask, incredulous.

The deputy nods.

"Sea-Doos can travel ninety," Joel adds. He is lining the victim's empty torso shell with a plastic "entrail bag." He will pour the examined organs into this bag, replace the breastplate, and sew closed the Y-incision, thus prepping the body for transport to a funeral home.

When most people think of drunk driving accidents, Dr. Cohle notes, they think of automobiles, but many people die in drunk driving accidents involving other types of vehicles, such as snowmobiles and quads. Jet Ski accidents result in several morgue patients each year. "We had a case where an intoxicated woman driving a Jet Ski collided with a boat and was killed in the collision. The boat's propeller severed her leg, which police recovered later."

Dr. Cohle turns to Joel. "We need to take a look at that leg." The story reminded him of today's other morgue business.

The leg he is referring to is the leg of one of the apartment fire victims, recovered separately from the torso as police sifted through the ruins. This morning they need to photograph the leg for the official record, which Joel can accomplish while he waits for Dr. Cohle to finish the examination of the body organs. Joel disappears into the refrigerator and emerges a few seconds later carrying a translucent plastic bag inside of which is something bundled in a white sheet.

He sets the bag on the vacant autopsy table, which he has covered with a blue sheet. He unwraps the bag, unfurls the sheet inside, removes the leg, and places it on the blue sheet. On the wall behind him, the x-ray portrait of another fire victim—the one who appeared to swallow nails—hangs on the x-ray box like a ghostly painting.

Joel stands on a stool and snaps several photographs of the leg with the morgue's digital camera. The charred leg is jet black and bent at the knee to form a V. Shards of skin hang from it in strips. Without the foot, which is clenched like a fist, at first glance it would not look human.

While Joel photographs the leg, Dr. Cohle finishes his examination of the snowmobile rider's body cavity organs. A thorough examination reveals nothing out of the ordinary—no forensic smoking gun like severely blocked coronary arteries—except for some bruising on the lungs. The victim sustained no rib fractures to explain this bruising, but such bruising *would* accompany a closed head injury. No disease, such as heart disease or emphysema, which might have caused this death, was discovered either. In other words, nothing was found to contradict the possibility that if this victim hadn't died in a tragic accident, he would have lived a very long life.

This is expected. "I'm banking on some kind of head injury," Dr. Cohle notes to the deputy standing by his side. If McBride died when he hit the pine tree, the evidence would reside inside his head . . . which Joel has placed on a white "head block"—a plastic block placed under the neck and used to prop up the head so the skull can be opened. He cuts a line across the scalp with a scalpel and with a dry, tearing sound tugs the face down and forward and the scalp backward to expose the off-white skull. With a special tool called a Stryker Saw—a saw with an oscillating blade—he will cut off the skull cap (calvarium) and remove the brain.

A two-by-three-inch black blotch on the skull's surface coincides with the bruising on McBride's scalp, but this does not appear to denote a head injury significant enough to have killed the man.

A loud whirring sound fills the morgue as Joel works the Stryker across McBride's skull, creating small clouds of bone dust. After a few minutes, he has excised the semispherical calvarium, exposing the brain. If a head injury caused McBride's death, the evidence would now appear as thick, reddish-black matted blood inside the protective membrane—the dura—that lines the inside of the skull.

But what everyone in the room expected to see—hemorrhaging—does not exist. Joel removes the brain, places it in a stainless steel bowl, and sets the bowl on the workstation where Dr. Cohle will examine it. A study of the brain reveals no injuries. This is bad news: no apparent cause of death. It is as if a demon crept out of the shadows and into the moonlight, reached into Bryan McBride's body, and stole his life. Despite the absence of brain injury, Dr. Cohle explains, McBride could have died from a concussion, which can for a time paralyze the brain stem, especially if the concussion coincides with alcohol consumption. A concussion is usually a mild head injury and represents one end of the spectrum of craniocerebral trauma; severe skull fractures represent the other. A concussion can in fact kill by "stunning" the brain stem, causing cessation of breathing in addition to loss of consciousness.

A concussion, however, is not a common cause of death. Another possibility: this victim died of an alcohol or drug overdose or a combination of the two.

Now the cause of death will hinge on the toxicology report, which will be complete in a few days and will indicate the presence and level of substances in the victim's system when he died. With a high blood-alcohol level, McBride would have been more susceptible to hypothermia, which could have caused his death. Like drowning, hypothermia leaves no conclusive evidence for the ME to find and it becomes a cause of death only if all others have been eliminated.

Doc shakes his head as he glances at the snowsuit on the floor; such thick clothes would make hypothermia an unlikely scenario, and *if* his brother's story is true, the victim lay on the ground unconscious for only about an hour—not enough time to freeze to death. High enough levels, on the other hand, would allow for the conclusion that he died of a drug or alcohol overdose, which would explain the crash.

Or perhaps he ingested poison, which would raise the potential of homicide.

Thus, the autopsy procedure this morning will end with no answer to the question of what killed Bryan McBride, just speculation about how he died. *If* the victim on the table was Bryan McBride . . .

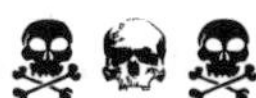

Everyone has skeletons in the closet. For some, they consist of lovers taken behind the back of a loyal, loving, and unaware spouse. For others, they consist of bottles containing whiskey, Vicodin, or Valium. For still others, they consist of a criminal past or sexual fetishes . . . hundreds of skeletons could appear on this list.

The Kent County Morgue has thousands of them.

Apart from the anatomical skeleton that resides against a support pillar and greets all who enter with his wry cat-who-ate-the-canary smile, the morgue's closet contains many other skeletons: stories of deceit, greed, and murder; of love triangles, serial crime, and accidental deaths. These stories, stories of the victims who passed through the morgue, are the medical examiner's skeletons, and his file cabinet, his closet.

To write *Cause of Death: Forensic Files of a Medical Examiner*, I observed and even assisted to some degree Dr. Cohle and his forensic team in conducting dozens of autopsies. I know what occurs during an autopsy. Those experiences brought me into the morgue;

now I wondered what lay inside its closets, what fascinating stories occurred in forensic pathology beyond the limited scope of my first-hand experience.

As I listened to the Kent County medical examiner talk about car accidents and watched as Joel dealt with a charred human leg, I began to wonder about the skeletons in the ME's closet. If we opened the Kent County Morgue's file cabinet, what skeletons would emerge? What stories would they tell?

So Stephen D. Cohle, the Kent County chief medical examiner and a veteran forensic pathologist with nearly twenty-five years of solving forensic mysteries, and I decided to open the closet (which consists of several file cabinets actually). To open the ME's closet is to open a Pandora's box of sorts. In Greek mythology, a vindictive Zeus filled a box with disease, famine, and pestilence and gave it to the incessantly curious Pandora with instructions not to open it. Of course, the wily god of gods knew that she would open it and unleash these bad things on the human world. And open it she did.

The ME's box, however, does not contain plagues and disease but victims who perished at the hands of angry spouses, serial killers, alter egos, demons (the mental sort), and their own negligence. For true-crime junkies, the box represents a treasure trove of stories, each of which would make an excellent script for a *CSI* episode or even a movie. Indeed, the stories that emerged would send any scriptwriter scrambling for his pen.

In the following chapters, these skeletons tell their stories and, collectively, they tell the true-crime stories of the Kent County chief medical examiner and his team of forensics experts. Dr. Cohle has been solving forensic mysteries from his base in Grand Rapids—the second-largest city in Michigan—and while a majority of his cases took place in Michigan, many have implications that transcend state borders ("Hey, You, Get Off of My Cloud," for example, and "Scorecard"). As a whole, they represent a cross-section of crime in mid-America. Yet none of these cases is mundane; each has a unique forensic twist—the one commonality uniting them in this collection.

In fact, the word *mundane* does not belong in any sentence about the business of the morgue.

Some of the stories the skeletons will tell:

A woman's body floats to the surface of a small lake connected to Lake Michigan. Time and Mother Nature's creatures obliterated all but speculation about her cause of death and identity, leaving two questions: who is she and how did she die? The badly decomposed remains don't match those of any missing persons, and only after months of intense searching do forensics experts discover that the body took a unique journey before it was recovered. ("The Sea Shall Give Up Her Dead")

While driving through his fields, a blueberry farmer notices a charred ring of earth with a metal chest at its center. As he approaches the chest, he makes a macabre discovery: charred human remains. The skull fractures leave little question that someone murdered this man, but who, and why? To answer these questions, investigators must first answer another: who is he? ("No Tombstone for 'Jack': An Untitled Story in Five Acts")

Someone drugged and strangled two young farmers attending a convention, but the killer left a telltale forensic clue. The trail goes cold until police arrest a drunk driver in California. In the trunk of his Toyota they find what became known as a "scorecard"—a list of victims—and with it the story of a serial killer who did his ghastly work in California begins to unravel. But did this serial killer also kill in Michigan? ("Scorecard")

People die at acute care facilities for the elderly. It is a sad fact of life. But did two nurse's aides help the Grim Reaper collect as many as eight victims at the Alpine Manor? And if so, who masterminded the plan? ("M-U-R-D-E-R?")

A man believes that the Mafia has infiltrated his local police force, and when the police come to disarm him, a standoff results.

When the smoke clears, one man—a decorated veteran police officer—has sustained fatal gunshot wounds. A jury would ponder the question: murder or self-defense? ("The Right to Bear Arms")

Police come to arrest an outspoken critic of government on suspicion of solicitation. He barricades himself in his home. After a lengthy standoff with state and local police in which one trooper (despite shield and body armor) dies of gunshot wounds, the man's house erupts in flames. Investigators find no trace of his body; somehow, he managed to escape. Days later, they discover and confront him, and the confrontation leads to his death. He sustained dozens of gunshot wounds but never fired his weapon, raising the question, did the police act with appropriate force? ("Rebel Yell")

Two libertarian, pro-hemp advocates run a marijuana-friendly campground until they cross an ultraconservative prosecutor bent on ending their bacchanalian parties. They pledge to die before they leave their campground, which is exactly what happens. Yet, did they have to die? Did authorities go too far? ("Hey, You, Get Off of My Cloud")

She is everything to him: the object of his obsession. Did his obsession lead him to rape then murder her with a baseball bat? Jurors would hear her story from beyond the grave—a story about a sexual obsession out of control, but would they listen? ("Obsession")

He's been known to slap around his women. She's got a sharp temper and once hit a boyfriend in the head with a cast-iron skillet. They're lovers, and their love spat turns deadly, but was it murder or self-defense? ("Punch Drunk")

He loves his wife and will do anything to keep her. She doesn't feel the same. An argument results in her death, but did she push him into a homicidal rage? ("It's Not a Weapon; It's a Tea Mug!")

At a party, a husband and wife begin to discuss past romantic encounters. Enraged, he slaps her across the face. She falls back, dead. But could a slap in the face kill her, or did something else cause her death? And was her death an accident or a murder? ("A Slap in the Face")

Their marriage is crumbling, but they decide to take one last family trip. She will never return home. The pool of blood suggests that she died from injuries caused by an accidental fall from a boat dock. So how did she wind up facedown in the lake? Was her death an accident or a murder? ("Ghosts of Arcadia")

A prostitute kills her "john" over payment for services rendered. She appears to be suffering from multiple personality syndrome, which raises the question, which one of her personalities pulled the trigger? ("I Did It, but *I* Didn't Do It")

A mother calls 911 because her child has stopped breathing. She doesn't know it, but the sleep monitor her doctor prescribed has a memory chip. Would the monitor's memory chip preserve evidence of a tragic accident . . . or a murder? ("Loved Him to Death")

A teenager with a history of drug use and assault murders an unsuspecting youth who wandered by his parent's house. He perpetrates the most unbelievably horrific mutilations on his victim's corpse and videotapes himself doing it. Why would he do such as thing? He told authorities he heard voices in his head directing him, but did he, and if so, what role did the voices play in the macabre story? ("Head Case")

Faced with several conflicting versions of how the murder occurred, the prosecution must try to extract some truth from the tangle of deception that results when a body is found buried in four hundred pounds of concrete. The cause of death is simple—gunshot wounds to the head—but who pulled the trigger, and is an innocent man in prison for the crime? ("Sex, Lies, and Cement")

A check written on the day two elderly ladies disappeared leads to their killer. Faced with overwhelming evidence, the murderer makes a chilling confession but leaves out one vital detail: what caused the damage to one of his victim's hands? ("The Hand That Feeds")

Two murder victims surface from a shallow grave. The murder investigation uncovers a vast drug network and the identity of their killer. He claims he acted in self-defense, but was his claim just an elaborate ruse designed to conceal a brutal, premeditated murder? ("I Shot the Drug Dealers, but I Swear It Was in Self-Defense")

A call to the police reveals the location of a dead body. Police find the body of a woman—reported missing by her husband days earlier—frozen into a snowbank. Police chip the body from the ice; the body then must thaw in the Kent County Morgue before the autopsy can take place. The difficulties authorities experience extricating and thawing the body would be just the beginning of their headaches. Months of finger-pointing and allegations create an almost impenetrable quagmire for prosecutors as they attempt to answer the question, who murdered the ice woman? ("Who Murdered the Ice Woman?")

Indeed, the stories these skeletons tell could fill immense volumes. Yet this collection offers an alternative to the long-winded and incredibly detailed true-crime novels that line the shelves of bookstores and libraries. If the true-crime novel, with its exhaustive and often irrelevant detail, is a cup of cappuccino best sipped at a café accompanied by a leisurely hour of conversation, these intense stories are espresso shots.

And like shots of espresso, the stories these skeletons tell are strong; they contain graphic detail culled from the ME's case reports and interviews with forensic experts. And each contains some unique forensic twist. If you dare open the closet, perhaps even step inside, if you pay Charon to take you across the river Styx to the other side, and if you listen, the skeletons will tell you fascinating tales of intrigue, deception, and murder.

# 1. identity crisis

To paraphrase the great green ogre Shrek, identity is like an onion; it has layers.

People carry their identity in bits and pieces. Any one of these bits and pieces does not create a three-dimensional image of the holder; rather, each represents a puzzle piece. When the pieces are assembled, a more detailed image appears.

Consider the items found in the author's wallet as an example: driver's license, Social Security card, credit cards (two), bank card, car warranty card, museum membership card (two), zoo membership card, scuba diving certification card ("C" card), and family photographs. Any one of these items contains a name. One or two add a date of birth, which indicates that the owner is thirty-something.

The other items would provide Sherlock Holmes with enough evidence to complete a personality profile of the subject. From them, one could deduce that the owner likes to go to museums, he occasionally rents DVDs from Blockbuster, he frequents 7-11 and has a weakness for Slurpees (a free Slurpee punch card), he knows how to scuba dive, he drives a Honda Accord, he sometimes gambles and is superstitious (how else would you explain the casino poker chip?), and he lives with three women (the family photograph of his wife and two daughters).

The driver's license photograph provides another layer of identity: physical appearance. Height: five feet seven and a half. Weight: 195. Corrective vision. Eye color: blue. Not an organ donor. He is singularly homely. He has red hair; in his youth it was fire engine red but it is now just a few strands of strawberry blond covering the top of his head. Holmes would deduce that he is employed as a physical laborer or that he spends a fair amount of time in the gym each week (he has wide shoulders). The family photograph provides more information: he is slightly taller than his wife, whose thick mane of curly auburn hair presents a sharp contrast to his bare pate, which glistens under the photographer's light.

The modern crime scene investigator and forensic scientist could find another layer of identity in the man's wallet. A strand of hair trapped in a crease contains his DNA. And the paper items in the wallet contain an invisible albeit specific identity marker: his fingerprints, which any detective could lift with a little graphite.

For the forensic scientist and medical examiner, the subject's body provides another layer of identity: a unique combination of physical markers such as evidence of past injury or body modifications. A cursory examination of this subject reveals the lack of tattoos. An x-ray would reveal that he has never broken a bone (knock on wood) but that his lower right leg has a well-healed scar that runs from mid-shin to the knee, where as a nine-year-old he cut his leg open on an iron spike. His teeth contain a number of fillings—evidence that at one time he spent some time in a dentist's chair.

Investigators who must establish a victim's identity can search through any one of these layers to match a name with a body. Sometimes, however, Mother Nature and her creatures obliterate a victim's identity. Crabs, crocodiles, sharks, and other species may consume portions of a victim's body. Or murderers may destroy these layers of identity. These forces can create a headache for investigators who find themselves with a full-fledged identity crisis when they must piece together clues from what pieces remain. Or they must enlist specialized forensic scientists to search through the physical detritus left in the wake of mutilation or physical decomposition to find a name for John or Jane Doe.

Authors and screenwriters often have their fictional heroes and heroines struggling with an identity crisis. In Martin Cruz Smith's novel *Gorky Park*, made into a movie starring William Hurt and Lee Marvin, Moscow militia detective Arkady Renko must solve the murders of three victims left in the snow of Gorky Park—Moscow's version of New York's Central Park. Yet the wily killer has obliterated his victims' identities. After shooting them, the killer skinned their faces and fingertips and shot them in the mouths to shatter their teeth. The killer, realizing that investigators identify suspects by probing the relationships of the slain, left his victims without identity and the authorities with an identity crisis. Renko manages to identify the victims, in part because he enlists the aid of a prominent forensic anthropologist who reconstructs their faces with clay.

In *The Whole Nine Yards*, Nicholas Oseranski, a dentist who is aware that investigators often use dental records to identify a victim, hatches a plan to fake the death of contract killer Jimmy "the Tulip" Tudeski by replicating his dental restorations in the mouth of a dead person. He takes x-rays of the Tulip's teeth and creates the appropriate restorations (bridges, fillings, caps) in the dead subject, who they then burn up in a car. When investigators study the teeth of the charred remains, they will conclude that they have discovered the Tulip. Case closed.

While fiction sharply differs from reality in that wily killers and nature's minions often leave a body that takes *months* and sometimes *years* to identify, such authors and screenwriters typically borrow from actual cases reported in newspapers—cases like the following, in which victims, their identities shattered by the elements or murderers, left investigators with vexing identity crises and the ME with more skeletons in his closet.

## The Sea Shall Give Up Her Dead

### The Prayer for the Burial of the Dead at Sea

> *We therefore commit his body to the deep, looking for the general Resurrection in the last day, and the life of the world to come, through our Lord Jesus Christ; at whose second coming in glorious majesty to judge the world, the sea shall give up her dead . . .* [1]
>
> —*Book of Common Prayer*, 1892

She is a cruel mistress: dark, beautiful, exotic, and temperamental. One can become lost gazing at her beauty, and one can become lost in her cold embrace. Lake Michigan is vast, lined on her east coast with seemingly endless yellow sand beaches that disappear into the distance. From her waters rise sand dunes—great hills of sand that sit on her eastern shores like high-rise buildings capped with verdant deciduous and evergreen forests. The beaches rival any on Earth, yet one must tolerate the lake's frigid embrace—"liquid ice"—during all but the exceptionally hot summer months when vacationers can swim without wetsuits.

For years, Lake Michigan represented a liquid highway on which three-masted schooners and, later, steamships transported cargoes such as timber, giving rise to port cities located where tea-colored rivers mixed with the deep blue water of the "Big Lake." She is the only one of the five sisters who resides entirely inside the borders of the United States, making her America's lake. Now the old port cities have become tourist destinations for nature junkies who disappear in the deep forests, hiking or biking miles of trails through state and national forests, kayaking or canoeing miles of rivers that snake throughout Michigan's lower peninsula, winding toward the lake; freshwater sailors who tack in the unpredictable winds; and fishermen who pull salmon and pike from the depths.

Her mood can change with little if any notice; a hailstorm can appear in mid-August, monstrous swells in October, a blinding snowstorm in November. And with dangerous undertows, she reaches out and pulls unsuspecting swimmers into her depths. An undertow that pulls swimmers away from shore renders them virtually powerless; the frantic swimmer thrashes, but for each foot forward, the current pulls him three in the opposite direction.

Each year, she claims victims who venture into her waters during the "in" season of May through September. Most become victims as a result of hubris or negligence: swimmers who venture too deep or ignore the red flags posted to warn of dangerous surf; boaters who drink too much and fall overboard or collide with others. She keeps some of them, and some she returns . . .

On March 25, 2004, one returned in Pigeon Lake—a small inland lake just north of the port city of Holland, Michigan, and connected to Lake Michigan by a narrow channel. A few private homes sit perched on the shores of Pigeon Lake, but the largest resident is a Consumers Energy plant that occupies much of the area around the lake.

At approximately ten in the morning, a couple who lived on the south side of Pigeon Lake saw what looked like a dead animal floating in the water. A closer look from their dock revealed a horror about thirty feet offshore: a human body in an advanced state of decomposition that had obliterated everything—age, height, weight—everything except for the victim's gender, leaving a mass virtually unrecognizable as human. She was nude and without jewelry, leaving police no idea about her identity: no driver's license, Social Security card, or credit cards, and no signet ring containing the victim's initials, either.

The only certainty was that her body emerged with questions: Who am I? What am I doing here? How did I die?

These questions—questions that would vex investigators until an unbelievable clue led them to unravel the riddle of the Pigeon Lake floater—would remain unanswered for eighteen months. Until that clue emerged in the most unlikely place, the woman represented a forensic riddle.

While Jane Doe traveled to the Kent County Morgue for an autopsy, police—led by Ottawa County Detective Dave Blakely—began their investigation. The last event that occurred at Pigeon Lake was a New Year's Day celebration during which a few intrepid people, perhaps warmed by a few shots of liquid spirits, water-skied on the lake. Perhaps a water skier consumed one too many celebratory beverages and drowned, except no one was reported missing after the celebration.

Perhaps a resident or someone visiting a resident or renting a house on Pigeon Lake fell onto a dock, hit her head, and rolled into the lake, except no one associated with the homes along the lake was reported missing either.

The advanced state of decomposition suggested that the victim spent some time underwater before surfacing. Since the 2,500-foot-long boardwalk was closed to the public on October 15, it appeared likely that Jane Doe entered Pigeon Lake sometime prior to that time.

Another possibility existed: Jane may not have entered the water in Pigeon Lake. Instead, she could have met her end in the Big Lake, and her body traveled in currents through the channel into the smaller lake.

Or perhaps a mermaid had died and floated to the surface: an implausible if not farcical conclusion, but one as good as any that would appear in the succeeding months.

Lying nude (as found) on the stainless steel autopsy table in the Kent County Morgue, the victim looked more like a monster than a mermaid. Time and the elements had obliterated the victim's body. Such damage is consistent with victims, such as drowning victims, whose bodies remain submerged for long periods of time.

Drowning is a violent process; the victim, desperate for a breath of air, thrashes in the water, kicking, scratching toward the surface. This struggle causes a depletion of ATP (adenosine triphosphate) from the muscle tissue, causing a more rapid onset of rigor mortis (stiffening of the muscles). The body sinks, but decomposition causes the formation of methane gas inside the body cavity, and after a time the body surfaces (hence the name *floater*).

The environmental conditions dictate the length of time for a body to become a floater. In the warm, tropical water of the Caribbean Sea, the process takes a few days; extremely cold water can stall the formation of gas, so in icy waters such as Lake Michigan in mid-winter, the process could take months. If Jane Doe entered the ice-cold water of Lake Michigan sometime in the late fall or winter when the water temperature at the bottom is in the high thirties or low forties, she could have remained submerged for a long time—a likely possibility that would explain the extensive damage to her body and the advanced state of decomposition when her body did surface in late March. Jane Doe likely entered the water when it was cold and spent a lot of time on the bottom, during which time the elements caused extensive postmortem damage.

When submerged, the weight of the head and torso causes the human body to lie at the bottom in an inverted position, which accounts for the damage often found on a victim's face and arms, which usually dangle along the bottom and are the most exposed to postmortem damage. Postmortem abrasions and cuts often appear on the head and arms, caused as currents move the body along the bottom; sand, mud, or seaweed can become lodged in the victim's nose and mouth (but not lungs). Marine life such as crabs and turtles that feed on the body can also cause extensive damage.

Jane Doe's appearance suggested that animals had fed on her body for an extended period of time. Several areas of tissue were missing, and the sharp, defined borders around the absent tissue suggested animal activity. Much of her upper left arm was missing, including the radius bone; portions of skin and underlying muscle of her right arm were absent. Much of the right side of her face, scalp, and portions of her chin were gone. Most of the right ear had been damaged by animal activity, and the left was missing entirely. The absence of both eyes gave the body a ghastly, almost inhuman appearance.

Jane's lower extremities also suffered from her apparently lengthy stay underwater. The absence of much of the skin and muscle of her right thigh exposed the femur, and much of her right calf was missing. The elements had reduced her weight significantly. When she died, she weighed an estimated 170 to 180 pounds. On the morgue scale, she weighed 135.

Jane had also sustained numerous rib fractures and a large cut over her right eye. Dr. Norm Sauer, a forensic anthropologist and professor at Michigan State University, examined Jane and confirmed the presence of several fractures in the bones of Jane's face.

The large facial laceration and the fractures suggest that Jane had gone into the water as the result of an accident, such as a fall during which she struck her face on a hard surface, lost consciousness, and drowned. Or a more insidious possibility loomed: her death could have been a homicide in which someone struck her and threw her into the water.

Or perhaps she didn't drown at all. Perhaps someone stabbed her to death, or strangled her, and tossed her remains into the lake to conceal the crime. If so, Mother Nature obliged. The advanced state of decomposition might have obliterated signs of trauma, such as stab wounds, which would point toward a cause of death other than drowning. One thing was certain: Jane did not sustain gunshot wounds. Evidence of gunshot wound tracks would have remained.

Because Jane Doe was found in a lake, drowning as a cause of death would seem the most likely possibility, yet this conclusion is not a sine qua non. Despite the fact that the autopsy revealed no other cause of death, drowning does not present a forensic quick fix for cause of death, since, contrary to popular belief, drowning leaves no telltale forensic clues to guide the forensic pathologist.

Drowning can occur in one of two ways. The victim holds his breath as long as possible before, desperate for air, he breathes in a deep draft of water. The water enters the victim's lungs and death follows. This is called wet drowning—the most common form. A small percentage of drowning victims die as a result of dry drowning, in which water suddenly flooding the victim's throat causes the airway to close—a laryngospasm. Because a person can drown without aspirating water into the lungs (dry drowning), the absence of water in the lungs does not exclude the possibility that the victim drowned. Conversely, the presence of detritus in the lungs, such as sand or mud, would indicate that the victim breathed in some of the sediment in the water and therefore likely drowned.

Since drowning leaves little to no forensic evidence—no forensic smoking gun for the ME to find—the autopsy of a drowning victim is a process of excluding all other possibilities. This is called a "diagnosis of exclusion." If no other cause of death emerges during the autopsy, such as a lethal level of narcotics in the victim's blood at the time of death or a radial skull fracture indicating a fatal head injury, and if the circumstances warrant such a conclusion, drowning becomes the cause of death.

With no other clear cause of death, the medical examiner must rely on the circumstances surrounding the death to make a determination. Context, in other words, is everything in a diagnosis of exclusion. This case, though, lacked context, because the death occurred apparently without witnesses and the victim lacked an identity.

In addition, the manner of death (murder, accident, or suicide) involving drowning victims is difficult if not impossible to establish. For example, if the autopsy of Jane Doe revealed that she sustained a blow to the head—a blow that would not have killed her but left her unconscious—the question as to *how* she received the blow would arise; the circumstances (her body found floating in a lake) dictate that she drowned, but did she fall, strike her head, then topple into the lake (an accidental death)? Did she hurl herself against a hard object and then fall into the lake (suicide)? Or did someone hit her and throw her unconscious body in (murder)? Although homicidal drowning is rare, because of the difficulty in establishing manner of death in cases involving drowning, it is a stratagem sometimes employed by murderers attempting to simulate an accidental death.

Jane Doe's case had entered the Kent County Morgue as fragmented as her body: no witnesses to her death, no identity, no context . . . the advanced state of decomposition may have obliterated signs of the true cause of death, or Jane may have drowned, but without context, cause of death could not be established. If someone saw Jane drinking while sitting on the end of a Pigeon Lake dock, and if the toxicology report indicated that she had not ingested a fatal amount of alcohol, one could reasonably infer that she passed out, fell into the water, and drowned. Jane's toxicology report, however, revealed just a trace of alcohol (14 mg/dl), and no such context existed.

Cause of death? Indeterminable. Manner of death? Indeterminable.

Unfortunately, the autopsy raised more questions than it answered.

Did Jane Doe enter the water in Pigeon Lake, or did she enter the water in Lake Michigan, carried by currents through the channel into Pigeon Lake? And *when* did she enter the water? Likely months prior to discovery, based on the advanced state of decomposition. And *if* Jane Doe drowned, what circumstances led to her death? Why was she nude? Did she have an accident while skinny-dipping, or did someone strip her body before tossing it into the water? Or did she commit suicide by throwing herself naked into the frigid water where she would succumb to hypothermia within minutes and drown? Suicidal drowning, though, like homicidal drowning, is a very rare occurrence. And how did she sustain multiple rib fractures, which seemed suspicious for an accident or a suicide?

The answers to these questions most likely hinged on the answer to another question: who was Jane? If investigators could identify her, if they could replace the name Jane Doe on the autopsy report with a real name, perhaps they would be closer to finding out what happened.

Investigators did have a vague description to aid them in their search for her identity; a superficial examination during the autopsy presented a few clues about Jane's antemortem life that investigators could use in attempting to establish her identity. Extensive dental work suggested she made frequent visits to her dentist, and an x-ray revealed that she once broke her ankle and had it surgically repaired. Now, investigators needed to find a missing person who fit the profile: a woman, fifty to sixty years old, five feet seven, 170 to 180 pounds, with a history of cavities who once broke her left ankle. *If* authorities could discover her identity—*if* they figured out who Jane was—they would have a good chance of discovering how she died and how she ended up floating in Pigeon Lake.

Jane's teeth would provide the most important clue of all.

Teeth are like fingerprints—each person's identity is preserved in his or her teeth. Multiply the number of teeth by the number of possible dental "fixes" and the number of possible materials used in those fixes, and you have a virtually infinite variety of results, making teeth almost as useful in identifying an individual as fingerprints. If a twelve-year-old boy falls on concrete during a game of driveway basketball and chips his tooth, the moment will be preserved in the cap that his dentist used to repair the damaged tooth. Like this hypothetical boy, Jane's fifty-plus years of dental work left a specific, identifiable pattern. Someone would have a record of this work. The trick was to find that someone.

Because she had had extensive dental work, and because Jane's teeth presented the most likely chance of pinpointing her identity, a forensic odontologist was consulted. Dr. Roger Erbaugh traveled to the Kent County Morgue to fill out a postmortem dental chart for Jane Doe. On the chart—essentially a diagram of two arcs representing the upper and lower jaws—Dr. Erbaugh sketched the dental work in Jane Doe's mouth. If and when investigators produced a likely candidate for Jane from a missing person's report, Dr. Erbaugh could confirm or deny the identification by comparing the chart he sketched at the Kent County Morgue (the postmortem dental chart) with dental records from the missing person's dentist. With the premortem and postmortem dental charts placed next to each other, the comparison is simple: similarities and differences become evident, like a shiny gold filling in a person's front tooth when she smiles. Dr. Erbaugh characterizes this part of the process as an easy one that any layperson could complete.

When the Kent County medical examiner's office needs help in identifying a body—when a victim's identity is not 100 percent certain—Dr. Erbaugh is consulted. He works about ten to fifteen such cases a year in which he confirms or disproves a victim's identify based on dental records. He made the positive identification of Dorothy Perkins (see "The Hand That Feeds"), and now he would lend his expertise to helping identify the Pigeon Lake Jane Doe. For Dr. Erbaugh, forensic odontology offers a fascinating sideline to his "day job" at the dental practice he began after he graduated with a doctor of dental science degree from the University of Michigan's School of Dentistry in 1976.

Dr. Erbaugh's résumé of solving mysteries of identity began during a conversation with a high school friend whose father happened to be the head of pathology at Blodgett Hospital. Within a month, he received a call with a request for help identifying a victim who was doused with gasoline. This began a thirty-year sideline in forensic odontology. Specialized training for forensic odontology followed: he attended the Armed Forces Institute of Pathology in Washington, DC, where he received basic training in identification techniques and bite mark analysis specific to odontology. Dr. Erbaugh is also a member of the American Society of Forensic Sciences.

Dr. Erbaugh's fictional counterparts spend much of their time analyzing bite marks; for example, the *CSI* forensic odontologist might pair a victim with a sociopathic serial killer through some dental idiosyncrasy left in a bite mark. Dr. Erbaugh's role in the forensic process, though, typically involves the identification of remains. On occasion, investigators will ask him to match a perpetrator with a victim through the identification of a bite mark. For example, in one case, a man bit a prostitute. Because the man had many missing teeth, Dr. Erbaugh could confirm that the bite marks on the prostitute came from his jaws. And once in a while he will get a case involving child abuse, in which a physician or investigator might consult him to determine who might have made the bite mark on the abused child's body.

Pairing bite marks with the teeth that made them is a tricky, highly subjective process, and one that Dr. Erbaugh prefers to avoid. For example, investigators consulted Dr. Erbaugh in a strange case that illustrates the slippery nature of bite mark identification. A man stabbed a woman thirty times in the face with a pair of scissors but claimed it was in self-defense because she bit him. The perpetrator had a sharp cut on the web of his hand he claimed was a bite mark that represented his defense for stabbing her thirty times. After studying the wound, however, Dr. Erbaugh determined that the abrasion was not a bite mark at all; it was a wound caused by the scissors. It was self-inflicted. Such cases are vanishing from the CSI landscape, though; better DNA evidence has eliminated the need for bite mark identification.

The process for identifying a victim usually begins with the disarticulated jaws, which are removed from the corpse and sent to the forensic lab at Dr. Erbaugh's dental office. If investigators suspect a match between a victim and a missing person, they will send dental paperwork, such as x-rays and a dental chart, along with the jaws so Dr. Erbaugh can make a comparison. If they match—mystery solved. If not, authorities must follow other leads.

If authorities have no idea of the victim's identity, however, they cannot supply the dental charts, and the process would begin with only a description of the victim's teeth. If the victim's face (and thus identity) has been obliterated by severe damage or decomposition, like the Pigeon Lake Jane Doe, the Kent County medical examiner might contract a forensic anthropologist to study the remains and generate a biological profile. A facial reconstruction artist would then create a likeness based on the biological profile.

Because Jane's head would travel from the Kent County Morgue to Dr. Norm Sauer's forensic anthropology laboratory at Michigan State University in East Lansing, the face had to be kept intact and the jaws could not be removed. To study the jaws, then, Dr. Erbaugh traveled to the morgue to examine the teeth in situ, or in their original position. (Ten months later, Jane's disarticulated jaws would arrive at Dr. Erbaugh's lab where he would take postmortem x-rays.)

"I'm just looking at generalities," Dr. Erbaugh says when describing the process of matching antemortem and postmortem dental charts.[2] Generally, he looks to match specific, definable features with antemortem records.

The next phase of identifying a victim through his teeth involves taking x-rays and describing the teeth by the universal numbering system for dentistry and sketching any dental work or restorations on a chart. Adults generally have thirty-two teeth (including wisdom teeth). The numbering sequence begins with the upper right wisdom tooth, which is number one, and follows the arc of teeth to the upper left wisdom tooth—number sixteen. The sequence continues to the lower left wisdom tooth—number seventeen—and continues around the lower arc to the lower right wisdom tooth—at thirty-two, the last in the sequence. The postmortem dental chart of an adult who has had his wisdom teeth removed would indicate that numbers one, sixteen, seventeen, and thirty-two are missing. If a victim has had the number one tooth removed, description would begin with tooth number two, which is a molar.

A victim's teeth present a wealth of information that can be used for identification. "You have to think of each tooth like a cube," Dr. Erbaugh suggests. Each tooth has six sides. One of those sides is the root; the other five are the biting surface, lingual (facing roof of mouth), buccal, distal (backside, away from the midline), and mesial (toward the midline). Thirty-two teeth multiplied by five surfaces on each tooth multiplied by the various types of restorations (such as bridges and crowns) multiplied by the various filling materials dentists use to repair damaged teeth (such as amalgam, tooth-colored composites, porcelain, and gold)—the combinations number into the thousands and make it virtually impossible that any two people could have identical dental charts. Thus, teeth are as useful as fingerprints when identifying a John or Jane Doe.

The type of material used for dental work can indicate where the victim received dental treatment. Russian dentists, for example, typically use stainless steel, and their work often does not meet standards required of dentists practicing in America (the filling and the material used may not meet exactly). And the sense of aesthetics differs: Russian dentists, perhaps sacrificing looks for lower cost, might use steel crowns in the front of teeth rather than porcelain that would conceal the repair. Such information can provide the vital link between a Jane Doe victim and a possible identity. If the Pigeon Lake Jane Doe had stainless steel caps, investigators would have one more clue to her identity—she likely either lived or traveled in Russia.

If identification comes from matching specific, definable features on antemortem and postmortem records, what happens if the victim never had any dental restoration work? Just about everyone has had a cavity that needed filling, but a younger victim may have died before having the dubious pleasure of experiencing the dentist's drill and the laughing gas. In such situations, the forensic dentist can use the shape of the teeth and the roots to make an identification, if she has access to antemortem dental x-rays.

Dr. Erbaugh's highest profile case serves as an interesting illustration of the process used in identifying a victim through his teeth. Two Indiana college students were involved in a hideous car accident. One of the women, Whitney Cerak, supposedly died in the accident, but Laurie Van Ryn survived and returned to her Michigan hometown, where she received treatment at a rehabilitation center. Because hospital personnel had questions about the identity of the patient they were treating, the director of the hospital called the pathology department at Spectrum to ask for advice. The pathology department suggested a forensic odontologist to confirm the patient's identity.

Enter Dr. Erbaugh.

Dr. Erbaugh called Van Ryn's dentist and made arrangements to pick up her dental records, then he went to the rehab center. He made an initial, cursory examination of the patient's teeth in the dark of the patient's room at the rehab center. A comparison with Van Ryn's dental records produced a shocking revelation—they were not the same! This finding raised an interesting question: who died in the Indiana car accident and who survived?

This initial identification needed verification, so the patient was transported to Dr. Erbaugh's office for x-rays and a complete examination. Dr. Erbaugh verified his earlier finding: the young blonde in the chair at this office was not Laurie Van Ryn!

The next morning, the hospital called Dr. Erbaugh. They had obtained dental records for Whitney Cerak and wanted him to examine them. He compared the records with those he assembled the night before, and they were the same: Laurie Van Ryn was Whitney Cerak. Indiana investigators had mixed up the identities of the women. How had this happened? The two women, both with long, straight blond hair and similar facial features, looked like sisters. Someone simply jumped to the wrong conclusion.

The real Laurie Van Ryn had been buried approximately a month earlier in a Mecosta County cemetery under a headstone with Whitney Cerak's name. The body would need to be exhumed, but under Michigan law, a body cannot be exhumed without a death certificate. There was, however, no death certificate for Laurie Van Ryn, only for Whitney Cerak. Once the red tape had been cut, Dr. Erbaugh traveled to the funeral home holding the remains to make a positive identification of Laurie Van Ryn.

Teeth, Dr. Erbaugh explains, are valuable in identifying human remains "because they are pretty indestructible." Teeth survive the ravages of time; skulls unearthed after being buried for centuries usually have well-preserved teeth. Murderers, real and imagined, have attempted to cover up their crimes by obliterating their victim's identity. If fictional detective Arkady Renko in *Gorky Park* consulted Dr. Erbaugh, he could likely make an identification based on what was left of the victims' teeth despite the killer's best efforts to prevent this possibility.

Teeth generally survive fires, although when a fire becomes extremely intense, the moisture inside the teeth vaporizes and they explode. These types of scenarios, which Dr. Erbaugh has seen many times, present difficulties for the forensic odontologist. They don't occur often, though. Even intense fires often do not completely destroy a victim's teeth. The lips burn away and the front teeth explode, but the back teeth are sometimes protected.

In certain circumstances, however, a fire can destroy all of a victim's teeth, leaving only the root tips for identification. When a fire obliterates all of a victim's teeth, it also obliterates any certainty in identification. A house fire would usually not generate sufficient heat to do this type of damage; a burst gasoline tank would. To destroy the possibility of identification, therefore, a murderer would have to either remove all the victim's teeth or create a fire hot enough to obliterate them.

Whatever or whoever killed the Pigeon Lake Jane Doe left a vital clue to her identity intact: teeth—the one part of Jane Doe's body not ravaged by time, the elements, and marine life. After examining the Pigeon Lake Jane Doe's teeth and completing a postmortem dental chart, Dr. Erbaugh filled out a National Crime Information Center (NCIC) report. Michigan law requires the completion of an NCIC report for unidentified bodies and missing persons. The report, which includes a dental chart, is posted in a nationwide computer database for investigators working missing persons cases or attempting to establish the identity of a victim.

While the forensic professionals studied Jane Doe, sheriff's deputies circulated computer messages about Jane throughout Michigan as well as other Great Lakes states including Illinois, Indiana, Ohio, and Wisconsin. Their efforts generated a few leads. A migrant worker disappeared in January 2003, but she proved not to be Jane Doe. No one matching Jane's description had gone missing from the neighboring Allegan and Kent counties, either. A woman from Marshall fit Jane's description, but the advanced decomposition of the body suggested that Jane entered the water long before the Marshall woman was reported missing.

One promising lead came from Macomb County on the eastern side of Michigan and across the state from where Jane surfaced. The lead involved a resident of New Haven—a wealthy suburb of Detroit. Judith Matisse left her home on May 19, 2003, in a Chevrolet Impala and vanished. Her daughter reported her missing. Her height (five feet seven), weight (145), and age (fifty-five) fit the profile.

Police found her husband, James, in his car two days later in the parking lot of a New Haven church, the victim of a bizarre suicide. He had strangled himself with a plastic zip-tie. He left a suicide note in the car. The couple owned and operated a business together—Unlimited Services—but the investigation revealed evidence that suggested they lived anything but a perfect life together. James Matisse had filed for a divorce in April 2003, perhaps motivated by jealousy over a relationship between Judith Matisse and a convicted rapist incarcerated in a state prison. Judith Matisse, investigators alleged, may have even used company funds to finance the convict's appeal, whom she met as a volunteer at the prison. An ugly picture seemed to form as a result of James Matisse's suicide and Judith Matisse's disappearance: investigators came to believe that the missing woman was the victim of a murder-suicide engineered by a jealous husband.

Four months later, on September 16, 2003, a towing company discovered Judith Matisse's Impala parked on a side street near Comerica Park in downtown Detroit, home of the Detroit Tigers. Murderers often park their victims' cars in public places as a way to create a red herring for investigators. Harry Bout (see "Sex, Lies, and Cement") and Keith Prong (see "The Hand That Feeds") both transported the cars of their victims to airports to create false trails with the hope that when police eventually found the cars, they would believe the missing persons simply hopped jets to some distant locale.

Someone—James Matisse, if the sinister murder-suicide theory was correct—parked the car in an ingenious place. The streets in the vicinity of Comerica remain clogged with parked vehicles during home stands from early May to late September—the professional baseball season. A car left on the streets there could sit for weeks if not months unnoticed. Investigators found one annoying clue that suggested the car had sat abandoned for four months, long enough for insects to move into the abandoned vehicle: one beehive in the trunk and another by the front passenger door. Judith Matisse had also left her purse in the car, odd for someone who voluntarily walked away from the vehicle.

If James Matisse had not committed suicide, he would have found himself in handcuffs, under arrest on a potential murder charge: motive, opportunity, but no body and no weapon. Police had no idea where Judith Matisse had gone. She had simply vanished. Now, investigators hoped, the discovery of Jane Doe would plug the hole in what had become a vexing mystery, and Ottawa County sheriff's deputies could bring closure to their case as well. Jane's profile fit Judith Matisse, and since the Matisse couple traveled throughout West Michigan on company business, the appearance of her body across the state made sense if James murdered her and dumped her in familiar territory. What didn't make sense was why, if Judith Matisse entered Pigeon Lake in late May, her body didn't surface until the following March. In May, the water of Pigeon Lake would not have been cold enough to slow the formation of gas and keep her from becoming a floater.

In following the lead to Pigeon Lake, though, Macomb detectives had followed a red herring. On March 31, 2004, Dr. Erbaugh compared the postmortem dental chart of Jane Doe with dental records of Judith Matisse. They didn't match. Jane Doe, whoever she was, was *not* Judith Matisse. As of this writing, the body of Judith Matisse has not been found; in August 2004, she was officially declared dead.

By the end of March, despite casting their net throughout the Great Lakes states, Ottawa County sheriff's deputies had fielded five inquiries, none of which solved the mystery of Jane Doe's identity. They even investigated a missing California native who disappeared in the mid-1990s. It began to look like no one was missing Jane Doe. Perhaps no one was; as strange as it sounds, maybe no one had filled out a missing persons report for her. How could this happen? How could someone disappear and no one miss her? Maybe she was murdered and her killer did not want her to be missed. Or perhaps a mermaid *had* died and floated to the surface.

The case went cold until Dave Eddy—a Michigan state police cold case investigator—took the case to a missing persons training conference held in Florida and sponsored by the US Department of Justice. Eddy discussed the Pigeon Lake Jane Doe with other attendees. The conference would provide the denouement that would lead to the unbelievable solution of the mystery.

Eddy, a detective sergeant in the violent crimes unit who also investigates cold crimes, became interested in the case when he saw a facial reconstruction of the Pigeon Lake Jane Doe done by a state police artist.[3] He contacted the Ottawa County Sheriff's Office, and he and detectives David Blakely and Venus Repper began a joint investigation. Over the course of their investigation, they used a national missing persons database to generate possible matches between Jane Doe and missing persons from the Great Lakes states of Illinois, Indiana, Michigan, and Wisconsin. Their search resulted in three hundred potential matches for women the same age, weight, and height of Jane Doe and who went missing any time after May 2003 based on an estimate that she had been in the water for approximately nine months.

The investigative trio narrowed their search several times before they came across an intriguing lead: a woman named Barbara Biehn who went missing from Racine, Wisconsin, on December 22, 2003—directly across Lake Michigan from Pigeon Lake. The date fit the circumstances; if she went into the lake in December, the icy water would have slowed the formation of methane gas and kept her from surfacing until the following spring.

However, one element seemed to make the match unlikely. Police found her car abandoned on a causeway in Wisconsin, so if the missing Racine woman was Jane Doe, she must have floated *across* Lake Michigan and into Pigeon Lake—an unlikely if not impossible scenario. Even though she fit the profile, no one had connected the missing Racine woman with the Pigeon Lake Jane Doe because of this seemingly impossible scenario; how could a body float over a hundred miles?

At the missing persons conference, Detective Eddy discussed the feasibility of a match with other investigators and forensic experts, including a forensic dentist from California who suggested they compare dental records of Jane Doe with the missing Racine woman.

Eddy also consulted an expert at the National Oceanic and Atmospheric Administration who confirmed the possibility—albeit an extremely unusual one—that underwater currents and winds could move a body the almost one-hundred-mile distance from Racine to Pigeon Lake. The extensive damage to the body from animal activity and the fact that cold water can slow the formation of gas that would bloat and float the corpse suggests that Jane Doe spent a significant time underwater. Because the extreme cold temperatures of the water in the depths of Lake Michigan can retard the process of decomposition, bodies may lie at the bottom in various states of decomposition, creating an interesting image of a mermaid population on the floor of Lake Michigan.

Forensic anthropologist Dr. Norm Sauer (see "No Tombstone for 'Jack': An Untitled Story in Five Acts"), however, believes that she made the trek across Lake Michigan on the surface, pushed across by the currents.[4] At some point on this unlikely journey during the winter months, Jane may have encountered ice formations and may even have become stuck in one, which could have caused the multiple rib fractures.

While the national database, the NCIC, did not contain Barbara Biehn's dental records, the Racine police missing persons file on Biehn contained another reason to believe that she was Jane Doe. Biehn, her file noted, had undergone a surgical repair on her left ankle. So had Jane Doe, and the hardware used to correct the ankle contained serial numbers that investigators could match to the hardware used to correct Jane Doe's left ankle.

Racine police also obtained Biehn's dental records from her dentist and forwarded them to detectives Blakely and Repper, who would once again consult their forensic dentist with the hope that he could remove any question about Jane Doe's true identity and thus end the mystery that began in Pigeon Lake a year and half earlier.

On October 18, 2005, Dr. Erbaugh compared the dental charts: Jane Doe's postmortem chart that he had completed in the Kent County Morgue eighteen months earlier and Barbara Biehn's antemortem dental records from Racine. They matched. Jane *was* Barbara Biehn. Period.

Three days before Christmas in 2003, Barbara Biehn, from Racine, Wisconsin, left her husband a note that she was going shopping, and disappeared without a trace. Her car was found parked on the side of Christopher Columbus Causeway, her purse, keys, and money still inside. She would surface three months later a hundred miles away, directly across Lake Michigan from Racine in tiny Pigeon Lake, her body nude and decomposed.

The positive identification came five months after Jane Doe was buried. The badly decomposed corpse found in Pigeon Lake had entered the ground of a Michigan cemetery as Jane Doe on May 19, 2005. Across Lake Michigan two days later, Biehn's family, who believed her dead but knew nothing of the Pigeon Lake Jane Doe and her connection to their lost loved one, held a memorial service in Wisconsin on May 21, 2005. Jane Doe and Barbara Biehn, while the same person, had two different funerals within days of each other.

Despite the positive identification, Biehn's death leaves a few unanswered questions. How did her body make it into Pigeon Lake? Did she drift through the narrow channel connecting it with Lake Michigan? According to Detective Sergeant Eddy, investigators discussed another intriguing possibility: at the time Biehn's body appeared, the Consumers Energy plant on Pigeon Lake took water from Lake Michigan through an intake valve that did not have a protective grill. The summer before her body surfaced (in 2003), a female scuba diver ventured too close to the intake valve, and it swallowed her . . . literally. A gentle yet forceful current took her on an unnerving journey in total darkness through the intake pipe only to be spit out later in a reservoir. Perhaps Biehn's body took a similar journey. Investigators explored this possibility, but according to Detective Blakely, it is an unrealistic scenario because the intake pipe enters into a reservoir that is separated from Pigeon Lake by barriers.[5]

And what happened to Barbara Biehn along the Columbus Causeway? This is a question that may never be answered. Did someone murder her and toss her into Lake Michigan, or did she commit suicide? All of the evidence seems to support the fact that she took her own life, although the extreme decomposition of her body and subsequently no clear cause of death fail to remove the question mark behind the word *suicide*. And the fractured ribs also raise the specter that someone beat or stomped her to death . . . it has happened (see "Punch Drunk"). The rib fractures, however, could also have occurred during her unlikely journey across the lake. According to Dr. Sauer, a forensic anthropologist who studied the case, the fractures could have been caused by contact with ice.

While the rib fractures are suspect, other circumstances seem to support the notion that Biehn had committed suicide. She suffered from depression, and had attempted suicide before. She was also locked in a battle with breast cancer, and the chemotherapy prevented her from taking antidepressant medication. Perhaps Barbara Biehn slumped into a deep depression and decided to end her suffering.

The chemotherapy also created an interesting red herring for investigators. Detective Blakely notes that Jane Doe didn't have hair.[6] Initially, investigators believed that contact with Lake Michigan's sandy bottom caused the lack of hair, when in fact, the chemotherapy was responsible. Another interesting question about the case may never be answered: what happened to Barbara Biehn's clothes? They have never been found. Did she strip and then jump into the icy lake? While the absence of clothes appears to give the case a sinister undertone, this fact can be explained by her long journey across the Big Lake. The clothes may have come off while her body floated across.

If Biehn did commit suicide, though, she avoided the most common method chosen by women: overdose. The toxicology screen revealed no chemical culprits. And she didn't shoot herself either, as we already concluded. In fact, it appears she chose an extremely rare method of suicide: she threw herself into the icy clutches of the Big Lake and possibly froze to death or drowned. If her deteriorating physical condition did lead her to one final and ultimately successful suicide attempt, it would be a secret she would leave at the bottom of Lake Michigan.

In Barbara Biehn's case, the sea did give up her dead, but she didn't give up the decedent's secrets.

Cause of death: indeterminable.

Manner of death: indeterminable.

## Notes

1. Many variations of the prayer given for the dead at sea exist. This one is from *The Book of Common Prayer and Administration of the Sacraments*

*and Other Rites and Ceremonies of the Church according to the Use of the Protestant Episcopal Church in the United States of America* (New York: James Pott and Company, 1892).

2. Dr. Roger Erbaugh, personal interview with Tobin T. Buhk, July 14, 2006.

3. David Eddy, Michigan state police detective sergeant, violent crimes unit, telephone interview with Tobin T. Buhk, August 23, 2006.

4. Norm Sauer, PhD, professor of anthropology at Michigan State University and forensic anthropologist, personal interview with Tobin T. Buhk, September 27, 2006. At his office on the campus of Michigan State University in East Lansing, Dr. Sauer discussed his experience with this case and the John Doe found in a blueberry patch (see "No Tombstone for 'Jack'").

5. Dave Blakely, Ottawa County detective, telephone interview with Tobin T. Buhk, December 3, 2007.

6. Ibid.

## No Tombstone for "Jack": An Untitled Story in Five Acts

### Act 5: The Burial

No elaborate funeral processions.

No tearful eulogies from relatives and friends.

No singing of "Auld Lang Syne" at the wake following the burial.

No sobbing spouse to lay flowers at the headstone or sprinkle a can of the decedent's favorite beer over his grave.

No street names or other landmarks to memorialize the fallen.

In fact, no headstone to preserve the name of the occupant of the cement crypt six feet underneath it. No witty or somber saying or favorite quote serves as a pithy summary of a life shortened by a hammer one day in May 2002. The omission of a headstone makes sense. This victim died without an identity. What would be etched onto its surface? "Here lies John Doe. Age: between thirty and fifty. Height: between five feet six and five feet ten. European descent."

No, no tombstone for him.

Just a lonely section of brush away from the lawn where the "other half" lives. Or rather rest. If John Doe was a golfer, he could appreciate the irony of being laid to rest in the rough. If he spent any time in poverty, he might feel comfortable on the other side of the tracks. If a foreigner, he might understand the notion of an invisible barrier, the feeling of being a stranger in a strange land. That is what he is, buried in Lakeshore Cemetery, likely hundreds if not thousands of miles away from where and what he once called home.

No relatives to say good-bye.

Only six strangers, who watch as the cemetery workers lower the simple box into the hole in the earth. Not even a pine coffin but one constructed of cardboard and particleboard—a coffin less elaborate than the one his murderer arranged for him four months earlier. The state of Michigan provided $234 for the gravesite and $289 to cover the cost of transportation, the coffin, and the reverend.

A local reverend gave a short eulogy to the victim as four Ottawa County sheriff's deputies and a funeral director watched, the soundtrack of a heavy late summer rain shower provided courtesy of Mother Nature.

The Kent County Morgue held the remains of the body on one of the shelves in its freezer since the discovery in May, but the tiny refrigerator—unlike the walls of sliding drawers that typify morgue depositories on television shows—is only about the size of a small bedroom. Pressure from overcrowding forced this victim to an unmarked gravesite off the beaten path in a corner of Lakeshore Cemetery.

Despite the best efforts by forensics experts throughout the state, the occupant of that pine box remains nameless except for the generic tag "John Doe." It isn't for a lack of effort.

This small rural graveyard in Michigan's Grand Haven Township represents the final stop on the victim's odyssey that began with a macabre discovery four months earlier. His is a story in five acts. Untitled. A work in progress.

## Act 1: A Macabre Discovery

The Greeks conjured a myth to describe the changing seasons. Persephone, the gorgeous daughter of the earth goddess Demeter, became the obsession of Hades, god of the underworld. Hades wanted Persephone and he would not accept rejection, so he turned to subterfuge. He kidnapped the young beauty and married her in the underworld. Demeter searched for her missing daughter, and her sorrow led to cold, harsh weather. Crops could not grow, and people went hungry. Eventually, Zeus forced Hades to relinquish Persephone to save humankind from starvation.

The wily Hades, however, had a trick—three pomegranate seeds—up his sleeve. He fed them to his wife, who as a result was forced to return to the underworld one month for each seed she consumed. When her daughter returns to her husband, Demeter grieves, and Earth's climate changes into winter, a season often associated in literature and the arts with death or dormancy.

When Persephone ventures back to Earth, to her mother, Demeter's joy becomes Earth's spring, the season associated with birth. It's easy to see Demeter's joy in the panoply of colors that is Michigan in the spring.

In Michigan, April showers bring blueberries. The United States leads the world's production of blueberries, and Michigan leads the nation with approximately a third of the total production. Most of the blueberry production comes from the counties that run up Lake Michigan's east coast. Harvest season spans from July to September, during which hired hands pluck around fifty million pounds of blueberries each season. Like the birds that find their way back to Michigan when the snows melt, groups of transients travel north to pursue steady labor as agrarian workers, spending most of their time in the blueberry fields and apple orchards.

In May 2002, amid the chirping birds and the hushed cacophony of the country, a blueberry farmer discovered a gory scene in the middle of a forested area between his blueberry fields: a steel travel trunk sitting in the middle of a charcoal circle. The box was about a foot in height and two and a half feet long, its battered, contorted, and charred skin still shiny despite the evident damage from the fire. It looked like a metal hope chest. The faint smell of gasoline suggested the accelerant used to ignite the blaze. Or rather, funeral pyre.

Inside the box were the burned remains of a man. His legs dangled over the rim, and his head was tilted at an awkward angle, like someone had jammed it into the box to make it fit. His mouth hung agape, like he died while gasping for breath or in the middle of a scream. His arms were held up in front of him, like a boxer. From his appearance, one could conclude that he died in the midst of a violent struggle, yet the posture resulted from the fire used in an attempt to obliterate his remains, and with it his identity. When a human body is burned, the fire dehydrates tendons, and they shorten and flex.

While the fire didn't obliterate this man, it did obliterate his identity. Nothing remained to indicate who lay in the box: no driver's license, no Social Security card, no supermarket discount card or credit card; any piece of identification this man carried went up in smoke. No face, either. In short, no identity.

The farmer had just found the individual whom investigators refer to as "Jack in the Box" (also the title of a documentary produced by a local college's film class). The designation gives law enforcement officers a name for the nameless victim—a surrogate identity to replace the generic "John Doe" and a persona to replace the objective tag of "victim."

While an exhaustive search of the crime scene did not produce anything to establish Jack's real name, investigators did uncover some tantalizing clues. Chemical tests indicated that the gasoline used to start the blaze came from Amoco. With no Amoco stations in the vicinity, it seemed reasonable to conclude that at least the gas and maybe the victim came from some distant location.

Tests of the box failed to produce any fingerprints, but the box did contain more clues left by a sloppy killer or killers: a fiberglass Craftsman claw hammer, its handle melted from the intense heat of the fire; four pieces of a baseball bat; a T-shirt, which subsequent investigation revealed was manufactured by a defunct company in Southern California; and pieces of a nylon rope and a plastic Wal-Mart shopping bag. And perhaps the most interesting clue of all: fragments of a Timex watch, frozen in time when the fire started, preserving the exact moment when this man lost his identity, when the fire transformed him into the subject that investigators named "Jack in the Box."

While Ottawa County detectives pondered these clues, Jack would travel east to the Kent County Morgue, where an autopsy would uncover more clues about his death.

## Act 2: The Last Doctor Jack Will See

From the scene, investigators transported the remains of John Doe, or "Jack," to the Kent County Morgue to determine manner and cause of death. The first step in the autopsy procedure involves weighing and measuring the victim. He was a slight man, standing between five feet six and five feet seven inches tall and weighing approximately 135 pounds (fire typically reduces the weight of victims, so in the morgue his remains weighed 108).

Did Jack's killer burn him alive? This question is answered by examining the victim's airway, the bronchi of each lung, and the larynx. The presence of soot in these areas would indicate that the victim was breathing and thus alive during the fire. No soot was found. And the victim's blood contained less than 5 percent carbon monoxide—a normal level. If the victim had been alive during the fire, this level would be higher. Jack was dead before he went into the fire.

But when did he die? While the fire obliterated some evidence the ME might have used to pinpoint time of death, an examination of the internal organs revealed that he died within two days of when the body was discovered. If a much longer period had elapsed between the death and the discovery, the organs would not have been firm but soft from decomposition.

Although charred remains present difficulties in conducting an internal examination, Jack's cause of death became clear upon examination of his skull; several sharp, forceful blows with a heavy, blunt object left four depressed fractures in his skull. The shape and contours of the fractures left little room for speculation: the head of a hammer fit the craters on the skull perfectly. Specifically, Jack's assassin used a claw hammer to dispatch his or her victim. Investigators recovered a claw hammer from the scene, its head 27.5 millimeters in diameter and consistent with the depressed fractures: the hammer's round head neatly fit into the craters it created in Jack's skull.

The hammer illustrates the maxim that form follows function; various types of hammers are designed for specific purposes. Claw hammers, so named because of the curved "claw" opposite the head, are used to pound in and, when necessary, straighten or pull out nails. A killer or killers struck Jack on the head with such a hammer, causing the four depressed skull fractures. The fifth fracture—the linear fracture—resulted when Jack was struck in the back left side of his head with some other type of blunt instrument, such as a baseball bat, like the one investigators discovered in pieces at the scene.

These injuries present one possible reason for the presence of the plastic Wal-Mart bag and the pieces of nylon rope. Jack would have bled profusely, and his killer or killers may have fastened the bag around his head with the nylon rope in order to contain the blood.

The cause of death: blunt force trauma. The manner of death: homicide. In early spring 2002, someone murdered this man.

But who? The fire destroyed the victim's face and fingerprints. Whoever killed Jack recognized the fact that obliterating a victim's identity also obliterates the suspect's identity, particularly if the victim and his killer knew each other; a lack of identity makes the task of finding suspects difficult if not impossible. With a lack of suspects, investigators usually begin by delving into the victim's biography, including his movements before death, as a way of identifying possible perpetrators. In this case, though, investigators had no name, no address, no biography to investigate. To solve this crime, investigators would need to replace the generic victim name "John Doe" with the victim's real name.

Investigators did have one clue about the man's identity: extensive dental work suggested Jack had paid frequent visits to a dentist. He would see one more: forensic odontologist Roger Erbaugh (see "The Sea Shall Give Up Her Dead"). The disarticulated jaws of the victim traveled to Dr. Erbaugh's forensic laboratory, where he created a postmortem dental chart of Jack's teeth. Sometimes killers, aware that dental remains are almost as unique as fingerprints, will attempt to destroy a victim's teeth through tremendous heat. Perhaps a desire to obliterate Jack's identity by obliterating his teeth caused his killer to create a gasoline-fed fire. If so, he failed.

Jack had several fillings and a few gold crowns. His four upper front teeth were false—they were part of an upper dental plate construction. The work was not recent; experts estimated that the work took place at least a decade earlier and most likely occurred in the southern United States or Mexico. This was not inexpensive dental work; the sum would have amounted to thousands of dollars. This led to speculation that the victim came from an affluent background.

Yet without an antemortem dental chart for comparison, Jack's teeth would help investigators make a match only after they identified possible victims. Thus, this tidbit of information is like a puzzle piece. Now investigators needed to find the puzzle into which the piece fit. Without the larger picture for reference—the puzzle frame—the colors and fragment of an image on the puzzle piece make little sense.

## Act 3: *Bones*, but Not the Television Show . . .

From the Kent County Morgue, Jack's remains traveled southeast to Dr. Norm Sauer's forensic anthropology laboratory at Michigan State University. Dr. Sauer joined the faculty of Michigan State University in 1973 and earned his PhD in physical anthropology a year later. For the past thirty years, he has split his time between the world of academia with its ivy-covered brick walls and complicated research, and the world of forensic science with its baffling mysteries and real-life tragedy.

Dr. Sauer has applied his expertise in forensic anthropology to many high-profile cases. He worked in Manhattan, assisting medical examiners in the identification of human remains just days after terrorists knocked down the World Trade Center. From Manhattan, he traveled to Shanksville, Pennsylvania, where Flight 93 crashed, helping to identify victims of the plane crash. He even helped search for Jimmy Hoffa's remains on a farm in southeastern Michigan.

One of his most challenging cases came in 1993, during the investigation of a missing teenager. Rose Larner, a teenager from Lansing, Michigan, disappeared in 1993. Despite a full-fledged investigation, police found no trace of the girl. Then a break came in 1995, when a witness named Billy Brown came forward and told the story of what happened to the missing teenager.

During a weekend of drugs and sex, one of three partiers murdered Rose Larner, dismembered her body in a shower, burned and scattered some of the remains, and took a significant portion of the remains to a northern lake on which Brown's family owned property. In a large fire, they burned the rest. Investigators managed to locate the firepit (which had since been covered over). Sauer then led an archaeological dig of the site and recovered eight small, fingertip-sized pieces of human bone.

Microscopic sections were made from several of the bone specimens recovered during the excavation so they could be examined under a microscope. The sections consisted of very thin slices—about 1 millimeter thick (an inch equals about 254 millimeters)—mounted on glass slides. Under a 100× magnification, several features unique to bone become visible. These features consist of lacunae, canaliculae, lamellae, and osteons. The size and type of osteons in these slices indicated that they came from human bone. An examination revealed that the bone fragments found in the pit had indeed come from a human. The FBI conducted a DNA analysis, but the samples were too burned to produce a successful DNA sample.

Consequently, the bones were never positively identified as Rose Larner's, yet the circumstances of the case—including the testimony of Brown—were so compelling that prosecutors ultimately won a conviction.

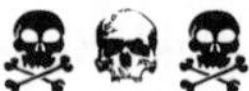

On a warm afternoon in September 2006, almost four and a half years after the discovery of Jack, Dr. Sauer is at work in the forensic anthropology laboratory, which consists of several rooms on the third floor of a Michigan State University building.[1]

The forensic anthropology laboratory's central room is about the size of a two-stall garage. In this room, Dr. Sauer and his partner Dr. Todd Fenton solve the most vexing forensic mysteries. Together, they work about sixty cases a year.

The first thing one sees when entering the laboratory is a long table, on the surface of which the anthropologists study remains. This morning, a white towel covers the table, and across its surface is strewn a collection of various bones including two human skulls. Police, Dr. Sauer explains, found the bones in the attic of a recently deceased man, who apparently had a collection. Some people collect stamps, others coins or baseball cards; this man collected bones, and his accumulation contained both animal and human bones.

In one corner of the room stands a skeleton. Its tea-colored bones indicate that, unlike its plaster-cast cousin in the Kent County Morgue, it is real. Dr. Sauer studies the skeleton; he can read its physiology like a book. He points to the pubic region and explains that the skeleton is male. With time to study the skeleton, he could discover its physiological biography, including its ancestry.

The forensic anthropologist's most common involvement in criminal investigations is the positive identification of unknown remains—in other words, helping police find the real identities of victims. In a typical case, they will receive remains and study them to generate a biological profile, which they submit to investigators. When investigators find a potential victim, they will return to the forensics anthropology lab with x-rays taken before the victim died (antemortem). Drs. Sauer and Fenton will make a comparative study of the remains and the x-rays and determine the feasibility of a match.

Dr. Sauer presses a videocassette into one of three players/recorders next to two large tables with lamps dangling over a white surface like tentacles. These machines allow Dr. Sauer and his forensic team to superimpose photographs over skulls to make comparisons.

The blue screen on the television disappears, and an image—a police booking photograph of a woman named Wendy Curry—appears on the screen. As the tape rolls, the photograph disappears and a skull—possibly hers—appears. The two images become one, with the ghostly image of the skull superimposed over the police booking photograph. To make a positive identification, Dr. Sauer studies key "landmarks," which include five "points of orientation": corners of eye orbits (ectocantion: attachment sites for corners of the eyelids); chin (gnathion); subnasale (under the nose). This equipment is also used in cases when police ask Dr. Sauer to match or "exclude with confidence" suspects by comparing surveillance video and other photographs/video.

The Wendy Curry case provides a good example of the forensic anthropologist's typical involvement in a criminal investigation. On September 3, 1998, police recovered the skeleton of an unidentified woman in Muskegon County. Investigators brought to Dr. Sauer the skull and some photographs of a possible victim, including three booking photographs—frontal and right/left lateral—and some family photographs.

Dr. Sauer superimposed the images over the skull, and despite all of the images provided, could not exclude her; in other words, the remains likely belonged to Wendy Curry. The process, Dr. Sauer explains, is usually an attempt to exclude.

"We go into a case assuming the person in the photograph and the victim are the same person," Dr. Sauer explains. "Our attitude is to prove that it is not that person. If we cannot, then that raises questions." The better the data, the stronger the conclusion. The idea is called "falsification": something cannot be proven true but can be proven false.

With the victim's identity established as Wendy Curry, police now wanted to know what had happened to her. Investigators suspected that damage to the first metacarpal of the left hand represented a defensive wound, as if she had raised her hand to shield herself. An examination of the wound, however, indicated that it came from postmortem animal activity and thus provided no evidence of foul play.

Wendy Curry's ribs, though, told a different story. Dr. Sauer stands next to the skeleton to illustrate the nature of Wendy Curry's rib fractures. Seven rib fractures occurred at about the time she died (perimortem). He points to the skeleton's ribs and draws an invisible line in the air to illustrate that the seven fractures appeared in a line, suggesting they were caused by the same event, like something heavy fell onto Wendy Curry's chest. An additional thirty fractures occurred before death (antemortem). These fractures suggest that Wendy Curry died a horrific and painful death when her attacker stomped her to death. This type of injury has happened before (see "Punch Drunk").

In fact, it had happened to Wendy Curry before. The forensic evidence suggested that Wendy Curry had suffered similar injuries in the past; both sides of her rib cage demonstrated fractures in various stages of healing. Some fractures contained bulbous sections where the bone healed, indicating old fractures, perhaps years old. The bulbous spots where the bone healed look like the knots on a tree branch. Some of the fractures had recently begun to heal, and some had occurred at about the time she died.

The forensic anthropologist can follow certain clues to determine if the fractures occurred perimortem, or at about the time of death: (1) No evidence of healing (healing occurs in about two weeks); (2) Evidence of the "green stick effect." Dr. Sauer explains with an analogy: a dead branch from a tree will snap, but a branch from a living tree won't break. Its edges will bend. Bones have the same kind of patterns. Living bones don't always snap; sometimes they bend—the "green stick effect." Wendy Curry's ribs contained evidence of green stick fractures, indicating the fractures occurred when alive or recently dead. (3) Lack of differential staining. The staining on all of the surface was the same. If the surface of a bone is exposed to the elements, some differential staining/discoloring would appear. Differential staining indicates differential exposure.

The rib fractures provided the key evidence in obtaining a criminal conviction because they indicated a manner of death; they told a violent saga of domestic abuse that ultimately led to murder. Her killer, a live-in lover, was convicted of first-degree murder and sentenced to life in prison without the possibility of parole.

Dr. Sauer would also apply his expertise to the vexing identity crises that developed with the blueberry farmer's macabre discovery.

After an examination of the remains found in the metal box, Dr. Sauer produced a biological profile for the John Doe called Jack discovered in Grand Haven Township. The profile is a vital stop in Jack's odyssey from oblivion to identification, because the profile provides a snapshot of the victim that can be used to find or dismiss possible matches with missing person's reports. When the remains left Dr. Sauer's forensics laboratory, police could rule out anyone not of European ancestry and taller or shorter than the range of five feet six to five feet ten, and anyone younger or older than the range of thirty to fifty years of age. While the biological profile is admittedly vague, it does allow investigators to narrow their search.

It also provides vital information for forensic artists, who must bring a face to the faceless.

## Act 4: A Face from Facelessness

From Dr. Sauer's laboratory, Jack's skull and biological profile traveled to Michigan state police trooper and forensic artist Fernando Martinez.[2] When all other means to identify a victim fail, investigators turn to someone like Martinez to help identify a victim. For twenty-five years, Martinez, one of five forensic artists employed by the state, has used his artistic ability to help identify the state's unidentified victims by creating two-dimensional likenesses of them. Such drawings circulate among law enforcement agencies, which in turn circulate them through the media in an attempt to secure a victim's identity. These are the faces that appear in newspapers, postcards, and on milk cartons.

Trooper Martinez also on occasion draws facial reconstructions of living subjects using photographs instead of skulls. For the Michigan State Department of Corrections, he has drawn age enhancements of escapees who managed to evade capture for years. These updated images helped identify and capture convicts whose visages have been altered by time. When creating such a drawing, Martinez explains, he relies more on family members than photographs. Sometimes, family members of murder victims will even ask him to draw a likeness of their lost loved one as he or she might appear today, although he typically rejects such requests because the survivors, he suggests, need to let go.

Now retired, Martinez spends his time riding his Harley Davidson around Michigan, satisfying his artistic urges by snapping photographs of various subjects with his Canon SLR 20D and attending photography workshops. He has not left law enforcement behind entirely; he pursues security gigs around the globe, including a one-year tour of duty in Kosovo and a three-month stint in New Orleans as a security contractor. The US military, he explains, contracts base security to private firms such as Halliburton; in Kosovo, his job consisted of manning a machine gun in a guard tower. In a New Orleans devastated by Hurricane Katrina, he provided security for construction crews who were helping to make the city rise from its own rubble.

Forensic art, he explains over a plate of buffalo wings and a Sam Adams Boston lager, is part art and part science. Martinez began as an art student before leaving to join the state police, who made good use of his artistic ability by providing him a dual role: law enforcement officer and a forensic artist. Martinez trained as a forensic artist under leading experts, including forensic art guru Karen Taylor, at the Federal Bureau of Investigation's base at Quantico, Virginia.

The process seems simple, but it is anything but. Two-dimensional facial reconstructions typically involve two perspectives, frontal and profile views, although Martinez notes that during his tenure in the state police, he specialized in frontal views only.

At the forensics anthropology laboratory at Michigan State University, Dr. Sauer cleans any remaining flesh from the skull by boiling it in a stainless steel oven with borax soap, leaving the skull an off-white color. After the skull leaves Dr. Sauer's laboratory, the forensic artist adds flesh markers, which is a trade name for pencil erasers of various lengths, to indicate likely depth of tissue based on several factors including the subject's age, sex, and ethnic background. Because the subject's race dictates the placement and depth of the tissue markers, the biological profile becomes a vital element. Race, for the purposes of forensic artists, consists of three general categories: Caucasoid, Mongoloid, and Negroid. Together, these tissue markers provide an outline of the victim's face. After the skull is boiled, though, oils continue to ooze from the bone, which makes it greasy, and sometimes, Martinez notes, the markers slide off and need to be reapplied.

Next, the skull is photographed to obtain the proper perspective: a one-to-one perspective with no left-to-right or top-to-bottom deviation, which can cause distortion and thus render a drawing inaccurate. The forensic artist places a sheet of vellum paper over the photograph of the skull, and with the skull as the background, begins to sketch the face on the vellum overlay. The tissue markers suggest the outline and shape of the face, and various features on the skull dictate the placement of the eyes, the nose, and the ears. After several drafts, a face is produced.

Often, Martinez suggests, the skull will tell the subject's life history. For example, abuse of alcohol and drugs like methamphetamine, which leads its user to consume a large quantity of sugar, leave a telltale clue: rotten teeth. Such specific, potentially identifiable features will dictate how he depicts a subject. If the subject had some significant dental feature, such as a gold cap, he might draw the face as smiling. To smile or not to smile, in other words, depends on what the smile reveals.

Some aspects of human anatomy, Martinez explains, remain the same no matter what the ethnic background of the subject. For example, the eyeball remains the same regardless of race. Forensic artists are taught that they should equate the size of the human eyeball to the size of a US quarter. So when making a forensic drawing, Martinez places a quarter over the vellum in a spot equidistant between the two points in the eye's orbit where the eyeball connects.

Ethnic background does provide specific characteristics the forensic artist can use to create a realistic likeness. Fernando Martinez removes a sheet of lined paper from a black leather portfolio to demonstrate. With a few rapid sweeps of his wrist, he creates a realistic eye. He circles in the eyeball, its top edge tucked under the eyelid. One defining trait of men of Middle Eastern descent, he explains, is a raised iris, or an iris that partially disappears under the top eyelid. At Quantico, years before the 9/11 tragedy sparked hysteria about Middle Eastern terrorists, forensic art instructors showed students mug shots of men of Middle Eastern ancestry, and every one possessed raised irises.

Other groups of people have their physiological idiosyncrasies as well, and knowledge of these traits is vital to the forensic artist. If he knew that the subject of a drawing was a male who came from the Middle East, Martinez would likely draw the eyes to include the feature unique to this group of people. This subtlety could make the difference between a realistic drawing and a nonrealistic one, between a victim's identification and oblivion.

Still, this is forensic *art*, which involves a tremendous amount of subjectivity. Martinez could render a drawing of a skull this week that might bear marked differences to a rendering of the same skull next week. An amount of subjectivity is understandable yet somewhat troubling for the forensic artist. A family member cannot identify a loved one if he or she does not see that loved one in the two-dimensional facial reconstruction. Therefore, if an identification of a victim through one of the artist's drawings represents success, then a lack of identification represents a failure, and a vexing one.

To date, no one has come forward to identify the man whose murderer struck him several times on the head with a hammer, placed his body in a metal box, and incinerated him with gasoline, obliterating his facial features and thus his identity. The lack of a positive identity, Martinez explains, makes him feel like he did something wrong, even though he had very little to go on: the skull and three lines in a biological profile.

"In a majority of cases," he explains, "I had some hair." Strands of hair provide the forensic artist with an idea of the length, texture, and color of a subject's hair. For Jack, however, Martinez had to work without a hair sample. Hairline, style, and color became mere guesswork. And a lack of identification has left him wondering if he made the wrong guesses.

For this reason, Martinez would like to make another sketch of Jack. Maybe another sketch would help place a name on the tombstone at Jack's grave. Maybe not.

Maybe no one is missing the man from the blueberry field, which would make this a rare case of an identity that remains forever unsolved. Each year, migrant workers travel north to areas where they can find employment picking fruit. Did Jack travel north with a caravan of people who did not report him missing because, as illegal immigrants, they did not want to call attention to their community? If so, why would anyone want to kill a harvest worker attempting to pluck a living from West Michigan's blueberry bushes? Did he witness something? Did he fall victim to a marauding serial killer? Was he the sacrifice of a group of Satan worshipers?

Investigators made inquiries at local migrant camps, which produced no leads. This case is flooded by question marks covering every file page about the body found in the Grand Haven blueberry field in the spring of 2002.

One can imagine the scene of this murder on a balmy night in May in some distant field or forest. The figures appear as mere outlines, their frenetic movements framed by the moonlight and set to the shrill chanting of crickets. The crack of the hammer hitting bone . . . crack,

crack, crack . . . and one outline falls to the earth and becomes a black, shapeless mass.

The killer wraps the victim's head with a white plastic funeral shroud and conceals it with nylon rope. The bag quickly turns pink from the blood still oozing out of the victim's head wounds.

The killer drives down the highway in the darkness with his horrible secret in the trunk, looking for a desolate place where he can conceal the crime without detection (investigators believe Jack was murdered in one area and dumped somewhere else; the discovery site is not far from a major highway). He finds a dark, forested spot out of sight of the headlights moving down the highway. Down the dirt two-track he travels until he finds a forest glade.

He drops the box onto the earth. The pungent stench of gasoline fills the night air as he douses the metal coffin.

And then a bright orange glow lights up the scene. The flickering light playfully dances off of the trees and brush and makes the entire scene appear alive. The killer, still obscured by darkness, appears as a shadow. A chalk outline. As anonymous as the victim whose funeral pyre he has just lit.

What is known: the victim stood between five feet six and five feet ten and at the time of death was between thirty and fifty years old. The extensive dental work indicates that he made frequent visits to a dentist. The damage to his skull suggests that his death was no accident. What is not known: his identity.

Jack needs an identity for many reasons, including the need to identify suspects in his murder, because a killer walks free, possibly a threat to others, and has eluded justice in this heinous crime.

And Jack needs a headstone containing a name. Although the grave lacks the traditional marble gravestone etched with the victim's name and a touching epitaph written by a bereaved relative, it no longer lacks a marker. A county commissioner paid for a bronze plaque with the inscription "UNIDENTIFIED MALE / MAY 2002 / KNOWN ONLY TO GOD." It is the final piece of dialogue in this untitled story.

Jack's grave sits in the pauper's section of the cemetery on a bluff under a large tree, a few feet away from the rough, untrimmed thresh bordering that part of the complex. It is a nice spot, where rays of the sun fall onto the green grass through the canopy of leaves overhead. When the author visited the site in August 2007, someone had placed a floral arrangement by the marker—a reminder that someone, perhaps a complete stranger, remembers the tragedy that occurred one dark night in a blueberry field. The floral arrangement is also a reminder that someone, somewhere, knows Jack. It is just a matter of finding that someone.

The story of Jack's death is a play in five acts. Untitled. It is a work in progress.

## Notes

1. Norm Sauer, PhD, professor of anthropology at Michigan State University and forensic anthropologist, personal interview with Tobin T. Buhk, September 27, 2006.

2. Fernando Martinez, Michigan state police forensic artist (retired), personal interview with Tobin T. Buhk, October 25, 2006. Over a plate of buffalo wings and a few beers, Mr. Martinez provided a brief lesson in forensic art and discussed his experiences.

# 2. series

In the Zoo of Criminology, the most visited species is the serial killer.

When you first enter the Zoo of Criminology, you find to your right the Island of High Jinx. Visitors can lose track of time and spend hours here, watching bunco in action as scam artists concoct schemes and attempt to fool their fellow scam artists to deprive them of valued items such as food or cartons of cigarettes (in this analogy, they are the human version of spider monkeys, although this is an insult to spider monkeys).

To the left, you will find the Burning Circle of Arsonists. The zoo gives these pyromaniacs various items to burn, but you might want to remove your coats before you enter, because it gets hot in there.

Beyond the Burning Circle you will find the Ring of Thieves. Please secure all personal belongings before entering this exhibit. The zoo is not responsible for any lost or damaged items.

You may want to visit these areas first, because the majority of visitors will head straight to the zoo's most visited section: the Serial Killers. Because they are very dangerous, each is confined to his own cage. Here, you will find many fascinating subspecies, their names as colorful as their modus operandi: the "Lonely Hearts Killer" (sometimes referred to as the "Black Widow"), the "Cannibal Killer," the "Lust Murderer," the "Thrill Killer," the "Missionary Killer," the "Visionary Killer."

Indeed, in the Zoo of Criminology, the most visited species is the serial killer. Their horrific crimes have captivated the public, whose appetite for books and films about serial killers appears insatiable, a type of bloodlust by proxy of media. True-crime junkies inject themselves with "hits" of serial crime in nonfiction works about Leonard Lake and Charles Ng, Ted Bundy, John Wayne Gacy, Eileen Wuornos . . . the list is endless. In the film *Copycat* (about a fictional serial killer who models his murders after the murders of famous serial killers), Sigourney Weaver's character notes that more books have been written about Jack the Ripper than Abraham Lincoln. Subsequently, every bookstore in America carries at least one title about Jack the Ripper (and probably several), whose name has become synonymous with serial murder. The serial killer appears in fiction as well in print, television, and cinema. Thomas Harris's Hannibal Lecter, or "Hannibal the Cannibal," is one example.

Because each serial killer has a modus operandi that he or she usually repeats for each kill, the medical examiner plays a key role in the hunt, capture, and ultimate placement of the killer in "the zoo" for study by academics, law enforcement officers, and the lay public.

And even in a midsize, Midwestern town, over the years, serial killers have contributed skeletons to the ME's closet . . .

## Scorecard

Until a chance arrest, the story of their deaths had a beginning and an end but no middle . . .

Every murder is a story, and as such, contains a beginning, a middle, and an end. For those who investigate murders, including the medical examiner, the discovery of the body and the subsequent autopsy represents the beginning of the story. The search for clues and suspects: the middle. The trial, conviction, and sentence: the end. This is the sequence of most police procedural shows such as *Law & Order* and *CSI*.

For a murder victim, though, the last chapter of his life biography occurs in a different order: the beginning consists of the background, such as how he knew or met his murderers. Did he become intertwined in a love triangle that turned deadly? Did he wander across a crime in progress on the way back from a routine trip to the pharmacy? The middle consists of the context of the crime. The end, the murder and the disposition of the body. Homicide investigators must therefore work in reverse, beginning with the last page of a victim's biography.

The last page in the biographies of Dennis Alt and Chris Schoenborn occurred on a chilly morning in December 1982. Working in reverse, investigators pieced together the beginning of their end, tracing the two men to a hotel in downtown Grand Rapids. Their autopsies provided details about their end and suggested a possible context for the crime. For five months, though, investigators could not piece together a definitive picture of what occurred during the hours between the time they disappeared and the discovery of their bodies. Until a chance discovery that occurred in another state, the last chapters of their biographies had no middle.

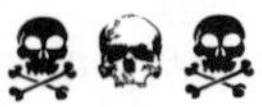

On the frigid morning of Thursday, December 9, 1982, at about 9:50 in the morning, a utility worker stumbled upon a ghastly sight in a rural area west of Grand Rapids. Two dead bodies lay near a water tower: one partially clothed, the other completely nude, but both lying on their backs and frozen from hours of exposure to the harsh Michigan winter. Despite the fact that neither man had a wallet or identification, before long, detectives managed to identify the pair.

The two men, twenty-four-year-old Dennis Alt and twenty-year-old Chris Schoenborn, had been missing for thirty-six hours. No longer. They had vanished only to reappear as the victims of foul play. The autopsies revealed that a grisly fate befell the two men, so the missing persons case had now become a murder investigation. The discovery of the missing men solved one mystery but led to another.

The bodies arrived at the Kent County Morgue in the exact state in which they were discovered: frozen. Only after the bodies thawed could the autopsy procedure begin. Dennis Alt—a man with a slight build at five feet eight and one hundred and thirty pounds—wore a tan V-neck sweater over a plaid shirt, a white T-shirt, and brown corduroy pants the night he died. The trousers and white Jockey underwear were pulled down below his waist to reveal his penis and testicles, suggesting a sexual component—perhaps an assault—to his death. The elastic waistband of the underwear had been tucked under Alt's scrotum, supporting the testicles and penis. The opening of his penis appeared enlarged. The pants pocket contained an enigmatic assortment of items: a single eyeglass lens, a quarter, a business card, and a handkerchief. The lining of the pocket was stained with purple ink.

An external examination of Alt's injuries suggested that a struggle occurred prior to his death. Several abrasions appeared on his face and on both ankles. The catalog of external injuries also included a four-inch contusion on his right thigh and a one-inch contusion on his right knee. Autopsy photographs taken at the time reveal dark purple smudges on his left thigh and underwear—ink that likely came from the same pen that left stains in the lining of his pocket. Did he carry a leaking pen in his pocket or did something else happen? A minor mystery to be solved later during the autopsy.

As for cause of death, the injuries, both internal and external, indicated that someone strangled Dennis Alt. Murder. Petechial hemorrhages covered the right side of his face, and a mark on his neck ran up the right side of his neck from under his chin to beneath his right ear. These external injuries likely occurred when someone applied pressure to Alt's neck and constricted the airflow, which within minutes caused death by asphyxia. The internal injuries provided conclusive evidence to support this cause of death: bleeding or hemorrhaging in the muscles of the throat.

The toxicology report indicated that Alt likely did not present much of a struggle to his killer: a combination of sedatives, specifically the prescription drug diazepam and alcohol would have left him groggy and lethargic or even unconscious.

Chris Schoenborn arrived at the morgue naked. Like Alt, his body contained a number of external injuries, including numerous abrasions on his lower legs and on his back between his shoulders and waist. And like Alt, he had been strangled, evident from the two pressure marks on the left side of his neck, which ran parallel to each other and extended from the middle of his neck to behind his left ear, and the extensive bleeding in the soft tissues of the neck.

The internal examination of the autopsy would uncover one other bizarre and horrific injury. Blood from Schoenborn's penis led to blood stains on his upper thighs and around the tip of his penis, indicating something out of the ordinary. A closer examination revealed the source of the injury: someone had inserted a ballpoint pen into the urethra of his penis and pushed it in as far as the pelvis. The pen, a white ballpoint pen just over six inches in length, contained in bright gold letters the inscription "Amway Grand Plaza."

The insertion suggested that, like Dennis Alt, Chris Schoenborn's murder contained some sexual component. Did the men voluntarily participate in some deviant sexual practice that involved the insertion of objects into the urethra? Their backgrounds made this seem very unlikely. Whatever the case, like Dennis Alt, Schoenborn likely experienced a diminished sense of awareness and pain, fortunately; the toxicology report indicated that he, too, had ingested a cocktail of alcohol and the prescription sedative diazepam.

The autopsy revealed the subtle clues of strangulation; someone, likely using some type of ligature like a belt or a cord, throttled the victims. And the toxicology screen suggested another facet of the killer's MO: the use of a prescription sedative. The missing persons case had turned into a murder mystery—a murder mystery with an end but not a beginning or middle.

Investigators would need to work backward, from the beginning of the story, to fill in the middle: the missing hours of the victims' last night, the missing pages in their life's biography. In reconstructing the story, investigators hoped to find the author of the murders. Or authors? Perhaps detectives would need to find two killers. That a two-person team committed the murders seemed a possible conclusion. One victim certainly would not sit and watch while a single killer murdered the other victim. Or perhaps a single killer bound his lethargic victims before finishing them off one at a time.

While the middle of the story remained shrouded in mystery, one thing remained clear. Sometime during the missing hours—the middle of this story—the two young men appeared to have been sexually assaulted, then brutally murdered. Then the killer or killers dumped their bodies in an area west of the city where a utility worker discovered them. But that is the end of the story. The inscription on the ballpoint pen suggested where to find the beginning.

The pen came from the Amway Grand Plaza, the most posh hotel in the county, so it seemed logical to trace the beginning of this tragedy to that setting. The Amway Corporation (now called Alticor), headquartered in the nearby suburban area of Ada, built a high-rise, silver-mirrored tower as an addition onto the old Pantlind Hotel in 1981. The tower stands erect like a silver index finger announcing the hotel's presence—the ultimate billboard. Standing next to the regal, early twentieth-century splendor of the Pantlind's original structure, with its period touches like giant potted ferns and ornate carved borders and decorative ceilings, the Amway Grand Plaza represents an example of the present meeting the past.

The tower's edifice seems to reflect Mother Nature's mood; a sunless sky in mid-winter gives the tower a look of coldness, of gray and blue tones; a sunset paints the tower a psychedelic orange.

In 1982, the hotel stood adjacent to the Grand Center Convention Center, DeVos Hall Performance Center—at the time the city's premier concert venue—and Civic Auditorium, where each year the Shrine Circus performed. The complex often played host to various events such as seminars, conventions, sporting events, and concerts ranging from the local symphony to pop stars. In early December 1982, the Grand Center and the Amway Grand Plaza hosted the annual three-day Michigan State Horticultural Convention.

Dennis Alt and Chris Schoenborn, along with hundreds who worked in the agricultural field, traveled to downtown Grand Rapids—the "big city," illuminated by its glitter and neon—to attend the horticultural convention. Both men, distant cousins who knew each other but did not spend much time together, worked farms on the fertile ridge along the western border of Kent County. Alt split his time harvesting fruit and milking cows on his family's fruit and dairy farm, while his cousin helped raise hogs and harvest fruit on his family's farm.

The young men looked forward to the "hort show," where they could see the latest farm equipment and perhaps enjoy a night on the town with their friends and neighbors who also made the trip. The older cousin, Alt, rode to the city with his mother, while Schoenborn drove his pickup truck.

The convention brought the two young farmers to the city where they would die a foul, premature death at the hands of an unseen monster who lurked in the shadows. Did this monster also attend the convention or stay at the hotel? This possibility brought the number of suspects into the thousands. Detectives interviewed several people who worked at the hotel and who attended the convention the night the two men disappeared. At some point, Alt and Schoenborn met their killer, and perhaps someone witnessed this liaison and could help bring the killer or killers into the light.

As investigators traced the two men's movements Tuesday night, they uncovered evidence that they had ended their night with a few cocktails—a fact established by their blood-alcohol level at the time of death. Although neither man had a reputation as a hard drinker or party animal, perhaps they decided to mix farm business with pleasure the night they disappeared—sometime in the very early hours of Wednesday, December 8. A group of men created a small disturbance at the Miss Apple Queen coronation—the Horticultural Society's beauty pageant. Not surprisingly, attendees noticed a group of young men in their teens and twenties whooping and hollering at the contestants. A worker also denied admittance to a few young men who attempted to enter the ceremony while carrying drinks. Either of these groups may have included Alt and Schoenborn.

During the night, both men also visited Tootsie Van Kelly's—in 1982 a popular Grand Rapids nightspot. The nightclub, which no longer exists, was inside the Amway Grand Plaza Hotel.

Like all hotels, the Grand Plaza caters to its guests with restaurants and nightclubs and complimentary pens bearing the Grand Plaza name, and, like bees to honey, hotel guests and locals alike flocked to Tootsie Van Kelly's, famous for its "Red Hot Mama" and seemingly infinite selection of beers from around the globe. In frigid December, it was a place to find warmth and the company of out of towners, like Dennis Alt and Chris Schoenborn, as well as hotel patrons visiting the city on business, or to see an act at the adjacent DeVos Hall.

At some point, Alt attempted to enter Tootsie Van Kelly's, but the manager denied him entrance because his staggering suggested he had already consumed enough alcohol. Schoenborn likely visited the bar sometime earlier on Tuesday evening, as the manager told investigators he thought he might have seen him inside but could not confirm that fact.

Later, though, the two cousins would return to Tootsies, or at least to the hallway outside of the nightclub. The last time anyone saw twenty-four-year-old Dennis Alt and twenty-year-old Chris Schoenborn alive was there around one on Wednesday morning. A Tootsie's employee saw both men at about this time talking to a third man outside of the bar. And then they simply vanished.

Here, the story skips a few pages—these pages are missing. Investigators could not ascertain what happened, or where it happened, with any certainty during the interval between the last sighting at 1 a.m. Wednesday morning at Tootsie Van Kelly's and 9:50 a.m. Thursday morning. The only certainty at this point in the investigation was that something bad had happened. Sometime during these lost hours of their lives, Alt and Schoenborn met with the foulest of play that involved alcohol, diazepam, a ballpoint pen, and ligature strangulation. Someone tortured and strangled them. So, to this point, the story of their deaths had a beginning and an end, but no middle.

When neither man contacted their families by mid-morning on Wednesday, family members drove to the city to find them, scouring the area for any clue left by the two farmers. They looked along the banks of the Grand River. They found nothing. Later that day, the two men officially became missing persons. Police managed to locate Schoenborn's pickup truck still parked where he left it in an underground parking structure.

Almost thirty-six hours later, a Consumers Energy meter reader made the horrific discovery of the victims' bodies, frozen and laying thirty feet from a water tower seven miles west of the city.

The missing hours represent a puzzle. The picture on the puzzle lay fragmented, the pieces scattered. Investigators knew that the picture would appear if and when they managed to find all the pieces. They had a few, but the piece that would suggest the placement of all the others remained missing: a suspect. The case went as cold as December in Michigan, and it would stay cold, the murders remaining unsolved until an unlikely arrest occurred in an unlikely place six months after the discovery of the bodies . . .

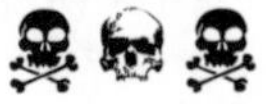

The surprise break in the Alt and Schoenborn murder investigations came with the arrest of a drunk driver in Orange County, California. Around 1 a.m. on May 14, 1983, Orange County Highway Patrol Sergeant Michael Howard and Officer Michael Sterling observed a Toyota Celica speeding down the highway, weaving in its lane, even crossing the solid white line onto the shoulder. Another drunk driver, it appeared, and a threat to the safety of others.

Suspiciously, the driver did not immediately pull to the side of the road when the patrolmen activated the red light. Instead, he slowed to thirty miles an hour and stopped weaving. They shined a spotlight into the car, and Sergeant Howard spotted the driver reach into the backseat and grab a dark cloth, which he placed on the front passenger seat.

The driver, thirty-seven-year-old Randy Kraft, pulled to the side of the road, stepped out of the car, and met Officer Sterling between the two vehicles. Sterling noticed that all but the top button of the driver's jeans were undone, and he detected the slight odor of alcohol. Since the driver was weaving, Officer Sterling escorted Kraft to the front of the Toyota and gave him a field sobriety test, which he failed.

Kraft, it appeared, had not partied alone that night. While Sterling tested Kraft's sobriety with a variety of physical coordination tests, Sergeant Howard noticed a reclined figure in the front passenger seat. With Kraft handcuffed, the officers wondered if Kraft's companion could drive the car home, so they asked him about the identity of the passenger. The man was a hitchhiker, Kraft told them.

Sergeant Howard inspected the figure by shining his flashlight through the passenger side window. The man appeared to be passed out, asleep, or unconscious, with what looked like a beer bottle on the floor between his feet (they found another bottle, similar yet broken, on the pavement by the driver's door). And although a coat covered much of the man's lower body, Sergeant Howard could tell that the passenger's pants were pulled down. Howard tried to awaken the man by shouting and knocking on the passenger side window, but the man would not wake up.

Howard then walked around the car to the unlocked driver's side. Inside the car, he found a folded knife and brown pill bottle labeled Ativan. In the backseat, he noticed a second pill bottle—an empty bottle of Valium—a cooler, and a leather strap. He reached over the driver's seat, grabbed the man's shoulder, and attempted to shake him into consciousness, but again, the passenger did not wake up. So Howard reached over the passenger, unlocked the passenger side door, and went to the other side of the car.

On the other side of the Toyota, he opened the passenger door and once again attempted to wake the man. But one cannot wake the dead. A closer examination revealed a shocking discovery: Randy Kraft's passenger had no pulse and his pupils remained fixed under the flashlight beam. He was dead. Sergeant Howard removed the jacket on the man's lap and discovered that his pants were pulled down below the waist, exposing his penis and testicles, which were propped up by the crotch area of the pants.

An autopsy revealed that Kraft's passenger had died from asphyxia when someone tightened something like a leather belt or strap around his neck and strangled him. Petechial hemorrhages in the throat structures suggested that the killer repeatedly tightened and loosened the strap. Thus, the death may have resulted from erotic asphyxia—a type of sex play in which the participants derive sexual pleasure from the deprivation of oxygen caused by strangulation—or the killer tortured the man before murdering him. The ligature marks on the man's wrists, though, indicated that someone bound him with something like a heavy rubber band, which made the sex play-turned-accidental death scenario seem implausible.

A toxicology screen revealed that at the time he died, the man had consumed alcohol (0.067 percent) and a prescription antianxiety drug called lorazepam, also known as Ativan. The combination would have rendered the man drowsy and lethargic. Investigators would discover that Kraft's passenger, a marine from a nearby base at El Toro, disappeared on May 13, 1983, when he went looking for a ride to a party he never attended. The forensic facts of this man's death should seem eerily familiar, like déjà vu—it's more than a feeling. The same forensic evidence appeared in the Kent County Morgue six months earlier.

The man, twenty-five-year-old Terry Gambrel, represented the last victim in the career of a very prolific killer who assembled a very lengthy résumé of murder in just over a decade of work. Sergeant Howard and Officer Sterling had just arrested a serial killer responsible for at least sixteen and probably several more murders, which may have included two unsolved homicides that took place in Grand Rapids, Michigan, six months earlier: the murders of Dennis Alt and Chris Schoenborn.

In fact, the manner of Terry Gambrel's death was not unique. The specifics of the murder—the killer's modus operandi—fit several other unsolved homicides in California. A Department of Transportation worker discovered the body of Eric Church—a twenty-one-year-old male of slight build (five feet eight and one hundred and thirty pounds). Church died as a result of ligature strangulation. A toxicology report revealed that before his death, he had consumed alcohol and a tremendous amount (2.5 milligrams per liter) of a drug called diazepam. This combination would have left Church comatose and could have killed him.

An off-duty Los Angeles police officer discovered the nude body of Geoffrey Nelson on a highway on-ramp on the morning of February 12, 1983. Skid marks at the scene indicate that Nelson's killer dumped his body from a moving vehicle, like he had done with Church. Nelson also died from ligature strangulation. And, like Church, Geoffrey Nelson had consumed a combination of alcohol (.14 percent at the time of death) and prescription drugs (diazepam and propranolol) that would have left him less than alert. One other thing: his killer had used a sharp instrument to cut off Nelson's penis and testicles. A lack of bleeding suggested that, fortunately, Nelson was already dead when this mutilation occurred.

Another victim, Rodger DeVaul, knew Geoffrey Nelson; a friend had last seen the two together on February 11, 1983. Two days later and a day after the discovery of his friend's body, a passerby noticed a dead body on a hillside by a road. Like his friend Nelson, the twenty-year-old DeVaul crossed paths with a serial killer who asphyxiated him. His wrists showed ligature marks that suggested that his killer had bound his wrists, and semen recovered from anal swabs indicated that someone had sodomized him. And like Nelson, DeVaul also ingested a modest amount of alcohol (0.07 percent) as well as propranolol and diazepam, which left him impaired and on the verge of unconsciousness.

The details of these three murders suggested that the California Highway Patrol, in arresting Randy Kraft, had captured a serial killer. Investigators obtained a search warrant for the Toyota a few hours after Kraft's arrest, and the car would produce a wealth of evidence pointing to Randy Kraft as the monster known as "serial killer."

Under the mats in the front seat were photographs of Rodger DeVaul, a man in corduroy pants that matched the pants Eric Church wore at the time of his death, and yet another victim named Robert Loggins Jr., whose body was decomposed to the point that cause of death became speculative (but an autopsy suggested he likely died of ligature strangulation). Under the car's passenger seat was a pink liquid substance that a criminologist later confirmed as blood. Gambrel's wounds did not bleed much, so the blood must have come from another of Kraft's victims, suggesting that Kraft conducted some of his dark work in the vehicle.

The trunk of Kraft's car produced more evidence, including a collection of photographs, one of which depicted a man sitting on a couch. The man appeared to be dead. Investigators also found a briefcase, inside of which was the mother lode: a cryptic list of entries sometimes referred to as a "scorecard." Coded entries on this list appeared to represent victims of Kraft's deadly machinations, including Church, Nelson, and DeVaul; the entries also fit several other unsolved homicides.[1]

Kraft's arrest prevented him from inking a cryptic entry for Terry Gambrel, but investigators believed that "2 IN 1 BEACH" represented the murders of Nelson and DeVaul. During Kraft's trial, the prosecution forwarded the opinion that Kraft met the two men on the beach, and at least one forensic detail supported this likelihood: blotches of blood around DeVaul's mouth and nostrils contained what appeared to be beach sand. During the murder trial, prosecutors would "decode" many more entries for the jury.

The evidence discovered in Kraft's car provided more than enough probable cause to obtain a search warrant for his house. Church, DeVaul, and Nelson all consumed alcohol and Valium the night they died; toxicological analysis confirmed that DeVaul and Nelson also consumed propranolol. Kraft's car contained the bottles for the drugs. In addition, there was blood on the seat, which suggested that Kraft killed at least one other victim. The evidence seized from Kraft's Toyota made a search warrant for his house a foregone conclusion.

Investigators made the first of three searches of Kraft's home during the afternoon of May 14—the same day that Sergeant Howard and Officer Sterling arrested Kraft for drunk driving.

By this time, word of the capture of a fiendish serial killer had reached Oregon. For serial killers, their modus operandi is the fingerprint they leave with their victims. It is this fingerprint, discovered during intense crime scene investigation and subsequent autopsies, that often leads to their discovery, arrest, and conviction. And it is often this fingerprint that connects the killer to his or her victims. Randy Kraft's fingerprint fit several unsolved homicides that occurred in Oregon, so investigators there contacted Orange County authorities. Kraft worked for the aerospace firm of Lear Siegler Corporation and on occasion traveled to offices in Oregon.

Serial killers often take "souvenirs" from their victims, and these mementos often become the rope that binds them to their victims and eventually the physical evidence that hangs them in court. The investigator who was in charge of the Kraft investigation and led the searches of Kraft's car and home, James Sidebotham, realized he had seen in Kraft's house several items described by the Oregon investigators that connected Kraft to the Oregon murders, although at the time of the first search, he did not realize the relevance of these items. A second search followed a second search warrant.

The second search of Kraft's home produced evidence that removed much of the doubt about Kraft's connection to the Oregon victims. One of the victims, Michael O'Fallon, owned a Kodak camera with his initials, MJF, etched onto it. Sidebotham confiscated the camera during his first search. During the second search, Sidebotham confiscated clothing that fit the description of O'Fallon's the night he died.

The second sweep also produced physical evidence that tied Kraft to three other Oregon victims, including clothing, tennis shoes, a shaving kit, and a pair of roller skates. These "souvenirs" provided a concrete physical link between the suspect and his alleged victims. All four of the murders fit Kraft's modus operandi: young men who consumed a combination of alcohol and prescription drugs and—except for one victim, whose death resulted from sixteen blows to the back of his head—died from ligature strangulation. And Kraft's business itinerary placed him in the vicinity where and when all four men disappeared in separate incidents.

In addition to the physical evidence obtained in Kraft's home, murders with Kraft's signature modus operandi brought his alleged Oregon total to six, including a twenty-nine-year-old named Anthony Silveira last seen on December 4, 1982—the last of Kraft's alleged victims in Oregon. Silveira's killer had tortured him (he jammed a toothbrush up his anus, and the presence of sperm indicated that a rape occurred) before strangling him and dumping his nude body beside a highway. When last seen, Silveira wore an army jacket with his name on it. Kraft was in Portland on Lear Siegler business between December 1 and December 4, 1982, before taking a flight to Grand Rapids, Michigan, where he spent December 5 through December 8 working at Lear Siegler's offices. He stayed at the Amway Grand Plaza. It was at the Grand Rapids hotel that Silveira's jacket would surface, but investigators did not realize the significance of this discovery until much later.

On December 8, 1982, a hotel security officer had discovered an army jacket with the name Silveira on it lying on a couch in a lobby area on the eleventh floor, about fifteen feet from room 1169: the room where Kraft stayed during his business trip. He turned it in to lost and found, but neither he nor the Michigan investigators at the time could possibly know the significance of the jacket: a "souvenir" that an alleged serial killer may have brought along with him on a cross-county business junket.

The news of the evolving Kraft investigation blew across America to Grand Rapids, where two murders fit Kraft's modus operandi. Dennis Alt and Chris Schoenborn disappeared on December 8, 1982, and were last seen at a bar in the Amway Grand Plaza. Now, the chance arrest of Randy Kraft along a highway in Orange County provided Michigan investigators with a suspect in the double murder.

A Grand Rapids investigator, Detective Sergeant Larry French, contacted James Sidebotham and described property missing from the two Michigan victims, including a jacket with a label bearing Chris Schoenborn's name. During a previous search, Sidebotham saw the jacket in Kraft's garage. After obtaining a third search warrant, he executed a third search of Kraft's house in Orange County, California, and recovered Schoenborn's jacket. The murders of Dennis Alt and Chris Schoenborn, it appeared, had been solved.

The manner in which serial killers murder their victims seldom changes. Allowing for slight variation, changing the place to Grand Rapids, Michigan, and the time to roughly six months earlier, the murder of Terry Gambrel becomes the murder of Alt and Schoenborn. However, the California Highway Patrol nabbed Kraft before he had the chance to dump Gambrel's body; if they hadn't, investigators would have been puzzled by yet another murder victim dumped in a highway ditch, and Kraft likely would have made more entries in his ledger as he continued his career as a serial killer. Gambrel's murder, coupled with Kraft's other victims, creates a composite sketch of Kraft's modus operandi and provides a possible sequence of events that occurred during the missing hours of Alt's and Schoenborn's lives.

With Kraft's MO in mind, it becomes possible to piece together the pages missing from the last chapters of Dennis Alt's and Chris Schoenborn's biographies. At some point, the two men came across an out-of-town businessman, who perhaps offered his victims beer spiked with the prescription drug diazepam, or offered the men pills to enhance their recreational buzz, and a lift in a rental car. Once the drug and alcohol combination left his victims sluggish and lethargic, the perpetrator enjoyed himself with his quarry. When finished, he strangled his victims and dumped them by a water tower in a rural area west of town before returning to the hotel with his souvenirs, including Schoenborn's "Mighty Mac" jacket.

In fact, the arrest for drunk driving that led to his exposure as a serial killer was not the first time Randy Kraft crossed the law. Kraft's criminal vita began with a mild infraction and escalated. In college, Kraft joined the ROTC and was a conservative political activist, but rumors about his alleged homosexuality and alleged taste for bondage circulated. He graduated from Claremont College in 1967 with a degree in accounting.

He also struggled with several physical demons that plagued him throughout his life. As a youngster, he suffered from a series of accidents, one time falling down a flight of stairs and hitting his head. As an adult, he relied on Valium to help with blinding migraine headaches and stomachaches. He also had a mercurial temperament.

His rap sheet begins with an arrest when he propositioned an undercover police officer while still in college in 1966. He attempted to make a go of a career in the air force, but the military was a poor fit for Kraft. Next, he worked as a bartender.

His problems with the law escalated with the alleged assault and rape of a sixteen-year-old boy who managed to escape Kraft's apartment. A search of the apartment yielded dozens of photographs depicting homosexual sex between Kraft and various partners as well as illegal drugs, but the lack of a search warrant kept Kraft from an arrest.

And then young men began to disappear, most strangled to death and most mutilated in some way, including bite marks and missing genitals.

Kraft's closest brush with the law came in March 1975, when his career as a serial killer almost came to an end. Boys beachcombing along Long Beach discovered a skull that proved to be the severed head of Keith Crotwell—a nineteen-year-old who went missing in that month while hitchhiking. Police traced the car that picked up Crotwell to Randy Kraft, who admitted meeting two men in a parking lot and giving one of them a ride but claimed that during their jaunt, the car became stuck in sand. Kraft went for help, and when he returned, his companion had disappeared.

Kraft was the chief suspect, but at the time, police had not found Crotwell's body, without which it would be impossible to fix cause and manner of death. A headless skeleton, missing both hands, turned up seven months later. The killer had wrapped the headless body, later identified as Keith Crotwell, in a carpet and deposited the rolled-up carpet inside of a pipe.

Kraft's chance arrest for drunk driving in 1983 brought an end to his criminal résumé and his killing spree.

After a lengthy preliminary hearing (seven weeks!) and a series of costly delays, the trial of Randy Kraft began in late September 1988—five years after his arrest. By the time the trial concluded on May 1, 1989, it was one of the most expensive murder trials in California's history. Kraft faced sixteen counts of murder for his Orange County victims, plus two additional counts for "inflicting mayhem" on Geoffrey Nelson (emasculating him) and sodomizing another victim. The presiding judge, Donald McCartin, however, barred reference to Kraft's alleged victims in Oregon and Michigan. Nonetheless, the case files against Kraft bulged with evidence. The prosecution presented to the jury no fewer than 157 witnesses and 1,052 exhibits, including the "scorecard" or "death list."

The "death list" provided a map and time line of Kraft's criminal activities, but prosecutors struggled trying to match victims to all of their respective coded entries. The list is in two columns. The column on the left side of the page contains thirty entries; the column on the right side of the page contains thirty-one. Four of the entries, prosecutors believed, represented two victims for a total of sixty-five. Investigators believed that Kraft did not make an entry for Eric Church, and the arrest apparently prevented him from making an entry for Terry Gambrel. These two victims bring the tally to sixty-seven. If the entries represented murders, then during his tenure, Kraft murdered enough people to fill a small lecture hall or restaurant.

At Kraft's trial, prosecutors had little trouble pairing the entries with the victims for whom he was charged. Circumstantial evidence and a virtually identical modus operandi tied the cases together, and the list tied them to Randy Kraft. The list and its victims, made public during the trial and the subsequent penalty phase, illuminated the depth of Randy Kraft's depravity.[2] A few examples illustrate the logic in the deciphering of the entries:

> PARKING LOT: After police tracked the Mustang that picked up Keith Crotwell, Kraft admitted to picking up a hitchhiker in the parking lot in the vicinity of where beachcombers found Keith Crotwell's severed head.
>
> HIKE OUT LB BOOTS: When murdered in early July 1978, Keith Klingbeil was hitchhiking (HIKE OUT). The pocket of his pants contained four matchbooks from a gas station in Long Beach (LB), and he wore boots (BOOTS). His killer had burned his left nipple with a cigarette lighter (an identical injury was inflicted upon Keith Crotwell).
>
> MC HB TATTOO: Robert Loggins, a nineteen-year-old US marine (MC) last seen alive in Huntington Beach (HB), had numerous tattoos (TATTOO).
>
> GR2: Kraft's business junket to Grand Rapids (GR), Michigan, placed him in Amway Grand Plaza Hotel, where Dennis Alt and Chris Schoenborn (2) were last seen alive. Investigators found Schoenborn's jacket in Kraft's garage.

The "death list" gave the jury a convincing piece of evidence, but it was not the prosecution's only evidence. The physical evidence recovered from the searches of Kraft's car and house linked Kraft to eight victims in ways hard to explain through coincidence and circumstance. The pièce de résistance consisted of a fingerprint from one of the crime scenes that matched Kraft's.

The print came from bottle shards recovered next to the body of Mark Hall. After a night of heavy drinking on New Year's Eve, 1975, Hall vanished. He reappeared a few days later. Off-duty police officers riding dune buggies in the mountains of Cleveland National Forest discovered his nude body about twenty-five feet from a road. An autopsy revealed Hall's horrific end—his killer packed his throat with dirt and leaves. Hall inhaled and swallowed some of the detritus and ultimately suffocated.

Although this would be a painful and slow death, Hall never felt a thing: at the time of death, his blood-alcohol level measured a staggering .67 percent (this is much higher than the typical "line of death" in ethanol overdose cases, which is .40 percent). Hall had consumed a sink full of alcohol and would have died from an ethanol overdose if his killer had not trumped this fate by suffocating him. In addition to the amount of alcohol, a toxicology screen indicated that Hall consumed a quantity of diazepam and two different over-the-counter cold medicines. The concoction left him unconscious.

The killer could play with his comatose victim with no resistance, and play he did, inflicting both antemorten and postmortem injuries on his twenty-two-year-old victim. He jammed a swizzle stick into Hall's urethra as far as the bladder, then cut off the penis and inserted it into Hall's rectum. With a cigarette lighter, he burned various parts of his victim's body, including his eyes and left nipple. Near Hall's body, as if a symbol of the young man's shattered life, lay shards of a broken bottle. Investigators managed to lift prints from the fragments, which matched Randy Kraft's right thumbprint. Hall's murder, prosecutors believed, appeared on Kraft's "scorecard" as NEW YEARS EVE.

Kraft maintained his innocence throughout the trial. He blamed the murders on other serial killers who had been caught and painted a portrait of himself as an innocent victim of circumstantial evidence. As for the list? The entries represented homosexual liaisons and other life events—a diary in code.

The jury did not believe this explanation and found Kraft guilty on all sixteen counts of murder and the sole count of mayhem but rejected the count of sodomy. Apparently, if suspicions about the "scorecard" are correct, the sixteen victims represent but a fraction of Kraft's total. The scorecard contained sixty-one entries, forty-five of which investigators managed to pair with victims, leaving twenty-two of the entries to speculation. For a period in the late seventies, investigators believe, Kraft changed the way he disposed of bodies: he continued to dump his victims' bodies along highways, but he placed them in garbage bags. How many victims remained undiscovered as trash collectors scooped up the bags and disposed of them in landfills or incinerated them? This question will likely remain unanswered. The total may also have included victims from at least three states.

At the trial, prosecutors could mention only murders committed in California, but during the penalty phase (which began on June 5 and concluded on August 11, 1989) they introduced evidence of eight alleged out-of-state victims: six from Oregon, collectively called the "I-5" murders (because most of the Oregon victims were found near this highway), and two from Michigan—Dennis Alt and Christopher Schoenborn. The jury recommended the death penalty, placing Randy Kraft on death row, which one day he will leave to die by lethal injection.

Although charges were filed in Michigan, Kraft would not answer for the murders of Dennis Alt and Chris Schoenborn in a Michigan court. While the case lacks the closure of a court conviction, the puzzle pieces fit. The modus operandi fits the other murders for which Kraft received life sentences: ligature or manual strangulation and drugging the victim with a mixture of sedatives and alcohol. The insertion of the pen into Schoenborn's penis seems congruous with the types of mutilation to the genitals that characterize Kraft's other crimes. The victims, young males, fit the profile of Kraft's other victims. In fact, at just over five feet eight and one hundred and thirty pounds, Dennis Alt seemed a mirror image of Eric Church.

And a witness saw the two cousins talking with someone who matched Kraft's description in the hall just outside of Tootsie Van Kelly's, indicating that at some point in the evening the boys came in contact with the serial killer from California.

This possibility is turned into a probability by other items that create a physical bridge linking Kraft and the two Michigan victims: the discovery of Dennis Alt's car keys in the hotel room Kraft occupied the night the two disappeared, the discovery of Schoenborn's jacket, with his name written in its lining, and a bottle opener found at Kraft's residence.

Did Kraft note the Michigan victims in his list? Did he concoct an acronym to remind him of his trip to Grand Rapids and the two young men whom he met at the hotel? Did the "2" in "GR2" stand for Alt and Schoenborn?

Although prosecutors could not raise these questions at Kraft's trial, they did at the subsequent penalty phase. They argued that the cryptic entry in Kraft's "death list"—"GR2"—suggested that his decade-long murder spree included two victims from Grand Rapids. This coded entry, the evidence suggests, may have been solved.

Other entries, however, may never be decoded, the last chapters in the victims' biographies remaining fragmented or unwritten. "ANGEL," "ENGLAND," "HARI KARI," and "OIL": what do they mean, or rather, *whom* do they represent? Twenty-two of the coded entries have not been linked to victims—twenty-two unsolved murders? Another troubling question remains: semen found in one of the victims and footprints by another victim's body suggest the possibility that Kraft worked in tandem with another killer at least some of the time.

The California Supreme Court reviewed Randy Kraft's trial and sentencing. During this appeal, Kraft challenged just about everything from the legality of the searches to the constitutionality of the death penalty, but the appeal would be in vain; the court upheld the death sentence. In the very near future, Randy Kraft will take the long walk to the execution chamber—the last chapter of his biography already written by a California jury. Like a vengeful mother, California will execute Randy Kraft for murdering so many of her sons.

In the meantime, he waits on San Quentin's death row. According to Kraft biographer Michael Newton, Kraft is an avid bridge player and used to while away the time playing bridge with death row neighbors and fellow serial killers Lawrence Bittaker, William Bonin, and Douglas Clark.[3] With a cumulative body count of forty-one confirmed and one hundred suspected, their card table contained the deadliest bridge foursome in the world. The executioner took Bonin in 1996, making him the permanent dummy in the San Quentin death row bridge games.

Soon, the game will lose another player. The last page of Randy Kraft's biography has already been written . . . by a jury in Orange County.

## Notes

1. The appeals decision of the California Supreme Court provides detailed information about Kraft's arrest and the subsequent investigation, including the various searches of Kraft's car and house.

2. Detailed information about the coded entries and how they match specific victims can be found in the lengthy decision of the California Supreme Court. The court's decision provides a thorough overview of the forensic details about each of the sixteen California victims for which Kraft was convicted. In its discussion of the penalty phase evidence, the court document provides detailed information about Kraft's alleged victims in Oregon and Michigan.

3. Michael Newton, "All about Randy Kraft: Death Row," Court TV Crime Library, http://www.crimelibrary.com/serial_killers/predators/kraft/10.html (accessed October 23, 2006). For a detailed probe of the Kraft case, readers are encouraged to consult Dennis McDougal's *Angel of Darkness: The True Story of Randy Kraft and the Most Heinous Murder Spree* (Grand Central Publishing, 1992).

# M-U-R-D-E-R? (Till Death Do Us Part)

A lesbian couple who snuffed out old people at a nursing home because it created a bond that would forever unite them, and who wanted to select victims whose initials collectively spelled "M-U-R-D-E-R . . ."

This story's synopsis sounds like the tagline to a movie premiere or like advertising copy from a debut novel. It sounds like something conjured by the twisted mind of a horror novelist or screenwriter.

Stories of murders that occur in a sequence provide fertile soil for writers because they appeal to the primal fears and morbid fascination of the American public. Novelists and screenwriters understand this fact, so they scour newspapers for true accounts that would make good models for great fiction. They find compelling storylines among the nation's headlines. They know that below the headlines lie true stories that are far more interesting, more bizarre, more disturbing than the most macabre stories conjured from imagination alone. They understand that "the truth is stranger than fiction." In 1988, the headlines in Michigan newspapers carried stories about a team of female serial killers whose crime seemed beyond possibility.

But is the case of Gwendolyn Graham and Catherine Wood a truth stranger than fiction or a fiction stranger than truth?

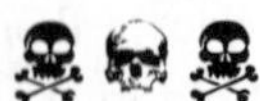

The large, yellow claw of a backhoe scratched through the earth covering the grave of Marguerite Chambers on Wednesday, November 30, 1988. A judge signed an order granting police the right to exhume her body from Rosedale Memorial Park almost a year after her burial because six feet below may be the evidence needed to convict a serial killer. So police officers hacked through the frozen earth to reach Chambers's body. Next to the grave, the bare arms of a tall maple tree provided an eerie backdrop for the day's drama.

It took about an hour to reach the coffin; inside a nearby garage, police broke through the cement vault with sledgehammers to remove the coffin inside it. Once they succeeded in removing it, the officers raised the coffin and placed it onto a flatbed truck, which took it to the Kent County Morgue.

People sometimes carry into the grave some memento from their surviving loved ones, such as a piece of jewelry or a letter. Sometimes they also carry into their graves secrets, and sometimes it becomes necessary to raise the dead to bring to light these secrets. Did the occupant of the coffin just raised from the grave conceal evidence of some deep, dark secret? Investigators hoped that the body of Marguerite Chambers could answer a vexing question: Did she die prematurely at the hands of her caretaker, or did she die of natural causes and become, after death, a murder victim only in the imagination of a twisted mind?

Marguerite Chambers died at the age of sixty. Like many elderly people who can no longer care for themselves, she lived in a nursing home as a "total care patient." Her death marked the end of a fourteen-year struggle with Alzheimer's disease, and by the time she died, she relied on others for everything. She could not feed herself. She could not walk. She could not talk. For Marguerite Chambers, the question of her death did not begin with "If" or "How" but "When." Because her death did not occur under suspicious circumstances, because she died of "natural causes," an autopsy was not performed. This morning, however, police had a good reason to interrupt her slumber: she might not have died a "natural" death. She might have been the first in a series of bizarre killings.

A second exhumation followed. Edith Cook lived a long life that ended just short of her centenary. At ninety-seven, she succumbed to her failing health and died from natural causes. Her death, like that of Marguerite Chambers, occurred without incident, thus no autopsy followed. Like Chambers, her later years proved less than comfortable. Chronic heart trouble (her death certificate notes cardiac artery disease as a condition from which she suffered) plagued her, so when she gasped for her last breath, her death seemed a natural consequence of her failing heart. Yet like Marguerite Chambers, Edith Cook's journey to the grave may have occurred prematurely.

Now, two years after their deaths, the women would travel to the Kent County Morgue for an autopsy to determine if their deaths occurred prematurely at the hands—literally—of nursing home employees.

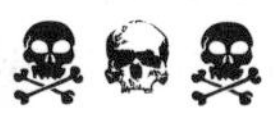

The murder investigation began a few months earlier, in October 1988, with a statement made by the ex-husband of an employee at a nursing home called Alpine Manor. Until Ken Wood contacted police about a bizarre story that seemed beyond the realm of possibility, no one suspected foul play at Alpine Manor. Wood's ex-wife, Catherine, worked as a nurse's aide at Alpine Manor in 1987 when Chambers and Cook died. Ken Wood's statement made his ex-wife appear to be an angel of death, not a Florence Nightingale.

Catherine Wood became pregnant and consequently a child bride at the age of seventeen in 1979. Although her marriage to Ken Wood had already disintegrated by 1986, their daughter presented a tie that ensured the parents would communicate from time to time. It was during one of these times, in August 1987, that she told her ex a story of murder.

Since the breakup of her marriage, Catherine Wood had become involved in a few homosexual relationships with coworkers at Alpine Manor, nicknamed "Gay Manor" for its contingent of homosexual employees. Her colleagues found the bleached blonde very attractive, despite the fact that at six feet tall and two hundred and fifty pounds, she was a large woman. It was during the night shift that she met and fell in love with a nurse's aide from Texas named Gwendolyn Graham.

Graham was something of a transient who changed residences and employment with some frequency. Born in California, Gwen moved to Tyler, Texas, as a young girl when her parents relocated there. She moved around a lot; as a teenager, she worked with a missionary group in parts of the United States and Africa. She moved back to California and traveled up the coast to Oregon and back before finding her way back to Tyler. She migrated north, following a friend who left Texas for Michigan in 1985. The winds carried her to Alpine Manor, where she began work as a nurse's aide in June 1986. Graham, who spoke with a slight Southern accent, was short at five feet three, but she walked tall; she was the type of woman who would become involved in a barroom brawl to avenge some perceived slight.

Wood's tenure at the nursing home began a year earlier than

Graham's. When she met Graham, Catherine Wood had been at the bottom of a downward spiral. She had divorced her husband of seven years and ballooned to over two hundred and fifty pounds. In the summer of 1986, she fell deeply in love with Gwendolyn Graham. The two became lovers and moved in together in September.

They may have appeared to be an odd couple, but in their demeanor, the two lovers appeared fit for each other. Coworkers at Alpine Manor characterized Wood as angry and brooding with a mercurial temperament. Ken Wood described her as "different people": a highly intelligent individual with a soft, sweet demeanor that concealed pent-up anger that would sometimes emerge from the depths.[1]

Gwendolyn Graham's personality seemed almost bipolar; she laughed one minute and yelled the next. At five feet one and one hundred and forty-five pounds, Graham seemed like a reverse image of Wood, who was an imposing figure. Despite her physical stature, however, Wood appeared to follow Graham's lead. She loved Graham deeply. She wrote poetry to her lover and, according to the story she told her ex-husband, she even became an accomplice to murder.

The couple's very active sex life involved bondage. They tied each other up. They scratched and bit each other. Sometimes their sex play involved dildos, sometimes other props were used to enhance their lovemaking. As recounted in *Forever and Five Days*—Lowell Cauffiel's exhaustive account of the case—Gwendolyn Graham explained that Wood often inserted ice cubes into her vagina, which to some might seem more like torture than pleasure, but she notes that she enjoyed the pain.[2] The two seemed to take pleasure in torture.

In the summer of 1987, the relationship bottomed out, and the two went their separate ways. Graham had become involved with another nurse's aide from Alpine Manor, and the new couple relocated to Tyler, Texas, where Graham got a job in another acute care facility. After the breakup, apparently, Catherine Wood decided to share her dirty little secret with someone she knew intimately: her ex-husband.

In August 1987, Catherine Wood made her confession to Ken

Wood. According to Ken Wood, his ex told him that she had helped her live-in lover smother six elderly patients at the nursing home. They planned on choosing victims whose first or last initials collectively spelled "M-U-R-D-E-R," but they abandoned this morbid version of Scrabble when they discovered that they could not easily find the right letters among their potential victims. They picked victims who could not struggle and whose deaths would not raise suspicion, so the initials in their names became a secondary consideration. According to Ken's statement, Catherine Wood characterized the murders as "fun."[3]

The sordid confession simmered for over a year before Ken Wood recounted the story for police in October 1988, because his wife had not obtained the psychological help he believed she needed. He told them that his wife confessed to participating in the murder of patients; a woman named Margaret was one of the patients. Margaret, in fact, was Marguerite. Marguerite Chambers.

The story led police to question Catherine Wood, who, not surprisingly, recounted a dissimilar version of the story she told her ex-husband—a version that removed her from the murders. She told them that when she entered Marguerite Chambers's room on January 18, 1987, she found Gwendolyn Graham in the process of suffocating the woman. Graham pushed a washcloth under her victim's chin while holding a second washcloth over her nose and mouth. According to Wood, Graham selected this method because it left no fingerprints, no bruising, in essence no evidence of murder.

Wood said that she did not attempt to stop Graham, but later the two discussed it. According to Wood, Graham said she committed the murder because the killing provided a type of release or catharsis of sorts. This feeling led to four more murders, according to a statement Catherine Wood gave to police in October 1988. Graham, Wood told investigators, also told her about a fifth murder victim—Edith Cook—whom she killed as an act of mercy to alleviate the woman's suffering.

Sometimes Graham told Wood about the killings ahead of time, and sometimes she told her about them afterward. Wood explained that Graham intimidated her into submission about the murders by leaving rolled-up washcloths where she knew Wood would find them.

Wood also told police that Graham took souvenirs from her victims. If true, Wood's statements suggested that perhaps a bridge of physical evidence linked some of the eight potential victims with Gwendolyn Graham, although Wood told police she discarded the totems when they broke up and Graham moved out.

Her story placed Graham inside a portrait labeled "serial killer." According to Wood, the soft-spoken, diminutive Texan was a vicious killer who murdered for sexual pleasure. She wanted to go to the police about the murders, Wood told her interrogators, but Graham threatened her, at one time shoving a loaded pistol into her vagina.

Throughout the fall of 1988, however, some of the details of Catherine Wood's story changed. At one time, she confirmed that the initial plan was to pick victims whose initials spelled "M-U-R-D-E-R," and during another interview, she claimed this was a fiction. During one interview, she told them that Marguerite Chambers represented the "M," and during another, she told them that Mae Mason did. She at one time claimed to have seen Graham murder Marguerite Chambers, and at another time denied witnessing the act itself.

Investigators found Wood's storytelling maddening; rather than providing a structured chronicle of the murders, she told the story in fragments as she shifted back and forth between events and dates. She couldn't remember some details or dates. The fractured narrative left a table covered by puzzle pieces, and detectives struggled to fit them together into a coherent picture. They tried to pin down Wood's story and its veracity with polygraph tests. The first test was inconclusive, but she passed the second. Most who interviewed her, however, found her manipulative.

Yet according to Ken Wood, Catherine Wood confessed to playing an active role in the murders, calling them "fun." Eventually, the story she told investigators evolved to where she admitted to playing a more active role. She even helped select the victims, she explained. They were supposed to take turns killing, in fact, but she could not bring herself to do it. Yet by her own admission she had participated, so she found herself facing murder charges for the deaths of both Marguerite Chambers and Edith Cook.

Incredulous detectives faced what seemed like a fantastic scenario. Wood's sordid tale indicated that Alpine Manor employed at least one female serial killer (and possibly two, if Catherine Wood acted as an accomplice) whose murderous résumé included at least five victims in a killing spree that began with Marguerite Chambers. This possibility raised suspicion about the cause of death for those who died at the home in the winter of 1987.

In fact, Chambers and Cook were just two of forty-four residents who died at Alpine Manor in the first half of 1987 (at the time, Alpine Manor housed about two hundred residents). Considering the severe medical problems of many residents in such homes, the number of deaths at Alpine Manor in 1987 was not surprising or uncharacteristic.

But Wood's story raised disturbing questions, and cloud of suspicion formed over eight deaths that occurred at Alpine Manor in the first half of 1987; at the time, the deaths were presumed from "natural causes," a fact reflected in their death certificates. Now, these eight elderly ladies represented the focus of a murder investigation.

- Marguerite Chambers, age sixty, died January 18, 1987, at 8:30 p.m.
- Myrtle Luce, age ninety-five, died February 10, 1987, at 2:30 p.m.
- Mae Mason, age seventy-nine, died February 16, 1987, at 4 a.m.
- Ruth VanDyke, age ninety-eight, died February 26, 1987, at 2:40 a.m.
- Belle Burkhard, age seventy-four, died February 26, 1987, at 4:25 a.m.
- Wanda Urbanski, age ninety, died March 2, 1987, at 10:50 p.m.
- Edith Cook, age ninety-seven, died April 7, 1987, at 2 a.m.
- Lucille Stoddard, age seventy, died May 1, 1987, at 7:48 p.m.[4]

Ruth VanDyke, like many of the others on the list, depended entirely on the staff of Alpine Manor. Deaf and blind by the time she died, she succumbed to a failing heart. Her son, a retired homicide detective, was with her when her heart stopped twice. He did not witness her death about an hour later, though, from what was presumed to be heart failure. She died within two hours of another possible victim, Belle Burkhard.

Mae Mason, like Marguerite Chambers, suffered from Alzheimer's disease. Unable to walk, she also depended on help from Alpine Manor's caretakers. Like Chambers, Cook, and VanDyke, she also supposedly succumbed to a failing heart.

The list provides some interesting information. All of the alleged victims, except for Luce, died in the evening hours between 7:48 p.m. and 4 a.m. The name of the first victim, Marguerite Chambers, begins with an "M"—in fact, the first three victims' names begin with "M"—not coincidentally, the first letter in the word "M-U-R-D-E-R." Serial killers typically kill according to some predetermined pattern, some sequence. Did the letter "M" somehow represent the beginning of some type of sequence that dictated the selection of victims as Catherine Wood initially led investigators to believe? Throughout the investigation, Wood's interrogators returned to the question about the selection of victims and the idea that the word "M-U-R-D-E-R" was an acronym intended to represent actual victims through their initials.

Wood's story left some in disbelief, and her tendency to vacillate on certain details, such as the "M-U-R-D-E-R" acronym, made her story even harder to believe. Police needed something concrete to support her story, such as forensic evidence uncovered during an autopsy. Physical evidence of a murder would go a long way to alleviating the doubts left in the wake of Catherine Wood's numerous and often inconsistent statements.

While the police suspected eight victims, they exhumed only two for autopsy: Chambers and Cook (three of the possible victims—Burkhard, Mason, and Luce—were cremated). Detectives hoped the Kent County medical examiner could uncover physical evidence of murder in the bodies of Chambers and Cook to support the allegations. Physical evidence would be very convincing in court. It would also solidify the story told by Catherine Wood, whose incessant story changes and history of prevarication made her a somewhat questionable source.

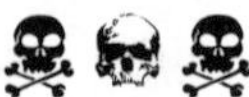

Later that blustery day, after police chipped through the frozen tundra of Rosedale Memorial Park, the remains of Marguerite Chambers arrived at the Kent County Morgue. In transporting her coffin, officers could hear a sloshing sound. Her crypt leaked, and water found its way inside her coffin. This was bad news.

Police knew that the autopsy might not provide any new information about the death they now considered suspicious. When a body is exhumed, the degree of preservation plays a vital role in what the medical examiner can find. Well-preserved bodies preserve forensic evidence, while forensic evidence tends to decompose with the body containing it. A body frozen in ice can preserve for years subtle markers of a premeditated murder, such as ligature marks, or of a struggle, such as bruises and abrasions. Bodies in an advanced state of decomposition would no longer yield such clues, particularly bodies left unprotected from the elements. In such scenarios, animal or marine life (see "The Sea Shall Give Up Her Dead") may obliterate portions of the victims.

Strict state and federal laws govern the burial of bodies (cremations occur under fewer legal restraints and stipulations). To protect the body from the elements, a corpse is entombed in several layers. These layers, like blankets, protect the body from animals that would feed on it. They also prevent the spread of disease by preventing the leakage of bodily fluids from the casket into groundwater. Some diseases, like hepatitis, could survive in a dead person's blood and could possibly remain infectious for some time after death.

The coffin, generally lined with copper or zinc, is screwed or nailed shut and then placed inside of a cement crypt or vault. The vault is then sealed and covered with earth. Sometimes, despite these protections, water penetrates the layers and creates quite a macabre scene for anyone who opens the coffin.

Marguerite Chambers's body, even though sealed in a cement vault, was exposed to the elements. The crypt leaked, and water settled inside the coffin. The moisture gave Marguerite Chambers a lime-green mask of mold that covered her face, the back of her neck, and part of her arm.

What does a body look like after a few years inside a coffin? Most people imagine a skeleton lying in a dark-colored, velvet-lined interior of a coffin, but depending on environmental factors, it can take years for a body to decompose entirely until it is reduced to its bare bones. Bodies suspended in frigid, near-freezing water or frozen in a block of ice can remain preserved for a very long time.

The coffin lining is often stained from bodily fluids; the body will swell as it becomes engorged with methane gas caused by decomposition. In this state, the body, whether male or female, bloats like an oversized puffer fish. Sometimes, the body tissues split, releasing fluids that can stain the coffin interior. And the putrid stench of decomposition can send even the most seasoned professionals to the bottle of wintergreen oil; a few dabs of oil over the mask can offer temporary respite from the smell. The putrid, pungent odor is considered one of the strongest and most disturbing odors in existence. When conducting the autopsy of an individual in an advanced state of decomposition, morgue personnel will typically double up their clothing, as the smell is so strong it can cling to the clothes and hair and create awkward social situations for the medical personnel who must emerge at the end of the day into the world of the living.

Exhumations offer roadblocks for the medical examiner other than the invisible menace of malodor. Decomposition in an advanced state can obliterate subtle signs of foul play, such as abrasions or scratches (see "The Sea Shall Give Up Her Dead"). And if the body is exposed to the elements, animal activity can make it difficult or impossible for the ME to discern stab wounds. Bullet tracks, however, generally survive.

The mortician who prepares the body for showing unwittingly creates other roadblocks to the postmortem examination of an exhumed body. Often, the medical examiner must undo the work of the mortician, who could not know when he or she embalmed the body that a backhoe would one day exhume what was buried. For example, the muscles of the jaw can become flaccid, allowing the mouth to gape open. Morticians will sew or wire the jaws together so that the deceased person will not appear to be sleeping with her mouth open.

In an attempt to find forensic clues that might point to murder, the work of Cook's mortician had to be undone. According to Catherine Wood, Chambers and Cook were suffocated with wet washcloths. If this was true, then their mouths might contain remnants of the murder weapon: fibers from the washcloths. In order to examine the mouth of Edith Cook, the wire the embalmer used to close her mouth, as well as the cotton placed in her mouth, had to be removed. And to detect the presence of any bruises or abrasions on her face, the makeup used to make her presentable had to be removed.

The bodies were exhumed so that investigators might discover possible evidence of a murder, but would any evidence be left to find? Some causes of death leave few clues, if any. Crafty murderers recognize this fact and sometimes choose a murder method that leaves no solid forensic evidence onto which the prosecutor can pin his case.

For example, suffocation of helpless, elderly patients with a rolled-up washcloth.

Generally, victims of manual strangulation will exhibit certain telltale signs: the ends of the delicate, horseshoe-shaped hyoid bone in the throat structure can be fractured, and bruising will appear in the throat structures. If the killer uses some type of soft barrier, however, these telltale signs might not appear.

If, as investigators believed, these elderly patients died when someone smothered them with a pillow or suffocated them by inserting something into their mouths, little or no forensic clues might appear during the autopsy. Such a death might leave petechial hemorrhages around the eyes or abrasions inside the mouth that may result from something like a rag being forced into the mouth, which would also leave cloth fibers . . . or it might leave no clues at all.

And since these two victims could not defend themselves, their deaths likely occurred without a struggle. If they were murdered, their killers chose them well. If they could have struggled against their assailants, their bodies, again depending on the state of preservation, could provide evidence of foul play: defensive wounds on the hands, like scratch marks or cuts, obtained when the victim attempted to shield herself from harm; bruises or patches of petechial hemorrhages on the chest or shoulders that would result if the murderer fell or lay on top of the victim; fractured bones of the arms or hands that might have occurred in a violent struggle.

For this reason, Belle Burkhard would have been an excellent candidate for exhumation. According to Wood's statements, Burkhard's arm had been injured during her murder, and some forensic evidence of this would appear on her body. Burkhard had been cremated, however, and any evidence of murder went up in smoke with her body, making the cause of her death only a point of speculation.

In the absence of specific indicators, the autopsy becomes one of exclusion: the medical examiner must rule out any other possible cause of death. The autopsy, then, might also fix the specific cause of death. When elderly patients die and an autopsy is not conducted, the cause of death becomes little more than an educated guess, with heart disease the usual culprit. Chambers's death certificate listed "myocardial infarction" as the cause of death; Cook's listed "cardiac arrest." A thorough examination of their bodies would reveal if the doctors who signed their death certificates made the correct educated guesses.

A thorough autopsy revealed no definitive evidence that the two ladies died from suffocation; no physical evidence of murder was found. But the autopsies did indicate that neither woman had significant heart disease, making the cause of death on their certificates wrong. Marguerite Chambers did not die of a heart attack. Edith Cook's coronary arteries contained some narrowing, but not enough to warrant the conclusion that she died from it, although it was a possible if unlikely cause of death.

Although evidence of a violent struggle would have provided powerful ammunition in court, investigators did not need forensic evidence from the autopsies to make their case; they accumulated enough other evidence to make arrests and file murder charges.

Consequently, the lack of evidence for natural cause of death for these two victims and the strong case the prosecution had assembled led to a change in cause of death from heart disease to suffocation for both Chambers and Cook. This is something of a judgment call for the medical examiner, and no judgment is ever infallible . . .

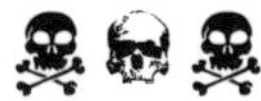

During their investigation, detectives traveled south to interview and ultimately arrest Gwendolyn Graham, who had relocated to her hometown of Tyler, Texas, shortly after the breakup with Catherine Wood and the alleged sequence of murders. Graham and her roommate had taken jobs at the Mother Francis Hospital in September 1987, but even though Graham was not linked with any suspicious deaths in Texas, hospital officials fired her when investigators told them of the murder allegations at a similar facility in Michigan. It is understandable that they felt uncomfortable with an accused murderess of total-care patients working in their nursing home.

Murder? Ridiculous, Graham claimed when detectives interviewed her. The "murders" were just stories she and Wood fabricated as a joke. A prank and nothing more. No one at Alpine Manor died from anything but natural causes. She even agreed to take a polygraph. Most of the test questions focused on Marguerite Chambers. The test results were inconclusive. Nonetheless, Wood's statements placed a figurative noose around Gwendolyn Graham's neck. In December 1988, the noose tightened. Detectives arrested her and brought her back to Grand Rapids, where she would face a jury, a prosecutor, and the star witness: her ex-lover.

A few days before Graham's trial began, Catherine Wood made a deal with the prosecution. The two charges of first-degree murder would be dropped if she pled guilty to one count of second-degree murder and one count of conspiracy to commit second-degree murder and testified against Gwendolyn Graham. Even though the plea bargain ensured that she would spend the next twenty to forty years incarcerated, she agreed. While some still had their doubts about Wood's sincerity (amplified by the differing versions she and Ken Wood told investigators), it seemed like a good deal for the prosecution; if Catherine Wood's testimony led to a conviction, the deal would take both of them off the street.

The prosecution painted a portrait of Catherine Wood as a physically formidable yet vulnerable partner in a relationship dominated by the malignant Gwendolyn Graham. The gentle giant fell prey to the sick whims of her lover. She made a good witness; she answered the prosecutor's questions with the fluidity of a person telling the truth.

In her testimony, she admitted playing a direct role in the killings: she acted as a sentry while Graham slipped into the unsuspecting victims' rooms and suffocated each of them with a rolled-up washcloth. They chose their victims carefully. They chose victims powerless to struggle or yell for help. In fact, as a test, Wood explained, they would sometimes pinch the nostrils of a potential victim and watch to see how much of a struggle the helpless woman could muster.

Wood was supposed to participate in the actual murders, taking turns with Graham, but Wood could not bring herself to kill, so Graham continued.

Wood, who loved Graham deeply, believed that the murders created a bond that would forever unite the two lovers. Their dirty little secret would keep them together—their unique spin on the sentiment voiced at a traditional Christian wedding: "Till death do us part." Catherine Wood even noted in her testimony that she wrote a poem to her lover in which "five days" represented the five murders that she believed would glue them together forever. Wood feared that if she did not acquiesce to her lover's murderous impulses, Graham would leave her for someone who would go along with her.

While the bodies of Chambers and Cook produced no forensic evidence of murder, the prosecution did have something concrete to present to the jury . . . sort of: Proposed Exhibits Number 1 and 2. Graham and Wood, like high school sweethearts, wrote notes and love poetry to each other. Among all the correspondence the lovers had exchanged, including letters, investigators found just two items that contained any reference to the murders, and both were found in Graham's mobile home in Tyler, Texas: a poem (Exhibit 2) and a love letter that contained a strange acronym at its bottom (Exhibit 1). The poem contained a cryptic line that, according to Wood, referred to the killings and their bizarre motive for them. "Forever and five days": the "five days" represented the five murders, each one of which bonded them together "forever." The "five" indicated that she penned the lines after the fifth murder.

The love letter contained the enigmatic acronym at the bottom: "IGTKM." Wood explained that the acronym stood for "I'm Going to Kill Madeline." She testified that she was supposed to kill patients as well, and for her first kill she marked for death a patient named Madeline Young. But she could not do it.

In her testimony, Catherine Wood depicted her ex-lover as a bully who used violence to subjugate her partner. The night Graham murdered Marguerite Chambers, Wood testified, Graham tied her up in their bed. Wood did not consider this suspicious, because their intimacy frequently involved bondage. On this night, however, the sex game went too far. Graham took a pair of socks, put them over her hands like gloves, and began to smother Wood. She stopped short of murder.

Indeed, jurors needed only to look at Graham, who wore short-sleeved shirts to her trial, to see confirmation of the violent tendencies Wood claimed her lover possessed. Circular indentations, like moon craters, dotted her forearms: burn marks. Wood told the jury that

Gwendolyn Graham would hold lit cigarettes to her skin to see how long she could stand the pain.

Wood's testimony made Gwendolyn Graham look like a pain-loving, masochistic, pervert turned serial killer. Wood's testimony, however shocking and damning, might not have sealed Graham's fate. The most damaging testimony to Gwendolyn Graham's defense may have come from other women who knew her. Her roommate in her Tyler, Texas, mobile home testified that Graham confessed that she killed patients in a nursing home. In fact, the roommate testified, even after detectives visited the pair in their mobile home, Graham reiterated that she *had* killed the nursing home residents. Several other witnesses testified that Graham had made similar admissions to them, although at the time they dismissed the story as a sick joke. Their testimony had one common denominator: the number of victims murdered. At various times, and to various people, Gwendolyn Graham told of five murders.

Graham's defense maintained that if any murders occurred, Catherine Wood committed them. *If* they occurred.

Graham testified in her own defense. The soft-spoken girl from Texas with a slight Southern accent seemed a far cry from the malicious deviant who browbeat the much larger Catherine Wood into going along with the murders. She came from a troubled past from which she bore scars, specifically scars on her arms. Her father, she alleged, sexually abused her, and as a teenager she burned herself with cigarettes as a way "to get" her father. According to Graham the marks were not, as Wood testified, the consequence of a masochistic game.

Now she faced abuse of a different kind: a dangerous ex-lover who had created a fiction to "get" her. She offered a more innocent explanation for the "murders": she claimed that the story of the murders was simply a joke that Catherine Wood was now using like a rifle to shoot the ex-lover who jilted her. She called it Wood's "head game"—nothing more than a sick joke in which she participated. The two would tell others that they committed murders when in fact no murders occurred, except in Wood's twisted mind.

Wood, she testified, often played such deviant tricks, like a malignant Loki bent on wreaking havoc. The story of the "murders" originated when a fellow Alpine Manor nurse's aide visited the couple at their home. Wood told the woman that she and Graham had killed patients, then escorted her to the bedroom where she showed proof: mementos taken from the victims (which Wood told police she threw away after the breakup).

Graham testified that she felt threatened by Wood. In her testimony, Wood had stated that Graham threatened her by ramming a loaded pistol up her vagina. This happened, Graham explained, but in reverse. It was Wood who made the perverse threat. Eventually she left Wood because she had had enough of Wood's head games.

She also offered a mundane explanation for the suspicious line of the love poem. The "five days" represented the five-month duration of their relationship. As for the acronym at the bottom of the love letter? She didn't remember its meaning.

Graham could explain everything. Unlike Wood, however, her story did not flow; she stumbled when answering the prosecutor's questions. According to Graham's defense attorney, the case came down to one simple question: who would the jury believe, Gwendolyn Graham or Catherine Wood?

But did it? Since other witnesses testified that Graham discussed the killings with them, the question for the jury really became, whom do you believe: Graham, or Wood and several others?

Under cross-examination, the defense questioned Dr. Stephen Cohle about the change in cause of death to suffocation. Although the autopsies of Marguerite Chambers and Edith Cook produced no physical evidence of suffocation, the cause of death was changed based on the lack of any forensic evidence proving the women died from heart disease as supposed and on information from investigators in this case. If that information from the investigators was inaccurate, the defense suggested, then the cause of death by suffocation could also be inaccurate.

The physician who certified death at Alpine Manor testified that he would not have changed the cause of death for these victims. He stood by his conclusion that Chambers and Cook died from heart failure. He also testified that he did not typically examine the bodies of victims after they died, so if Belle Burkhard had a suspicious arm injury as Wood claimed, it would likely have gone unnoticed.

The details revealed at the trial shocked the city, known to be a bastion of conservatism. Homosexuality, dildos, bondage, and masochism mixed with murder seemed incongruent with the Midwestern city's quiet demeanor and reputation as a great place to raise children. The trial seemed to suggest that the city itself had a Jekyll and Hyde nature: under the surface of family, church, and hard work there lay a subculture of sex lubricated by drugs and alcohol.

After discussing the evidence for five hours, on September 20, 1989, the jury returned a verdict: Gwendolyn Graham was guilty of five counts of murder—Chambers, Luce, Mason, Burkhard, Cook—and one count of conspiracy to commit murder. The court gave her five life sentences. At twenty-six years old, Graham entered the prison system where she will spend the rest of her life. She currently resides in the Robert Scott Correctional Facility—a prison for female offenders. Among her neighbors is Diane Spencer (see "Loved Him to Death").

Wood, at twenty-seven, began her term, but unlike her former lover, she could one day be free on parole.

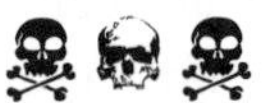

Graham protests her innocence to this day. She claims her jealous ex-lover fabricated the story about the murders. It is an interesting possibility: a vengeful and jilted lover who engineered a frame for five murders and in her testimony threw her ex-lover into it. In court, Wood appeared to be the injured ex-lover who would do anything for her paramour, including becoming an accomplice to a murder plan masterminded by her lover. But was she in fact the devious culprit who planned the killings and later planned the murder trial?

What if Graham was telling the truth? Is it possible that Wood and not Graham was the criminal mastermind who hoped that the murders would keep the couple together for life and that Graham committed the murders at Wood's direction? Is it possible that when the plan failed and Graham took another lover, Wood initiated the murder investigation to implicate Graham?

*If* the murders occurred. Graham's testimony suggested that they did not. The prosecution did manage to convince a jury without presenting physical evidence. In fact, three of the victims—Burkhard, Mason, and Luce—were cremated, so hearsay testimony was the only way to prove they died in any way other than natural causes. And during the trial, such testimony buried Graham.

Throughout the appeals process, Graham maintained her claim that no one died of anything but natural causes at Alpine Manor. The murders were a figment of her ex-lover's overly active imagination, conjured as payback for the fact that Graham replaced her with another lover. If true, Catherine Wood chose the perfect scenario for her fictitious crime—murders that left no physical evidence that could be uncovered at an autopsy.

Indeed, if Wood engineered a Machiavellian plan to frame Graham for murders that she masterminded, or that never occurred at all, she was willing to sacrifice her own freedom in the process: her deal with the prosecution sent her to prison for a minimum of twenty years, making her eligible for parole before she serves the lower end of her sentence. Wood's plea itself seems evidence of her resolve. This raises an interesting albeit disturbing question: was Catherine Wood willing to trade a decade of her life for revenge?

Apparently, the jury in Gwendolyn Graham's murder trial was not the only audience convinced of her guilt. She lost her appeal to the State of Michigan Court of Appeals in 1991, and another to the State of Michigan Supreme Court a few years later.

Unless some shocking revelation surfaces—some type of exculpatory evidence like a photograph of someone else smothering Marguerite Chambers or another of the victims from Alpine Manor, Gwendolyn Graham will spend the remainder of her life in prison.

Alpine Manor no longer exists. After the murders, the owners sold the complex, which has since become Saint Mary's Living Center. The change of ownership did not prevent the families of some of Graham and Wood's victims from filing suits against Alpine Manor, mostly for negligence for employing "dangerous and unbalanced employees" such as Graham and Wood.[5]

Despite any arguments to the contrary, the court of public opinion has convicted both Graham and Wood as a rare breed of serial killer: the female team. Their case appears in studies, typologies, and profiles of serial killers. Thus, if the murders committed at Alpine Manor did represent some type of perverted love pact, to some degree it worked; it married the names of Gwendolyn Graham and Catherine Wood, regardless of who plotted the deaths.

Perhaps the image of Gwendolyn Graham as a deranged serial killer places a face on a popular fear of murderous health workers who kill when they should protect. Perhaps she represents the real version of Annie Wilkes, the fictional nurse in Stephen King's novel *Misery*, who leaves the medical profession under the cloud of murder allegations and later tortures her favorite author, Paul Sheldon, after rescuing him from a car crash.

Were the murders at Alpine Manor also a fiction? Is this truth indeed stranger than fiction, or did Catherine Wood conjure a fiction stranger than the truth? While a jury, an appeals court, a state supreme court, and public opinion have convicted Gwendolyn Graham of murder most foul, for some, the question remains.

## Notes

1. Ken Wood, quoted by Ken Kolker and Susan Collins in "Friends, Co-workers Describe 2 Aides," *Grand Rapids Press*, December 6, 1988.

2. Lowell Cauffiel, *Forever and Five Days* (New York: Kensington

Books, 1992). Cauffiel's account of the case is definitive and probes the relationship between Graham and Wood in greater depth. Interested readers who want to know more about the case should consult his book.

3. Ken Wood, quoted by Susan Collins and Ken Kolker in "Suspect Relates Bizarre Tale of Killing," *Grand Rapids Press*, December 6, 1988.

4. A list of eight individuals whom police investigated as possible victims, along with cause of death listed on their death certificates and other pertinent biographical information, appeared in Susan Collins and Ken Kolker, "Suspect Relates Bizarre Tale of Killings," *Grand Rapids Press*, December 6, 1988.

5. Quoted by John Hogan in "Family Gets $50,000 in Nursing Home Death," *Grand Rapids Press*, October 31, 1992.

# 3. i fought the law and the law won

"Cross me again and I'll put a bullet in you," threatened "Gentleman" Tillman.

"You son of a bitch," yelled "Four Fingers" McCarver.

"I'd shoot Jesus Christ himself if he graveled me," Tillman retorted. He tapped the handle of his Colt .45—a gun the gambler bragged had cost him a hundred dollars when he purchased it during a winning streak.

The other four players at the table listened to the exchange uneasily. They had listened to the two men taunt each other for hours, taunts that seemed all thunder and no rain but that nevertheless escalated. They hoped that the thunder would pass without a lead rainstorm. The verbal insults started as figurative fingers poking the ribs, which became slaps, which became punches, and now literal fingers tapping gun handles.

Edward "Four Fingers" McCarver, a miner who had lost a finger in a mining accident, had enjoyed an uncanny run of luck, much of which came at the expense of "Gentleman" James Tillman, a gambler who earned his nickname for his infamous temper. One story, the telling of which Tillman appeared to encourage, depicted Tillman as a vengeful dental patient. When a dentist caused him pain, he retaliated by holding the man down and yanking out three of his teeth without anesthetic. And he hated to lose at poker, especially because when he left Virginia City, he planned to leave covered with gold and silver dust won from the miners of the famous Comstock Lode.

The appearance of Sheriff John Masters framed in the doorway of the Bucket of Blood saloon, just a silhouette against the setting sun behind him, did little to settle their collective nerves. Masters cradled a Greener shotgun in his arms like an infant; the sheriff in his advancing age had come to realize the value the Greener provided: a pattern of shot that even the fastest draw couldn't beat . . . or escape.

The lawman enjoyed a shadowy past—a former outlaw south of the border, some said—that served him well as keeper of the peace. Few wanted to tangle with Masters, whose physical appearance suggested that he felt comfortable imposing his will on others. His prominent brow ridge sported several scars, and both ears contained cauliflower lumps—trophies from past brawls.

Sheriff Masters eyed Tillman, who slumped down in his chair. Masters knew Four Fingers—the hard-drinking miner from Cornwall, England—as a part-time brawler with a quick temper who was responsible for one or more of the scars across his brow. Tillman, though, was a wild card; he knew the gambler only by reputation.

Patrons who had sidled up to the bar and hunkered over glasses of spirits abandoned their drinks, chased away by the specter of a wayward shot as both McCarver and Tillman had liquid courage after an afternoon of drinking—courage that could lead to bravado and errant shots.

The gamblers around the table listened to the eerie silence.

And then a "pop" like the cork exploding from a wine bottle broke the silence.

Several pops followed as the Bucket of Blood erupted with the racket of gunfire. A cloud of smoke formed around the card table as the smell of cordite filled the room.

When the haze cleared and the silence returned, Four Fingers lay facedown on the floor, motionless, with a pool of blood forming around him and blood oozing from three holes in the back of his blue gingham shirt.

The wild speculation began as soon as the smoke dissipated. No one saw anything, but everyone saw something, and each man in the saloon had a version of what led to Four Fingers's death. When the sequence of shots began, bar patrons, most drunk by the time of the incident, dove to the floor and out of the way.

Some maintain that Four Fingers drew on Tillman, missed his first two shots, then turned to run away when Tillman retaliated. In the haze, it appeared that Four Fingers and Gentleman James Tillman fired their weapons, despite Tillman's insistence that his gun jammed and he didn't fire the shot that killed Four Fingers.

The fact remained: someone shot Four Fingers in the back, and that someone, in the collective opinion of the eyewitnesses, was Gentleman James Tillman, who, it appeared, would have a date with a jury of angry townspeople and the hangman after the inevitable conviction. And the coward shot the hardworking miner in the back!

If a twenty-first-century medical examiner could travel to the Bucket of Blood of 1878, he would examine the bullet wounds in Four Fingers; the injuries to the victims represent clues that the medical examiner can follow to re-create the event.

Autopsy protocol dictates that each bullet wound is probed to determine its path, including point of entry and/or exit and the recovery of bullets and/or bullet fragments to determine who fired the fatal shot.

The victim sustained three gunshot wounds to the back, all three entering the right side, passing through the ribs and the right lung before exiting through the chest. The victim suffered another wound on his right side that ripped through his right kidney. Although these wounds may have eventually killed him, the fatal shot entered the chest an inch below the sternum, tearing through the heart. The shot passed through the heart at a slight upward angle but without left-to-right deviation. Since Four Fingers was standing when this shot struck his chest, the shot came from someone sitting at the table. A subsequent autopsy revealed a quantity of blood in the victim's pericardial sac. The bullet that entered Four Fingers's heart caused blood to flood the pericardial sac; as a result, the heart stopped beating. This bullet ended his life.

Case closed, or it would be, except for a little lead ball recovered during the autopsy—a .32-caliber lead ball. All of the handguns at the time of the shooting were the cap and ball variety; the size of the ball determined the caliber. Gentleman Tillman's Colt .45 used larger balls than the ball recovered. The other wounds most likely came from a larger caliber, but they did not ultimately lead to the victim's death. Tillman did shoot Four Fingers in the back, but this did not cause his death. In short, he did not murder the miner.

So who killed the man?

Another gambler sitting at the table, Thomas Chase, carried a Smith & Wesson .32 and told Sheriff Masters that for his protection, he held his .32 in his lap when the fight escalated. His hands were shaking; although he carried the weapon, he never had occasion to use it. The gun slipped from his hand and struck the side of his chair. After this, he heard the staccato succession of pops that were gunshots. This evidence suggests that inside of the cloud of smoke and cordite, the following scenario occurred: When Chase dropped his gun, it struck the side of his chair and discharged. The bullet traveled upward, striking Four Fingers in the sternum. After the shot, Four Fingers twisted. Tillman, believing that his nemesis had fired the shot at him, drew his .45 and fired four shots that struck Four Fingers in the side and back.

In a modern American court of law, a jury might find Tillman's four retaliatory shots as justified, since he believed that his adversary fired first and thus may have believed his life to be in imminent danger. Besides, the miner's death resulted from an accidental discharge of a handgun. If the lynch mob had its way and escorted the gambler to the tallest tree in town, or if the hanging judge scheduled a date for Tillman to visit the hangman, an innocent man, or at least a man innocent of the crime of murder, would pay.

The forensic evidence, if this scenario occurred a hundred and forty years later, would exonerate the accused. The wounds tell a story the witnesses could not or would not. Witnesses forget vital details, alter stories to fit preconceived notions, or lie to protect one or more of the parties involved. Or, sometimes, no witnesses exist. The pieces of forensic evidence, though, act as silent witnesses that find their voices in the morgue, where they tell the unadulterated story of what occurred. The medical examiner must understand their language and know how to listen to their stories.

Except for the location—the Bucket of Blood saloon is perched on the side of a mountain in the mining town of Virginia City, Nevada—this story and its characters are fictitious, although change a few names, locations, and circumstances, and such Wild West shoot-outs still occur. Sometimes hotheaded citizens clash with law enforcement agents and when they do, their disputes often send skeletons to the ME's closet.

## The Right to Bear Arms

*That jet has flown over my house three times today. Aerial surveillance. They're watching me, recording my every movement. Tracking my routine. Compiling a profile.*

*That car—a black Toyota Camry. No one in the neighborhood has one. He's slowing down as he passes. That same car passed a few minutes ago. I know it did. He's watching me.*

*The driver . . . never seen him before in my life. He's talking on a cell phone. He's calling them. The aerial surveillance. Telling them what I'm doing.*

*Who is that over there, across the street? Do I know her? No, never seen her before, but she's looking at me. What is that in her hand? A cell phone? She's making a call. She's calling them. In the car. They're looking for the right moment to get me.*

—The inner monologue of the paranoid

This inner monologue is humorous . . . unless it occurs in the mind of a person who has accumulated a weapons stockpile to protect himself.

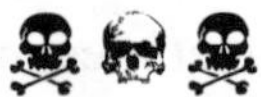

The four ionic pillars of the magnificent neoclassical mansion on Wellington Street give it a regal, majestic appearance, like that of an elegant lady. Her chin is slightly raised, suggesting a trace of haughtiness, almost a demure expression, as she is the most elegant in the neighborhood. Across from her on Washington stands another Victorian, its round turret or spire—typical of residences built in the late nineteenth century—giving away his true age; next to the lady at 230 Wellington, though, he is a mere child.

The Wellington Street mansion—at 8,247 square feet, the second-largest residence in Traverse City—sports all of the amenities a well-to-do Victorian family would require: a formal library, a billiard room, five fireplaces, a carriage house, and a five-stall garage. It came on the real estate market a few years ago at a price of $700,000. Today, the residence houses the Wellington Inn Bed and Breakfast. The inn's Web site contains a pitch that beckons visitors to the restored mansion: "Enter the stately mahogany and leaded glass foyer and be transported in time to an era of quiet and gracious living. A time when life was slower . . . when families entertained at home . . . and downtown was a leisurely stroll past elegant neighborhood homes."[1]

Like other stately homes, she can tell you fascinating stories, such as the story of her original owner—W. C. Hull, son of the founder of the Oval Wood Dish Company. As its name suggests, the company produced thin dishes made of wood. W. C. Hull had the home constructed across the street from his father's mansion.

She will also tell you, in hushed tones, another story—one that locals would prefer to forget . . .

Now she welcomes guests who would like to step back in time and sip of cup of hot tea in her period tearoom. Before she could host anyone, though, the old lady needed a facelift, as her porch was pocked with bullet holes. She received her wounds during one of the most violent events in the area's history—and the only cop killing in Traverse City's history. The small city at the end of scenic Grand Traverse Bay, known nationwide for its annual Cherry Festival, would be traumatized on May 12, 1998, by a standoff that would leave one of its officers fatally wounded. Residents of the area can still hear in their mind's ear the cracking of gunfire as John Clark and his army of firearms exchanged bullets with local and state police in an incident that led to the murder of Sergeant Dennis Finch.

For John Clark, the Wellington Street residence was his castle, both figuratively and literally. At the time of Sergeant Finch's death, Clark had stockpiled an arsenal for protection that would have given pause to the military of a small country. When Clark's confrontation with the police ended, investigators discovered the full extent of his weapons cache when they explored his house.

Clark's personal arsenal included

- 58,000 rounds of ammunition. That's 58,000!
- A .50-caliber Barrett rifle, capable of piercing tank armor or downing an F-14
- An AR-15 rifle (.223 caliber) with a 90-round magazine, including a flash suppressor. A flash suppressor is like a silencer, only instead of muting the report of a weapon, it suppresses the flashes of light that accompany a discharge. Clark likely used this weapon in the seven-hour standoff.
- A .560-caliber Weatherby Magnum—also called an "elephant rifle"—and many other types of guns

Investigators also found a few books in Clark's home: *Explosives for Sabotage*, a Central Intelligence Agency publication, and *The Ultimate Sniper*. They also found uncashed checks totaling $294,845.40 (more about this later)!

Some might consider the weapons cache as overkill. But John Clark needed the weapons because the Mafia was after him. He knew it. The "family" had taken over the city. He knew it. The Mafia had infiltrated the Traverse City police department. He knew it. And they knew he knew it, so now they wanted to silence him.

So when John Clark went out to rake the lawn on the morning of May 12, 1998, he was armed and ready, wearing a holster containing a loaded handgun. And on that morning, the Mafia would make its move. He knew it. Earlier that day, Clark was heard to say, "Today is the day that somebody is going to die."[2]

In many ways, John Clark has a fictional parallel in Jerry Fletcher, the taxi driver played by Mel Gibson in the 1997 film *Conspiracy Theory*. Fletcher sees a conspiracy around every corner. He sees black helicopters that hover over New York City and spy on people. From his apartment, he publishes a newsletter elucidating his various theories, he keeps consumables in padlocked containers in a padlocked refrigerator, and he places a glass bottle upside down on the doorknob after entering the apartment—a "poor man's alarm"—should unauthorized personnel attempt entry. For others, his theories are just that: wild machinations more suited to the suspense/thriller novel genre than a newsletter.

But for Fletcher, the black helicopters are real. He can see them. And they can see him. They're watching him. And then one day, they come after him.

For John Clark, that day came on May 12, 1998.

This type of paranoia was the subtext when Sergeant Finch confronted Clark early on May 12, 1998, except Clark's black helicopters were cars circling his house, watching him. Watching him. Mafia hitmen circling his house, watching him. As a police officer, Sergeant Finch and other officers—agents of the Mafia, according to Clark—had come to take him away or, worse, to assassinate him.

That morning, Clark's paranoia may have reached a fever pitch. Armed with a handgun, he approached some utility workers and voiced his opinion about the Mafia-police connection. The same day, the police received a call; John Clark had been observed raking his lawn while armed with a handgun in a holster.

A few minutes later, Officer David Leach arrived. Clark was

inside the house, so Leach knocked on the front door. He would later testify that he and Clark conversed—nonbelligerent small talk—but Clark became angry when Leach asked him to leave the sidearm inside when he worked outside.

Leave the house without a weapon? This was tantamount to sending a man to his death, given the ubiquitous presence of the mob. And the fact that a police officer suggested it, seeing as the Traverse City PD was in league with the Mafia, may have seemed like a conspiracy to John Clark.

Sergeant Dennis Finch arrived minutes later and began a discussion with Clark. The two knew each other, so perhaps Finch believed he could calm Clark, defuse the bomb inside of him—a bomb seemingly ticking toward detonation. Perhaps he could talk the weapon off of Clark's hip.

Finch, a thirty-year veteran of the Traverse City police department and a native of the area, joined the force in 1968 after serving four years as a marine that included time in Vietnam. During his career, he had come to know John Clark and the forty-eight-year-old's unique brand of paranoia quite well.

Clark didn't hide his opinions. On one occasion he appeared at a city commission meeting and voiced a complaint that local officials had become involved with organized crime. On another occasion, he spray-painted Mafia-related graffiti on the drive entering an exclusive neighborhood. He told a gunsmith that the CIA and FBI wanted him. The police report authored by Dennis Finch and filed after Clark's 1989 drunk driving arrest provides an interesting insight into his paranoia: Finch reported that Clark complained about the failure of the local authorities and the CIA to investigate "all the dead bodies that were in the woods that were hacked to pieces."[3]

In 1989, when Finch arrested Clark for drunk driving and resisting a police officer, the arrest turned into an altercation, compounding Clark's legal trouble. Finch testified at probate court that Clark had threatened him. The issue of Clark's mental health came up, but Clark managed to dodge the bullet of a mental health hearing. He instead agreed to an "alternative" treatment (the facts of which remain confidential but could include counseling and/or medication), which trumped a mental illness hearing.

Clark was free on a $15,000 bond, but a condition of his bond permitted officers to confiscate three firearms he possessed. He served thirty days in jail, two years probation, and lost his driver's license for two years. When he met the conditions of the bond and it was cancelled, though, police had no choice but to return the weapons.

John Clark had the right to bear arms. In 1989, he possessed a handgun permit (Michigan law permits the acquisition of rifles and shotguns without a permit), and the weapons were legal to possess. By the time of the 1998 shoot-out, Clark had obtained more handguns despite no longer possessing a permit to purchase them—one of the issues investigated after the standoff.

This was the subtext of the tragedy that unfolded that afternoon. Clark had two of the weapons from his arsenal on the porch—a handgun and an AR-15—while he spoke with Dennis Finch. Eyewitnesses describe Clark's demeanor on the porch as calm interspersed with moments in which he appeared agitated, shaking his hands in the air. Sergeant Finch had conversed with John Clark for ninety minutes when a patrol car arrived at approximately four in the afternoon. The arrival of the car may have triggered Clark's paranoia, given his feelings about the police-Mafia connection.

He retreated inside the house.

Sergeant Finch pulled his weapon, rushed onto the porch, and just made it inside the house. Officers present and neighbors who had gathered to watch the spectacle, and subsequently witness one of the community's heroes perish, claimed that as Clark reached for his weapon, Finch shouted at Clark to drop his gun.

The loud pops of gunfire shattered the silence in the neighborhood as Clark fired his weapon. Finch back-peddled onto the porch, and Clark sent a second volley of shots with an AR-15. By the time the first shot was fired, local area news had arrived and captured the scene both on film and in photographs (later used during the trial). The video captured Sergeant Finch's last act as a peace officer: just prior to the first shots fired, he yelled to Clark, "Put down the gun, drop it, drop it."[4]

When the smoke cleared, Sergeant Dennis Finch lay dying, his lifeblood dripping from the wounds caused by at least twenty-three rounds. He lay on the porch for twenty to twenty-five minutes between shocked police and John Clark with his AR-15. Officers yelled to Clark, pleading to let them remove Finch.

Just under thirty minutes after the initial shots, they would have an opportunity; a police officer provided cover and fired on Clark as he stood in the doorway, wounding him. Clark retreated back inside his mansion—his castle. A fellow officer dragged Finch from the porch and across Wellington Street with the aid of another officer. An ambulance rushed him to the hospital.

Clark fired another volley of shots after the officers evacuated their wounded officer and yelled for them to go away. The standoff had begun.

About three hours after the first shots cracked through the calm and silent veneer of the neighborhood, the Michigan state police emergency response team arrived, and in them, Clark would face a police army, complete with an armored vehicle.

The team—the Michigan state police version of SWAT—consisted of forty-four officers, two behavioral psychologists, a hostage negotiator, and an array of high-tech gadgets straight from *Mission: Impossible*. They used sophisticated monitoring devices, such as a telephone line that cannot be disconnected, to track John Clark's movements around the house. And they bathed the Wellington Street mansion in floodlights, which helped officers to see the scene but also provided an element of psychological warfare by creating a sense of isolation for Clark, like he was imprisoned inside a dome of light from which he could not escape.

During the next five hours, they would attempt to talk Clark into surrendering but without success. According to one eyewitness, he responded, "You'll have to come in and finish what you started," referring to the wounds he suffered when police returned fire earlier.[5]

The emergency response team obliged, ending the standoff when their commander drove the Peacekeeper—an armored vehicle (with an ironic name)—across the lawn to the front steps of the porch. Clark surrendered, and the standoff that began hours earlier reached a conclusion in the early morning hours of May 13 at approximately 12:45 a.m.

Sergeant Dennis Finch died of his wounds the day after the shoot-out, and while John Clark recovered from his wounds, investigators converged on 230 Wellington Street to scour the scene and the house. They accumulated evidence for the dual charges of first-degree murder and killing a police officer that Clark would face for his role in the tragedy that unfolded that afternoon.

Inside Clark's castle, which smelled of dogs and dog feces, they discovered tangible evidence of its occupant's paranoia . . . and more. Thirty-one spent 5.56-millimeter shell casings that matched Clark's semiautomatic AR-15 rifle lay strewn across the hardwood floor. They found his weapons horde. They found his books. Then they found a sinister surprise: a container that held a lump of what looked like plastic explosive. Police didn't find the alleged bomb during their first sweep because of the disarray and clutter, and the stench of the dog feces confused their dog during initial searches.

In *Conspiracy Theory,* Jerry Fletcher (Clark's cinematic mirror image) wired his apartment with an incendiary device. When the men in black helicopters came to his door (and broke the bottle he placed on the knob), he initiated this weapon of self-destruction and fled through a secret door while his apartment and all the evidence of his myriad conspiracy theories burned. Did Clark intend the bomb for a similar use as a defensive device? Or did he intend the explosive as an offensive?

Officers cleared the neighborhood while the bomb squad cleared the home. Ultimately, though, analysis at a state crime lab proved that the device was not a bomb.

Investigators also found another shocking item amid the ashes of John Clark's life: a pile of checks worth over $294,835.40. Clark, it appeared, had too much on his mind to bother with family finances.

Over the past few years, the small real estate empire accumulated by his father began to disintegrate. Unpaid property taxes in the amount of $123,000 led to a tax sale in which his family lost most of its real estate in the city. Bit by bit, the family lost other holdings in neighboring counties. Clark's obsession with the Mafia and apparent neglect of the real estate portfolio had brought his family's fortune, accumulated by his father, local real estate magnate John V. Clark, to the edge of ruin.

The price of self-defense, it appears, can be high, and Clark spent a good amount accumulating the weapons cache found by investigators in the Wellington Street home. The cost of the .560-caliber Weatherby elephant rifle and the .50-caliber Barrett would come close to $5,000.

While Clark recovered in the hospital and prosecutors prepared to charge him for homicide, Sergeant Dennis Finch traveled to see one last doctor at the Kent County Morgue. When a person is struck by multiple gunshots—in this case at least twenty-three bullets—cause of death may appear to be a foregone conclusion, but the autopsy of a homicide victim does more than determine cause and manner of death. It can ascertain the type of weapon used (if a bullet is recovered) and range of fire. Autopsies conducted on victims of multiple gunshot wounds thus involve a necessarily lengthy, painstaking process. Each bullet wound is probed to determine the paths of the bullets and which bullet or bullets proved fatal.

Replay the scene for a moment on your mind's television screen. John Clark retreats just inside the foyer as Sergeant Finch rushes up the stairs and onto the porch. Clark fires at Finch, who falls backward onto the porch. Other police officers spray the porch with gunfire, scarring the doorway and adjacent panels. Finch sustains twenty-three bullet wounds, but whose bullets? An early theory of Clark's defense held that Finch died from friendly fire; in other words, some of his fellow officers shot him by accident during the fray. So the type of bullets recovered from the body and the position of the entrance wounds could provide crucial evidence.

Sergeant Finch arrived at the Kent County Morgue and underwent an autopsy two days after the shooting. On the morgue table, his body provided evidence of not one but two battles. Bullet and bullet fragment wounds peppered his torso and told the story of the assault at the Wellington mansion, but external and internal examination would reveal the second battle waged that night at the hospital: physicians battled to save his life from the damage caused by the multiple gunshot wounds. By examining the battlefield, one can reconstruct the battle.

Dennis Finch sustained a minimum of twenty-three gunshot wounds and numerous bullet fragment wounds: thirteen wounds to the chest and abdomen, five in the left leg, two in the right thigh, and three in the back. Bullets traveled through the left lung, liver, left hemidiaphragm, fourth rib, and right kidney and testicle.

The surgical interventions, such as the extension of wounds for exploration, the sewing shut of others, and the removal of Finch's lower right leg, made difficult the interpretation of the wounds during the autopsy. These interventions and the missing lower right leg also made it impossible to determine the exact number of bullets that struck Sergeant Finch.

During the autopsy, twenty-three gunshot wounds and numerous additional bullet fragment wounds were explored. When a bullet from a high-powered rifle strikes an object, it often fragments. The numerous bullet fragment wounds in Dennis Finch's body indicate that he was struck by pieces of bullets after they initially struck some other object; these wounds were not counted among the twenty-three gunshot wounds and suggest that many more than twenty-three bullets strafed the victim. In fact, two jars that arrived with the victim contained numerous bullet and bullet fragments recovered by hospital personnel during their desperate attempt to save Sergeant Finch's life.

Most of the bullets struck Sergeant Finch in the front of his torso between his chest and hips, but entrance wounds also appeared on his back, suggesting that he may have sustained the wounds while twisting after receiving the initial wounds or even while lying on the porch. While no intact bullets were retrieved during the autopsy, the bullet fragments that were recovered matched Clark's AR-15 and not the weapons the police used. This forensic evidence, including the presence of bullet wounds in Finch's back, suggests that Clark, and no one else, shot his victim twenty-three times. Finch did not die from friendly fire.

The tremendous damage caused by the multiple gunshot wounds was evident in the external injuries Sergeant Finch sustained. Severe, uncontrollable bleeding in his right leg forced doctors to amputate the leg above the knee. Bullets shattered his lower left leg, fracturing both the tibia and fibula and blowing away much of the calf muscle.

Likewise, the internal injuries indicated the tremendous destruction done by the bullets and also documented the attempts to save the lawman's life. Diminished breath sounds on his left side led doctors to insert a chest tube to evacuate air and blood from the pleural cavity (the space in the chest where the lungs are situated). They performed a laparotomy, which resulted in a large quantity of blood being removed from the abdominal cavity. A gunshot wound to the spleen required a splenectomy; gunshot wounds to the liver, the diaphragm, and the stomach required suturing.

A wound left one testicle in pieces inside of the scrotum; consequently, doctors performed an orchiectomy. Bullets that passed through the left portion of his chest led to a rib fracture and perforations in the left lung, but his heart had sustained no damage. By the time he died, Dennis Finch had received approximately two hundred units of blood components. Despite the efforts of his doctors, though, Finch lost the battle.

Dennis Finch returned to the city he served lauded as a fallen hero. Blue ribbons memorializing his passing could be found everywhere, and the city law enforcement center was renamed in his honor. News of the event flooded homes in daily newspaper and television reports. His community would not allow Sergeant Finch to be forgotten . . . or his death to go unpunished.

John Clark faced dual charges: the killing of a police officer and a premeditated murder, both of which could bring life sentences without the possibility of parole. The defense, fearing that an unbiased jury could not be found among the inflamed citizenry of a grieving city, moved for a change of venue.

The presiding judge, however, believed that an unbiased jury could be found. John Clark would be tried in the same city in which he gunned down a thirty-year veteran of the police force and a veteran of the Vietnam War. A hero.

In such a case, one would expect a psychiatric evaluation to determine Clark's sanity and competency to stand trial. The evaluation would take place in the opposite corner of the state, at the Center for Forensic Psychiatry in Ypsilanti, an outlying community of the Detroit metropolitan area. Such an evaluation is conducted and submitted to the court, which then makes a determination about competency to stand trial. If found incompetent, the defendant is committed to a mental health facility until he or she becomes competent, which could take any length of time if it happens at all. The evaluation can take as long as eight weeks and slow down the litigation process, but prosecutors in Clark's case didn't need to worry about delays for long.

Appearing in front of a judge, John Clark trumped the psychological evaluation and denied his right to claim insanity or diminished capacity as a defense. Instead, he would assume a different defense strategy: he acted in self-defense! He feared for his life and believed that Sergeant Finch posed a threat when he rushed the porch, drawing his weapon. He protected himself. He was doing yard work that morning, not bothering anyone, and became hostile only after police arrived.

Legally, Clark could have acted in self-defense if the evidence proved that he believed Sergeant Finch was going to kill and not arrest him. To prove this, however, the defense would have to prove that any reasonable person in similar circumstances would likewise feel threatened. Another possibility, called imperfect self-defense, could also justify his actions as self-defense if evidence proved that Finch retaliated after Clark withdrew from the initial confrontation and renounced his hostile intentions.

An imperfect self-defense might go like this:

> "I'm going to put your lights out." The first man raises his arm but hesitates. After thinking for a few seconds, he says, "No, I'm sorry. I lost my temper."
>
> The second man, poised to defend an attack, slams his fist into the underside of the first man's jaw, knocking him to the floor.
>
> The first man leaps to his feet and lands a right cross; the second man loses his balance and falls, striking his head on a sharp corner of the coffee-table, sustaining a lethal head injury.

Add guns, and *if* something like this scenario occurred on the porch of the Wellington Street mansion, Clark had a good argument that he acted in self-defense. At one point during the standoff, Clark stated that "Finch put a gun in my face and came in after me," suggesting that he felt threatened, but would a reasonable person feel threatened in similar circumstances?[6]

Of course, the fact that Sergeant Finch sustained twenty-three bullet wounds seemed to dismiss any self-defense claim. And videotape taken during the incident showed that Clark fired at Finch in two volleys; after the initial shots were fired, Clark sent another cloud of hot lead at Finch with the AR-15. Other evidence, such as a statement Clark made—"Let's end this here and now, today"—also appeared to undermine Clark's defense.[7]

No one could ask Sergeant Finch what went through his mind in the seconds in which he decided to rush after Clark. He might have believed that Clark posed a threat to his community, and perhaps he saw an opportunity to wrest the gun from Clark. Did Sergeant Dennis Finch make a rational decision? Did his instinct take over during the fractions of a second during which he needed to decide to pursue or retreat? Right or wrong, rational or irrational, logical or illogical, the decision cost him his life.

In his closing statement, prosecutor Dennis LaBelle defended Sergeant Finch's decision. It was legally justified if Finch felt Clark posed a threat to the community or carried a firearm with unlawful intent.

But to prove premeditated murder, the prosecution had to prove that

Clark planned to kill. Did a statement he made that morning—"Today is the day that somebody is going to die"—suggest premeditation?[8]

Not according to Clark's defense. In his closing argument, attorney Neil Fink pointed out that Clark posed no real or even perceived threat to his community. He had no history of assault, and when he did cross the law during the 1989 drunk driving incident, he cooperated fully with the court.

John Clark didn't rant and rave and foam at the mouth, waving the loaded pistol in the air, firing into the sky, or aim at innocent passersby. He didn't plan to assassinate high-ranking members of the Mafia-controlled Traverse City PD. He simply conducted his yard work armed in case the Mafia or any of its deputies made their move. And he had the right to bear arms.

In fact (as the defense pointed out in closing arguments), neighbors didn't complain about Clark's behavior; they knew about his beliefs. He made no attempt to hide his conspiracy theories. Had the police not come calling on John Clark that morning, more than likely no shots would have been fired and no one would have died. Sergeant Finch went too far in attempting to arrest Clark, Fink told the jury; Clark, fearing for his life when Finch rushed toward him with his gun drawn, defended himself, and the shoot-out resulted.

After six days, without the testimony of John Clark himself, the jury would have to decide. They found John Clark guilty of second-degree murder and of killing a police officer. The second conviction ensured that he would spend the remainder of his life in prison.

Ultimately, the community would hear from John Clark, who commented before his sentencing. In his comments, which seem to underline the paranoia that defined his life in the years before the standoff, he stated, "I am greatly saddened by what I have seen happening to this community over a period of years. The people in this community . . . they want to believe that their police officers are honest that they're not corrupted that there's no criminal elements involved, but that's not the case here. And though I am saddened by it, I expected to hear police officers lie in my trial, and they did."[9] In his mind, he simply acted to protect his castle with his right to bear arms. The community just could not see the corruption, but he could. The Mafia had infiltrated it. He knew it.

The mansion at 230 Wellington Street experienced a rebirth of sorts. She became a fashionable bed and breakfast furnished in period decor, her interior restored to her original glamour. The visitor to Traverse City and the Wellington Inn can lounge in her tearoom and gaze through her stained-glass eyes with no idea about the events that occurred a decade earlier.

Now, John Clark's castle consists of a cell in a Michigan correctional facility. At least it will keep him safe from the Mafia members he believed hunted him . . . or it will keep them safe from him.

## Notes

1. Antiquities Wellington Inn, http://www.wellingtoninn.com/index.php (accessed March 30, 2006).

2. Quoted in Patrick Sullivan, "Clark Trial," *Traverse City Record-Eagle*, September 17, 1998, http://www.record-eagle.com/news/clark/17clark.htm (accessed March 30, 2006).

3. Excerpts of Dennis Finch's reports discussed by Barrie Barber in "Finch Tried to Get Clark Committed," *Traverse City Record-Eagle*, May 22, 1998, http://www.record-eagle.com/news/clark/22gun.htm (accessed March 30, 2006).

4. Quoted in Patrick Sullivan, "Jury Weighs Murder Case against Clark," *Traverse City Record-Eagle*, December 9, 1998, http://www.record-eagle.com/news/clark/9clarktr.htm (accessed March 30, 2006).

5. Quoted in Rich Wertz, "Man Charged with Open Murder in Shooting of Police Officer," *Traverse City Record-Eagle*, May 14, 1998, http://www.record-eagle.com/news/clark/14seige.htm (accessed March 30, 2006).

6. Quoted in Rich Wertz and Bill O'Brien, "Gunman Kills TC Officer," *Traverse City Record-Eagle*, May 13, 1998, http://www.record-eagle.com/news/clark/13shoot.htm (accessed March 30, 2006).

7. Quoted in Patrick Sullivan, "Jury Weighs Murder Case against Clark."

8. See note 2 above.

9. Quoted in Patrick Sullivan, "I Hope You Rot in Prison," *Traverse City Record-Eagle*, January 16, 1999, http://www.record-eagle.com/news/clark/16clark.htm (accessed March 30, 2006).

## Rebel Yell

The last chapter in Scott Woodring's life began with a great deal of irony: a devoutly religious man prone to quoting scripture in his letters and who condemned authorities for their laxity involving moral offenses was accused of soliciting a minor for prostitution at a gas station. This alleged offense would lead a man with a deep distrust of the "system" into a direct confrontation with state police.

Scott Woodring's worst suspicions of authority may have seemed justified when local officers appeared at his house to serve him a warrant. Although Woodring did not have a history of violence, they knew he had firearms, militia training, and a distrust of authority and US government. Despite warnings by Woodring's sister-in-law not to attempt an arrest at Woodring's house, three officers arrived to do just that on Sunday, July 6, 2003.

And those who watched as members of the state police tactical unit stormed Scott Woodring's home may have felt like they were watching a Wild West shoot-out. They observed in fascination and horror as the strange scene unfolded on Monday, July 7, 2003.

Local police had arrived at the simple, single-story residence a day earlier on Sunday to serve its occupant, Scott Woodring, a warrant for criminal sexual conduct. He had allegedly solicited a minor for sex in the nearby community of Hesperia. Next to the house, a giant radio antenna reached to the sky, like an extended index finger, warning the unwelcome to stay away.

Woodring met the officers with an unsubtle threat that was underlined by his radical and publicly expressed political views: he had a gun, he warned, after barricading himself inside of the residence. The state police arrived the next day armed to win the standoff that had developed. Perhaps anticipating fireworks, they evacuated people in proximity to an elementary school where they would spend the night. Woodring, they might have feared, had converted his house to a makeshift Alamo and would use it as the last stand for his radical political views.

Scott Woodring played an active role in promoting his beliefs. A member of a paramilitary organization called the Michigan Militia, his philosophy aligned with a broad, loose confederation of people who follow the antigovernment sovereign citizens movement—a belief system born in the 1970s with a group called the Posse Comitatus.

This group often leads members to attempt to form their own townships as a method of eliminating government jurisdiction. They call themselves by such names as preamble citizens, constitutionalists, freemen, and common law citizens, but regardless of the title, the beliefs remain the same. Typical items on the antigovernment sovereign citizen's agenda include a disagreement with taxes and gun control of any kind. Antigovernment is the heartbeat of this monster.

Those who follow the sovereign citizen movement often go to bizarre lengths to indicate their lack of respect for US government. Terry Nichols, an ardent member of this movement and an acquaintance of Timothy McVeigh (who was convicted and executed for his role in bombing the Alfred P. Murrah Federal Building in Oklahoma City), typically addressed letters with the acronym "TDC"—his way of telling people that he used the federal zip code system under "threat, duress, and coercion."

An individual named Paul Revere (not his given name) leads the Embassy of Heaven; another group, Ambassadors of the Kingdom of Heaven, disavow all governmental authority and sell fake license plates to followers nationwide to finance their cause. Another sovereign citizen leader created a version of English grammar even his followers find difficult to decipher. While these examples may appear humorous, the movement is anything but comical and has a very dangerous side.

Not surprisingly, individuals who attempt to circumvent the US government with such stratagems have a long history of tangling with authorities. Gordon Kahl, one of the leaders of the Posse Comitatus, killed two US marshalls who attempted to arrest him for a parole violation. When the murders occurred, Kahl had just left a meeting to establish a township. Kahl escaped, but four months after the incident, federal marshals tracked him to an Arkansas farmhouse. A shoot-out resulted. When the smoke and cordite dissipated, Kahl and a sheriff lay dead.

Until his standoff, Scott Woodring's battles with authority were relatively minor and peaceful; he was a citizen attempting to exert his influence within the system by stretching it, though never to the point at which it would break (Woodring never committed a felony). In the period between 1996 and 2000, he incurred eleven civil infractions or misdemeanors—violations of city, township, or state laws. He always paid any fines he received. Among other objections, he disagreed with license plate renewals and appeared in court to voice his opinion.

His civic activism and promotion of his beliefs would escalate and peak in 1996. Woodring attempted to assert his philosophy by running for Dayton Township supervisor, garnering 10 percent of the vote. Having failed to win public office, Woodring attempted to create a township as a vehicle to promote his beliefs. Across the country in the same year, a group called the Freemen attempted to establish Justis Township in Montana during an infamous standoff with federal authorities that lasted for eighty-one days. Likewise, Woodring attempted to establish a township in Newaygo County. In newspaper advertisements he promoted the Committee for a De Jure Township. This attempt failed as well.

Woodring's political activism, though, remained strong. Also in 1996, as a representative of the Michigan Militia, he attended the Third Continental Congress—a gathering of like-minded followers who wanted to establish a national militia.

He wrote letters to local newspapers in which he decried taxes and what he viewed as immoral behavior. "I have this against you, you permit Jezebel to teach My servants that sex sin is not a serious matter," he wrote in a letter titled "Indecency," submitted to Fremont's weekly *Times Indicator* about a month before his alleged solicitation.[1] In his letters, Woodring frequently quoted scripture.

Like many of his sovereign citizen predecessors, Scott Woodring's antigovernment sentiment would lead to a standoff with authorities with disastrous consequences.

The scene that took place at Woodring's house in early July 2003 must have presented a fascinating yet shocking tableau to the people of the small rural community of Fremont. The town was home to Gerber, the baby-food company, which had a large plant in Fremont and employed many locals, including Scott Woodring and his wife. Each year, the community of Fremont hosted the National Baby Food Festival. The thirteenth annual celebration of this festival would occur the week after the Woodring standoff. The locals, who lived amid sprawling cornfields, knew of Woodring's beliefs; some of them even shared his deep distrust for the US government, but few could have predicted the scene they witnessed, one more fitting for a big Hollywood blockbuster than small-town America.

On the afternoon of July 7, bystanders watched from a distance as an armored vehicle drove up to Woodring's residence. After negotiations failed, the state police decided to end the standoff. They lobbed canisters of tear gas into the house—a precursor to the state emergency response unit's invasion. A small SWAT unit—a tactical team trained to face gunfire—disappeared into the house with shields and body armor. A staccato rhythm of pops followed, and team members retreated from the same door they had just entered, this time dragging something difficult to identify from a distance.

The incident inside the house during those seconds occurred amid a haze of tear gas, smoke, and confusion, and would remain obscured by conjecture until an autopsy conducted at the Kent County Morgue determined who killed whom.

The poor visibility in the house from the tear gas and stun grenades made the task of the SWAT unit more difficult. Eight-year veteran Kevin Marshall entered first, moving through the haze behind a shield. Four members of the team had entered the house when the first shots were fired. One of the troopers behind Marshall fired one shot before his gun jammed. Another trooper thought the gunfire came from in front of them and to the right, so he fired several shots from a handgun where he believed the gunfire originated. Then he heard someone yell that the shots came from the floor, so he fired into the floor. Another trooper also fired at the floor and then sent shots through a wall into the stairwell leading to the basement.

During the fray, the lead man, Marshall, sustained four gunshot wounds, raising an intriguing and unsettling question: how did a trained officer, carrying a heavy shield and wearing body armor, sustain bullet wounds? Others present later reported that Marshall, while holding his shield, had turned to his right when the bullets struck him.

Team members dragged Marshall from the house. His battle against the four gunshot wounds began at the local Gerber Hospital and continued with an air evacuation to the larger Spectrum Health, Butterworth Campus Hospital in Grand Rapids. Just over two hours after entering Woodring's house, the thirty-three-year-old and father of two died on the operating table. Meanwhile, the standoff continued through Monday night and into Tuesday.

During the standoff, searchlights cut through the dark summer night while police snipers crouched among cornstalks. Through Monday night and into the morning hours of Tuesday, the strange, incongruous sounds of animals broadcast from a police van—a tidbit of psychological warfare designed to keep Woodring awake—drowned out the peaceful song of locusts typical for that time of year. Police had formed a double circle surrounding the Woodring residence, preventing Woodring from fleeing the scene.

While the standoff continued, Kevin Marshall's body traveled across town to the Kent County Morgue. A thick haze consisting of tear gas, smoke, and confusion in Woodring's house obscured the details of Trooper Kevin Marshall's tragic death; questions hung in the air, thick and palpable questions: how, if he carried a shield and wore bulletproof body armor, did Marshall sustain fatal gunshot wounds? And who fired the shots? The confusion in the house and the reports of fellow team members shooting in various directions gave the appearance of a friendly-fire accident. If the shots that killed Kevin Marshall came from something other than the large-caliber 9-millimeter and .40-caliber police-issued weapons, the fugitive would face a possible sentence of life in prison for murder.

Four bullets struck Trooper Marshall: two in the back and one in both his right wrist and right thigh. The position and wound tracks of these four bullet wounds were important, as they helped to clear the haze as to how Trooper Marshall sustained the wounds and from where the bullets likely originated; the bullet fragments would determine who fired the shots that killed Kevin Marshall.

All four bullets struck him from behind. One bullet struck his right wrist and, passing from the left to right, fractured the radius and ulna bones in several places. Another struck him in the back of the right leg; it entered the area of his right upper thigh/buttock. This bullet likewise passed from left to right and fragmented into three pieces when it struck the femur (large thigh bone) of Marshall's right leg, creating three exit wounds in his right hip.

These wounds, though, did not lead to his death. He died as a result of the two wounds in his back, one piercing the body armor he wore for protection and another tearing through a cloth piece of the equipment. The shield contained pocks from bullets, indicating that the shots came from in front of the troopers and not from the basement below, as some believed.

One bullet entered his upper left back below the left shoulder blade, moved in a left-to-right direction with a slight above to downward angle, and exited through the lower thoracic vertebral column. The other bullet that struck Marshall in the back entered the area of the lower left back by the base of his spine. The direction the bullet traveled was from below upward and slightly from left to right. The bullet fragmented when it struck his spinal column; one piece tore through the right adrenal gland and the right lobe of his liver, while the other grazed the surface of the left lung.

Since Marshall entered Woodring's house first as the lead man in a formation, the entrance wounds in his back seemed to support the idea that in the confusion, he sustained wounds fired by his SWAT colleagues. If so, his death resulted from a tragic accident but not a premeditated murder by a violent anarchist. A high-powered rifle, like a hunting or assault rifle, however, caused the wounds, not a handgun. Of the troopers who entered the house, one reported that his gun jammed; the third man who entered the house admitted to firing his weapon—a handgun. If their statements were accurate, then Marshall did not die by the trigger finger of another trooper. Another possibility existed: Marshall had his back turned to the shooter when he received the wounds.

One SWAT member reported that Marshall sustained the wounds while backing out of the house; he had turned toward his right when bullets struck him and fell forward onto his shield. The wound tracks seem to support a scenario in which the first bullet strikes Marshall in the wrist, and he turns to his right. With his back now facing the shooter, the next three bullets strike him in the back, all three—the two in the back and the one in the upper right thigh—passing from left to right. The bullet tracks from two of these wounds—from slightly upward—indicate that these bullets may have struck Marshall as he fell to the floor of the house.

The ballistic evidence also supported the notion that Scott Woodring had graduated from nonviolent protests to murder. Bullet fragments recovered during surgery and the autopsy were sent to the state police, who confirmed they came from a small-caliber weapon and not the 9-millimeter or .40-caliber weapons carried by police. Kevin Marshall did not die from friendly fire. This evidence made Woodring a fugitive cop killer.

The standoff ended the next day. On the afternoon of July 8, using armed vehicles borrowed from the Michigan National Guard, state police fired two percussion grenades in Scott Woodring's house. The type of percussion grenades the state police used has a side effect: they can cause fires. The house erupted into flames. The blaze was followed by explosions that may have resulted when the percussion grenades ignited ammunition. The house burned to the ground, leaving Scott Woodring and his unconventional philosophies in ashes. Or so the state police believed.

The state police siege drew criticism from some locals who shared Woodring's distrust of government and authority. After the standoff, some wondered how a warrant for a four-year felony justified burning down a man's house.

Perhaps the greatest ire came from Scott Woodring's relatives, some of whom watched, helpless, as troopers entered the house followed by the rapid, multiple bursts that sounded like champagne corks popping. They watched—a passive audience deprived of the opportunity to play a role in preventing a tragedy unfold—as the house caught fire and burned, Scott Woodring's Alamo reduced to ashes. Both Woodring's brother and sister offered their assistance to state police, who did not take advantage of what they felt was an opportunity to talk Woodring out from behind his barricade.

Ironically, for some, Scott Woodring's distrust of authority was underlined by what they saw as the reactionary and excessive force that led to his death. In their minds, the state police response oddly justified Woodring's beliefs. Now two people, one on each side of this dispute, had perished. Or had they?

A search through the debris resulted in a shocking conclusion: the absence of any trace of Scott Woodring. This led to the inevitable conclusion that, despite the double ring of officers surrounding the residence, he had managed to escape. Unless an automaton fired at the state troopers, Woodring must have been inside the house during the afternoon of July 7, but he could have escaped any time after the incident, likely under the cover of night.

In fact, both bystanders and police officers witnessed what likely was the escape of Scott Woodring through the cornfield during the evening of July 7. Several people saw a man, clad in dark clothes and carrying a rifle and a bag, crawling through the cornstalks. (The next day, July 8, police found a backpack not far from the Woodring residence that Woodring's wife identified as belonging to the fugitive; the backpack contained food and survival supplies.) Two local sheriff's deputies also saw a man walking along the north side of the Woodring residence at approximately 8:40 p.m. They notified the command post, but no action was taken for at least ten minutes.

A round of hindsight finger-pointing resulted—a dangerous suspect appeared to have murdered a state police trooper and slipped through the double net of officers surrounding the house. Among the excuses: local and state police units used different frequencies and when they did communicate, they used different and confusing nomenclature that resulted in a time lag between the sighting and a search around the house using a helicopter and an armored truck. They also did not extend their search beyond the house, and Woodring had escaped. Now they had to find a fugitive and potential cop killer who was likely armed.

A massive manhunt ensued. While few agreed with or condoned the murder of a law enforcement officer, many shared Woodring's suspicion of government, which raised the possibility of a Jesse James scenario in which sympathetic locals would shelter a fugitive who becomes a folk hero. For many, the standoff and subsequent destruction of Scott Woodring's house represented the worst excess of government power. A *Grand Rapids Press* article that ran July 10, 2003, captured the feeling in its headline: "Neighbors Reluctant to Condemn Suspect; They Share Fear of Government, but Want Him Punished If Proven Guilty."[2] The article discusses another fugitive, Eric Rudolph, who managed to elude capture in the North Carolina woods for five years. Scott Woodring's flight, though, would end a week after it began, and the *Press* article would become an eerie harbinger.

In the early morning hours of July 13, 2003, police received a tip as to Scott Woodring's whereabouts. He had not ventured far from his home and, according to the tip, could be found sleeping in a car parked in the driveway of a home just four miles from Woodring's house. At about 5:30 a.m., a tactical team of eight troopers in two patrol cars and two unmarked cars found Woodring in a Suzuki Sidekick. One patrol car pulled up behind the vehicle, and officers shined searchlights into the car to confirm they had found the fugitive.

After announcing themselves as state police, they requested he stay in the car. According to a state police press release from July 14, 2003, Woodring, attired in blue jeans and a black T-shirt (matching the description of the man seen fleeing the Woodring house during the standoff), ignored their commands, exited from the passenger door, then grabbed an assault rifle from the floor of the Suzuki. When Woodring turned toward the police with the rifle, five of the eight shot him.

Scott Woodring fell to the ground, dead, his body hit a minimum of thirty-two times with bullets and shotgun buckshot. The July 14 press release describes the last few moments of the fugitive's life: "As he exited, he withdrew a rifle and turned toward the troopers. Five of the eight troopers then fired."[3]

The gun Woodring carried—a Colt .223-semiautomatic assault rifle—contained a twenty-round magazine with one round chambered and the safety in the off position. Inside the car, police found another, larger .223 magazine and other items that Woodring used in his efforts to elude police: area maps, water, flashlight, and tools. They also found some cryptic writings that contained numerous biblical references.

The autopsy of Scott Woodring raised a disturbing question: how did he sustain multiple gunshot wounds in the back? Although the buckshot and the sheer number of wounds made it difficult to determine the entry and exit points for some of the wounds, the autopsy revealed that the majority of the thirty-two wounds were *in his back.* If one believes the police reports that Woodring pointed a gun at police (some statements have him raising the gun to eye level), at least some of the bullets and buckshot should have struck him in the front.

Scott Woodring lay on the stainless steel autopsy table in the Kent County Morgue in the blue jeans and black T-shirt he wore when police found him. His hands were cuffed behind his back.

He also had an interesting and somewhat enigmatic message written on his body. People adorn themselves with personal messages tattooed on various parts of their bodies, and victims arrive at the Kent

County Morgue often with bizarre messages inked into the skin. One victim, for instance, had "FUCK THE POLICE" tattooed on the inside of his lip—a message that most antigovernment advocates could appreciate. Scott Woodring had used black ink to scrawl his own message in the palm of his left hand—"IS 54:5"—as if giving himself a constant reminder of the biblical passage.

He had sustained twenty-six wounds in the back and six in the head and upper neck for a total of thirty-two. For classification and description, the thirty-two bullet wounds were placed into thirteen groups of single and multiple wounds. The bullets tore through many of the internal organs and created massive damage: eight wounds in the heart; nineteen wounds in both lungs combined; three wounds in the liver and stomach; one each in the left kidney and the pancreas; wounds in the brain as well as several other sites. Woodring's body was a veritable lead mine, with jacketed bullets, fragments of jacketed bullets, and buckshot recovered from various parts of his body.

Perhaps Woodring began to turn toward the officers, and in fear of the rifle he held or reached for, they discharged their weapons in self-defense, believing that he would point and shoot the weapon at them. He had allegedly killed a state trooper, so perhaps they feared a repeat of the shoot-out a week earlier.

The forensic evidence, though, did not support the idea that he turned or spun toward the officers before he was shot. None of the bullets or buckshot entered the side of his body, and none of the wound tracks ran the left-to-right or right-to-left course one would expect. The forensic evidence suggests the reality: a majority of the bullets that struck Scott Woodring struck him in the back.

The legal question to ask is: what would a reasonable officer do given the same circumstances? The Newaygo County prosecutor believed that the officers acted in a reasonable manner, as she considered the shooting justified. Justified or not, the thirty-two wounds would appear to the antigovernment contingent as overkill and, like the burning of his home, would seem to substantiate Scott Woodring's fear and distrust of government. Scott Woodring became a martyr for his cause.

What conspiracy theory would an antigovernment sovereign citizen movement follower conjure to explain Scott Woodring's death? Their theory: the government fabricated a charge to apprehend and/or murder a known antigovernment agitator. And the government was sloppy in its fabrication, attaching a charge for sexual solicitation to an individual who railed authorities for their laxity in dealing with moral transgressors.

The official justification: the antigovernment extremist refused to surrender himself to a legitimate government warrant and murdered a police officer in the ensuing conflict. Scott Woodring packed angst and an automatic weapon and consequently posed a danger to society when he eluded the police; they acted in their and society's better interest.

In the cryptic papers police found among Woodring's things in the Suzuki Sidekick, one biblical passage is prominent—Isaiah 54:5 (King James Version):

> For thine Maker is thy husband; the LORD of hosts is His name; and thy Redeemer the Holy One of Israel; The God of the whole earth shall He be called.

Scott Woodring felt the message important enough to write in the palm of his left hand. The first thirty-nine chapters of the book of Isaiah discuss the failures of two kings, Ahaz and Hezekiah, of the House of David, and cautions followers to depend only on Yahweh (God) rather than on other nations. The last portion of the book focuses on the notion of God as savior and redeemer.

The book of Isaiah, in its warning to avoid dependence on kings other than God, provides an interesting parallel to and symbol of the distrust in government that represents the heartbeat of the sovereign citizens movement. The black ink message on his palm is an adequate representation of Scott Woodring's beliefs, beliefs that led to the death of Trooper Kevin Marshall and ultimately himself. And as a representation of his death, it is a fitting epitaph.

## Notes

1. Excerpts from Scott Woodring's letters submitted to various newspapers, quoted in John Agar, "Standoff Suspect Called Dangerous," *Grand Rapids Press*, July 9, 2003.

2. Headline from *Grand Rapids Press*, July 10, 2003.

3. "Additional Information regarding the Investigation into Scott Woodring," Michigan state police press release, July 14, 2003, http://www.michigan.gov/msp/0,1607,7-123-1586_1710-71845—,00.html (accessed April 3, 2007).

## "Hey, You, Get Off of My Cloud!" (Over the Rainbow)

The sun passed below the horizon, leaving Rainbow Farm and everything on it obscured by shadows. One could still smell the smoke from the burning buildings. According to the local news reports, rain would soon douse the area.

Tom Crosslin and his companion, Brandon Peoples, neared the end of their short trek to forage for food. Peoples, a friend who had sneaked onto the farm through the one hundred and twenty-man army surrounding it, had decided to accompany Crosslin on the short trip to the neighbor's cabin to obtain provisions. They stopped when they reached the summit of Mount This—a small yet steep incline and the highest elevation on the farm. From this point, one could survey the entire compound below. So, if someone wanted to observe the goings-on at Rainbow Farm, this point would offer an excellent perch.

Perhaps Crosslin paused to contemplate happier times, in that moment revisiting one of his utopia's successes. Perhaps in that moment he saw the crowd of three thousand that he envisioned but never materialized, all gathered in the name of peace and personal liberty. After all, it was Labor Day weekend, when Rainbow Farm usually hosted the marijuana-friendly music festival Roach Roast. Not this year.

Perhaps he heard the echoes of Merle Haggard or Tommy Chong, who performed on the farm's stage, or the jeers and cheers as naked partygoers slid down the hill on a chute made from plastic sheets and lubricated with soapy water. It was Tom Crosslin's perfect world, his ideal society, his Shangri-la, his Xanadu, now reduced to ashes. His life's work, gone up in smoke.

Crosslin and Peoples moved along toward the house, with Peoples following a few yards behind, looking at the ground.

Crosslin cradled in his arms a Ruger .223-caliber Mini-14 semi-automatic rifle, which he would use if necessary to protect his utopia—or what remained of it—from a different sort of crowd that had now come to Rainbow Farm.

A sound from ahead broke the silence. Crosslin stared at the source of the sound for a few seconds—silhouettes framed by the diminishing light.

Like so many things involving this case, what happened next is a matter of perspective. The official version of the story has Tom Crosslin pointing his weapon at the silhouettes, and the silhouettes firing in self-defense—a simple matter of self-preservation: kill or be killed.

Rainbow Farm supporters believe that the agents fired on Crosslin without provocation. Some even use the word *murder* . . .

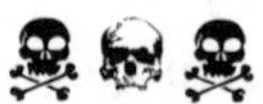

Everyone has a cloud—a place for contemplation and recuperation from the stresses of life. One man's cloud might be a leather easy chair he reclines in to disappear in the pages of an adventure novel. Another man's cloud might be a recreation room stocked with a pool table or foosball game.

The cloud is also a place to search for meaning and hopefully find it. Some look for it at the bottom of a bottle. Others look while in euphoria brought on by a syringe, a few pills, a white line on a mirror, or a weed rolled into a cigarette.

Tom Crosslin and Rollie Rohm's cloud consisted of thirty-four acres in southern Michigan's Cass County near the town of Vandalia. Rainbow Farm, as they dubbed their parcel of land, was their own personal cloud—their dream—where they could escape from a society that would judge them for their lifestyle choices. It was also a hippie utopia where they could congregate with others who held similar beliefs and breathe in all of the pleasures marijuana could offer, an idealized world unfettered by government regulation.

Many of the area's residents understood. The rural area of Cass County is peopled with libertarians for whom excessive governmental regulation represents the ultimate invasion of a person's individual freedoms. Their political platform revolves around what they view as an oppressive government overstepping its boundaries. The government has no right to restrict gun ownership. The government has no right to restrict marijuana use. And the government, under no circumstances, never, ever has any right to step on a person's cloud uninvited, much less dictate to a person what he should or should not do on his cloud.

For many area residents, their worst fears about government became actualized in early September 2001, when police surrounded Rainbow Farm. Yet this story polarized the locals, and as a result, two very different versions exist. In the eyes of the law and the prosecutor who led them, the end of Rainbow Farm resulted from a few extremists who had endangered society.

For those who believed that the government has already consumed too much of its citizens' freedoms, the police army, with its armored vehicles and heavily armed soldiers, laid siege to Rainbow Farm to eliminate someone who posed no threat and harmed no one; in this vision, the government forced these two men, Crosslin and Rohm, into a defensive position.

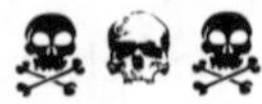

Grover "Tom" Crosslin was not one to allow others to step on his toes, so when the government came to invade his cloud, his response surprised no one.

As a teenager in Elkhart, Indiana, he dropped out of high school in the tenth grade in 1971 and took a job at a local carwash. When his boss shorted his check, he borrowed a friend's gun and retrieved his money at gunpoint, which cost him six months in jail. It would not be the last time Crosslin was involved with the law.

After his brief stint behind bars, he became associated with a biker gang and entered a short-lived marriage, doomed after a few years when he accepted his homosexuality. The lack of a formal education did not hurt him; he began a thriving business renovating old homes. The business evolved into real estate; Crosslin used land contracts to purchase his own properties. At his professional apex, Crosslin owned about twenty properties and had eighty employees. Crosslin had a big heart and a soft spot for hard luck stories; many on his work crews were men with pasts that they either wanted to recover from, escape, or forget.

His social life thrived as well. He often hosted extravagant parties for his work crews at one of his addresses: elaborate and popular social gatherings at which people ate, drank, and smoked marijuana. At some point, the thirty-four-year-old hippie real estate tycoon met Rolland Rohm, a sixteen-year-old with long, blond hair. Rohm seemed to be a younger version of Crosslin. At sixteen, he had already fathered a child and married a woman eight years older. Yet like Crosslin, his marriage had the lifespan of a june bug.

The pair appeared to be the ideal couple. They took long drives through the country and listened to golden oldies from the heyday of Motown. They picked and ate blueberries together. They fell in love.

Crosslin had not yet found his cloud, however, and his libertarian politics appeared in various symbolic gestures. In an early example of extending his middle finger to the local officialdom, he painted a house in vibrant pink and lime green to protest the building code. And the vanity plate on his white Rolls-Royce read "HEMP1."

In 1993, Crosslin's cloud appeared on the horizon about thirty miles to the north of Elkhart. When Crosslin had the opportunity to purchase the thirty-four-acre parcel of rolling land containing both forest and cornfield, he took it. For $35,000, he bought the piece of land that would become infamous as Rainbow Farm.

Their family became complete a year later when Rohm, bankrolled by his partner, won custody of his son, Robert. The three moved into the two-story farmhouse on Crosslin's property and lived as a family unit. Crosslin developed the property into a campground, which he hoped would generate adequate income to support his family.

Rainbow Farm, however, became more than their personal cloud. It became the grandiose vision for what the world could be with legalization of marijuana. Crosslin continued his tradition of throwing elaborate parties for his friends and family, which at Rainbow Farm evolved into major biannual celebrations of individual freedom à la hemp. One music festival, HempAid, took place every Memorial Day and signaled the beginning of the in-season for campers. The other, Roach Roast, took place every Labor Day and signaled the end of the season.

A crew had formed, all bent on living just beyond the grasp of the government, all who in spirit purchased a share in Crosslin's marijuana-friendly, libertarian Disney World. The farm's business manager lived in a white teepee. An event promoter, a carpenter known as "Whoa Boy," and a handyman known as "That Boy" joined the motley cast of regulars. Substitute marijuana for beer, and Tom Crosslin had created his own living version of a *Cheers* community where "everyone knows your name," with Crosslin behind the bar making the decisions.

In the eyes of a pro-hemp libertarian, excessive government regulation had turned the once lush paradise of America into a barren desert. Rainbow Farm represented an oasis of sorts, and many thirsty souls visited it and drank from the well of liberty by consuming marijuana despite the government's prohibition of it. They puffed on joints as they listened to musical acts on the stage. The snacked on hash brownies sold in The Joint—Rainbow Farm's own hemp-friendly café. They purchased souvenirs. They signed petitions for the Personal Responsibility Amendment designed to decriminalize marijuana.

At its apex, the Rainbow Farm campground complex included an annex that cost Crosslin $250,000 to build. The annex contained a coffee shop, a general store, office, laundromat, and showers. Thousands flocked to Crosslin's cloud to listen to bands, party, and smoke marijuana—free, it appeared, from government persecution. They thought nothing of parting with $65 for a three-day pass to stay on Tom Crosslin's cloud.

Rainbow Farm even maintained a Web site that proclaimed the farm's manifesto: "the medical, spiritual, and responsible recreational uses of marijuana for a more sane and compassionate America." Indeed, the festivals allowed Crosslin to give the finger to the government that he believed too often suppressed the liberties of its people. Thousands of middle fingers, actually. Crosslin had moved his civil disobedience from Elkhart to Rainbow Farms and intensified it.

To many, though, he wasn't a villain. Crosslin was a generous man who loved his community, and many in his community in turn loved him. The hippie philanthropist gave hay rides to local kids at Halloween and hosted Easter egg hunts. And his festivals provided a safe place to party.

No one overdosed; no riots ensued. Rainbow Farm maintained its own security detail that kept law and order. The festivals included soft drink stands and legitimate entertainment. Merle Haggard performed, as did Tommy Chong, whose pro-pot stand-up comedy titillated 2,800 people—the largest crowd assembled on Crosslin's cloud.

The festival promoters didn't advocate the use of other drugs, although sometimes the attendees used them anyway. In fact, for Tom Crosslin, the fight to secure individual rights provided the impetus for the festivals; the marijuana simply represented a symbol for that fight. At the major festivals, activists and pro-hemp politicians rallied support with speeches. Crosslin spoke out against the use of drugs other than marijuana. On the Rainbow Farm Web site and posted at its entrance were notices that anyone caught selling drugs would be removed. For years, people visited Rainbow Farm and used marijuana in peace. Crosslin's utopia, it seemed, was just that: a perfect world and a social statement about the decriminalization of marijuana. *High Times*, the pro-marijuana magazine, called Rainbow Farm one of America's best spots in the world to smoke marijuana.[1]

Crosslin's cloud rested on a rather tenuous foundation of legal technicalities. In Michigan, smoking marijuana is a misdemeanor, and police cannot venture onto private property for misdemeanors, which meant that Rainbow Farm was surrounded by an invisible wall that kept law enforcement from crashing the party. If partygoers gathered inside of a house or dwelling collectively to smoke marijuana, the landlord would be guilty of "maintaining a drug house"—a felony and big legal trouble that would likely lead to a police invasion. At Crosslin's campground, though, the partaking of marijuana occurred in open fields.

And until the 2003 passage of a federal law that changed the rules for concert promoters (the Illicit Drug Anti-Proliferation Act), event promoters in Michigan were not responsible for their guests' actions, including the use of illicit drugs. The very legal system that barred marijuana use gave Crosslin a bulletproof vest: virtual immunity from prosecution for marijuana use on his land. Or so it seemed.

Sooner or later the bacchanalian hemp festivals were bound to attract the attention of the local prosecutor, attention about as welcome as a bee at a picnic. Perhaps the scent that attracted the bees came when billboards advertising Rainbow Farm appeared off of a nearby highway.

Cass County prosecutor Scott Teter's politics put him at odds with the libertarians among the people whom he served. Elected in 1996, he established a reputation as a tough conservative when he erected billboards that read, "If your sex partner is under sixteen, they won't be when you get out of prison."[2]

In Teter's professional backyard—his jurisdiction—sat the hemp-friendly oasis. What occurred at the festivals represented the polar opposite of the antidrug stance the prosecutor took during his successful campaign for prosecutor. For the area's libertarians, the prosecutor was the portrait of government oppression. He would become Crosslin's nemesis, his archenemy. He would play Sherlock Holmes to Crosslin's Moriarty. Or the other way around, depending on one's perspective.

The prosecutor, whose passion some locals characterized as zealousness wrapped in legal text, came to believe that the rhetoric about utopia covered up the fact that the festivals had become an illicit pharmacy where one could purchase just about any drug imaginable. And, Teter believed, Tom Crosslin knew it.

In 1996, at Teter's initiation, police set up a sobriety checkpoint on the dirt two-track that was the only road leading to or from Rainbow Farm. They cited intoxicated drivers, which severely hurt Crosslin's festival attendance. The unspoken message sent by this action: the police were watching, looking, even searching for violators. Roach Roast and HempAid had just broken even, but with plummeting numbers willing to cross the invisible line between the law and the utopia beyond, Crosslin began to lose money. Rainbow Farm began a slow bleed and it had only so much lifeblood in the form of capital.

Despite what some characterized as government harassment, however, the festivals continued.

The feud between Crosslin and Teter escalated a few years later. In 1998, Teter sent a letter to Crosslin. In the letter, Teter explained that if undercover agents discovered "hard" drugs on Rainbow Farm, he would seize the property under drug forfeiture laws.

Those were fighting words indeed.

So Crosslin fired back. He penned a letter in which he hurled verbal vitriol at Scott Teter. He issued a threat of his own: "Our friends at the Michigan Militia have their ideas of how we should handle your threats."[3] The Michigan Militia is a paramilitary organization, and although members are officially anti-marijuana, several members had helped with security at Rainbow Farm. Crosslin removed any question of his resolve when he stated that "we [his family] are all prepared to die on this land before we allow it to be stolen from us. How should we be prepared to die? Are you planning to burn us out like they did in Waco, or will you have snipers shoot us through our windows like the Weavers at Ruby Ridge?"[4] This statement would prove eerily prophetic, as though Tom Crosslin had seen his own future. Thomas Paine once said that the tree of liberty must from time to time be watered with the blood of its patriots. Crosslin saw himself as a type of patriot, but would his blood water the soil of Rainbow Farm? The tone of his letter to Scott Teter seemed to suggest that he understood, perhaps even embraced, the possibility.

The letter also suggested that Crosslin would use violence if necessary to protect his cloud. He had turned to violence on one previous occasion. In 1995, he got into a bar fight and served some time in jail for assaulting a tavern patron with a length of PVC pipe.

The game was afoot, the fight under way. The proprietors of Rainbow Farm became engaged in a conflict with area prosecutor Scott Teter. A five-year feud resulted, with Crosslin and Rohm playing the Hatfields to Teter's McCoy. Scott Teter, though, was the real McCoy—a Boy Scout bent on protecting his constituents from what he saw as the evils plied at the thirty-four-acre hemp playground. Although some neighbors characterized Crosslin and Rohm as ideal neighbors, Teter felt that their festivals represented a danger to the community. Despite posted notices warning festival attendees against the sale of drugs, a cadre of undercover officers purchased just about every hard drug imaginable at Crosslin's festivals. They also filmed activity such as drug use occurring in the compound.

In attempts to stop the festivals and the drug use, Teter would fire a shot, usually some legal fine point, but Crosslin would dodge the bullet. For example, Teter tried to shut down Rainbow Farm because Crosslin did not possess the proper license to run a campground. Before he could, though, Crosslin obtained a temporary permit. Each shot weakened Rainbow Farm a little more, and the slow bleed that began with the sobriety checkpoint had threatened the life of Crosslin's experimental utopia. By 2001, he had drained his bank accounts in trying to keep his cloud flying and he took a mortgage on the cloud itself.

The feud would continue like this until the spring of 2001, when it escalated again. An incident occurred that seemed to underline the danger inherent in the festivals and to justify Teter's attempts to stop them from happening. The day after Rainbow Farm held a festival for eight hundred people, in a nearby community a seventeen-year-old died when his car collided with a school bus carrying a high school girls' softball team. A blood test revealed that he had marijuana in his system. He was wearing an entrance bracelet to one of Crosslin's shindigs. Teter had the catalyst, now he needed the justification.

He would find it in the bane of criminals everywhere—the IRS. He learned that Crosslin had allegedly paid his employees "under the table." Teter had finally found the leverage he needed to pry open Rainbow Farm's invisible gate. In May 2001, a group of armed officers searched the farm to find proof of tax violations. During their search, they found 301 marijuana plants and 3 guns (a 9-millimeter pistol and 2 shotguns), which placed Crosslin and Rohm in handcuffs facing several serious charges, including maintaining a drug house and manufacturing marijuana.

Following this discovery, Teter fired a shot that struck at the heart of Crosslin's family. Child protective services took Rohm's son from school and placed him in a foster home. Crushed, Rohm agreed to the criteria established to reunite him with his boy: move out of the farmhouse and attend drug rehabilitation. He tried.

Crosslin's prior convictions placed him in greater legal jeopardy than his partner. He faced a much longer prison term: up to twenty years. The state of Michigan, at Scott Teter's initiation, stood poised to seize the land and take Crosslin's cloud. And the party at Rainbow Farm was finally over; a judge issued an injunction forbidding Crosslin, free on bond, from hosting any marijuana-friendly parties.

Nonetheless, Crosslin threw one last party at the end of August—a small gathering. Little did he know that some of his guests were undercover agents who witnessed both Crosslin and Rohm smoking marijuana. With this violation, Crosslin faced the possibility of a revoked bond and immediate and long-term incarceration. The court ordered Crosslin and Rohm to attend a bond hearing, but neither man attended it.

Instead, Crosslin decided to make his final move; he decided to destroy his cloud. The hearing was scheduled for one-thirty, but

Crosslin had more important business. In a gesture that seemed to say, "If I can't have it, no one will," Crosslin torched the buildings that made up the complex. Every structure except the farmhouse and a few sheds went up in flames that threw jet black smoke into the sky. The billowing clouds, like a smoke signal in an old Western, signaled trouble on the horizon. Perhaps it was also Crosslin's way of giving the finger to Scott Teter and the government he represented.

The burning of Rainbow Farm suggested that Rohm and Crosslin would make their last stand on their property and fight the government to the bitter end on their own turf. "Stay away," they seemed to say, a sentiment punctuated with an exclamation mark when someone on the property fired at a news helicopter from South Bend, Indiana, hovering overhead. The bullet struck the chopper, which retreated and landed; no one was hurt. The bullet came from a .223-caliber rifle and would be a shot heard around the world. The armed revolt had begun.

Someone on Rainbow Farm had sent a powerful message: "Hey, you, get off of my cloud." Crosslin and Rohm repeated the message a few times during the next few days, shooting a volley at a fixed-wing police surveillance plane and showering a state police armored vehicle with lead raindrops.

By this time, county and state police officers had arrived, and the shot fired at the news helicopter would soon bring agents from the Federal Bureau of Investigation. An anonymous tip warned the local and state police that an ambush awaited them, so instead of storming the complex to arrest Crosslin and Rohm, they set up a perimeter around it. By Friday evening, the police force consisted of one hundred and twenty officers and agents including armored vehicles and snipers. Officials from the state and federal departments set up headquarters at an old school in the vicinity.

And so began the "Rainbow Farm standoff," aka the "Rainbow Farm siege," depending on one's perspective. *Siege* implies an assault from an unwelcome force, which, to Crosslin and those who believe the government unjustly strips its citizens of individual liberties, perfectly described the law enforcement army massing on the farm's borders.

The standoff lasted throughout Labor Day weekend. Crosslin and Rohm stayed inside the two-story farmhouse, vigilant of the snipers positioned around their land. They would make their stand as patriots, they believed, as citizens fighting for their rights. For their freedom they would become martyrs if necessary.

Even patriots must eat, however, so in the late afternoon hours, around four o'clock, Crosslin ventured out of the farmhouse. Accompanied by Brandon Peoples, a friend who had sneaked through the ring of police, he traveled down a dirt two-track road to a neighbor's cabin. At the cabin, Crosslin and Peoples gathered supplies including steaks and a Bunn coffeemaker. Some say they stole the provisions, some say the neighbor left the supplies for them—once again, a matter of perspective. But they forgot the coffee pot for the coffeemaker, so they made a second trip to the cabin a little after five o'clock.

They were headed back to the farm when they stopped on Mount This to survey the scene. And then Crosslin saw the silhouettes . . .

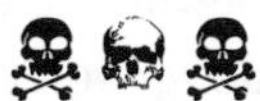

. . . Crosslin raised his Ruger to his shoulder, pointing it at the silhouette lying on the ground about twenty feet away. Two FBI agents then fired their weapons at Crosslin. One .308-caliber bullet struck him in the head while another—from a .233—apparently struck a nearby tree and fragmented, sending shards of hot lead at Crosslin. As a result, Crosslin sustained four bullet wounds, but it only took one: the bullet that struck him at the top right of his forehead, creating a 3/8-inch-diameter hole in his skull where the bullet entered. It exited at the back left side of his head with such force that shards of bone and fragments of the bullet or both strafed Peoples—who was a few yards away when the shooting happened—in the face. The bullet tore a gaping hole in the back of Crosslin's head, and a majority of his brain landed a few feet away. He sustained three other bullet wounds, but as for cause of death, they were superfluous.

In that instant, Tom Crosslin was pushed off of his cloud and he fell to the earth without having fired his weapon. He was dead before he hit the ground. His feud began with Cass County prosecutor Scott Teter, but the FBI ended it.

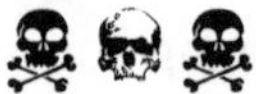

Police arrested and subsequently questioned Peoples before releasing him. An eyewitness—another agent nearby when the shooting occurred—reported Crosslin pointed his weapon at an agent stationed as an observer, and the agent then fired in self-defense—a story Peoples apparently could not confirm. A few yards away and looking at the ground, he heard but perhaps did not see the bullets strike his friend. When the bone and bullet fragments struck him, he believed himself shot and fell to his knees.

Autopsies become the required final chapter in stories ended by law enforcement weapons. In a community of libertarians for whom government agents are inherently suspect, the seige of Rainbow Farm left a wake of accusations about police abuse of power. Some people even suggested that the official version of events did not jibe with the reality, that the facts had been distorted.

During autopsies of gunshot wound victims, the medical examiner will examine the wound track to determine the path of the bullet, which can indicate the positioning of the shooter in relation to the victim. As part of the examination of the wound track, the forensic pathologist may use a long steel rod to gently probe the wound. He must use caution to avoid creating a false track. The probe is often photographed in the wound track for use in court testimony.

Defects on the clothes—the holes created by the bullets—are matched with the wounds to help verify the entrance and exit wounds, the position of the shooter to the victim, and thus the eyewitness account of the incident.

An autopsy cannot determine if Crosslin pointed his weapon at the FBI agent who shot him, but it can help re-create the shooting and either support or refute the eyewitness account of the incident. If the bullet that struck Crosslin entered the back of his head, for example, the shooter would have had to fire from behind him, which would indicate that Crosslin probably did not point his weapon at the officer.

Crosslin arrived at the Kent County Morgue dressed for a fight, wearing camouflage pants, coat, and boots. His left-front coat pocket contained a clip with thirty-nine unspent, full-metal jacket cartridges, evidence of his resolve to protect his cloud.

The powerful .308-caliber weapon used to kill Tom Crosslin left a macabre sight. The bullet that struck him in the forehead left his face and head severely damaged. A huge gaping wound obliterated the exact exit site. Generally, the smaller hole represents the bullet's point of entry—in this case the 3/8-inch in diameter hole in Crosslin's right forehead. The larger hole represents the exit wound. The appearance of the damage on his head leaves little doubt that when he received the wound, Tom Crosslin faced the man who shot him. Unlike his comrade in spirit, Scott Woodring, no one shot Crosslin in the back.

The bullet tore through Crosslin's brain, leaving only the cerebellum and brain stem. A special agent from the FBI brought to the morgue three boxes containing evidence collected at the scene: one box held a cracked pair of dentures, another held a piece of Crosslin's skull, and another held a 450-millimeter mass of brain matter—the remaining portions of the brain, retrieved from the site of the shooting.

Tom Crosslin sustained three other bullet wounds. Two bullet fragments hit the right side of his upper torso: one in his chest just behind his right armpit, and the other two and a half inches below it. Both wound tracks traveled from right to left and from below upward—consistent with the shooter firing his weapon while lying on the ground (according to reports, Crosslin raised his weapon and pointed it at the FBI agents when he spotted one of them on the ground). These wounds are consistent with the scenario that one of the agents fired a round that struck a tree and fragmented, the pieces then hitting Crosslin.

The forensic evidence also supports one other vital element of the eyewitness account. One bullet fragment, its copper jacket recovered from the area of the seventh right rib, would have passed through

Crosslin's right arm just above the elbow if he had been standing with his arms at his sides. But instead of a bullet wound track through it, the arm contained a graze wound, indicating that the bullet portion that struck Crosslin in the right lateral chest area first grazed his arm—an injury consistent with the victim holding his rifle level to shoulder, as the eyewitness described.

An additional wound resulted when a bullet fragment wound up in Crosslin's right hand and further fragmented into seven one- to two-millimeter lead pieces, recovered from the soft tissues.

The autopsy revealed nothing that would contradict the story that Crosslin raised his weapon and the agents fired at him in self-defense.

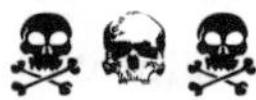

Meanwhile, Rollie Rohm waited at the house for his partner who would never return. Now, he faced the police army alone. He gave his terms: he would surrender the following morning at 7 a.m. if he could see his son, Robert.

Authorities arranged for Robert to visit his father at the house at 7 a.m. the next morning, but he would never complete the trip. The extraordinary saga of Rainbow Farm would not have a mundane ending but an extraordinary, mystifying ending. At approximately six o'clock Tuesday morning, September 4, 2001—just an hour before Rohm planned on surrendering to authorities—an orange glow appeared in the upper window of the house. The glow intensified, and soon flames engulfed the home. Rohm had apparently set fire to the last significant structure on the farm.

According to the official version of events that unfolded that morning, Rohm exited the house a half hour after the flames appeared, dressed in camouflaged garb with his face painted black. He carried a .223-Mini-14 and ignored repeated commands to drop his weapon. Instead, he crouched behind a tree and pointed the gun at an armored vehicle heading toward him. Two men in the vehicle had stuck their heads out in order to see, making them potential targets. To protect these men, two Michigan state police snipers fired at Rohm. One missed, one didn't, sending a bullet through the stock of Rohm's rifle and into his chest, killing him. A second bullet hit Rohm as he fell backward. His requested reunion with his son never occurred. Like Crosslin, he never fired his weapon.

Why would Rohm set the house on fire and exit carrying a weapon? Perhaps he did not want to go to prison. Perhaps he did not want to live the rest of his life without his partner of eleven years. Perhaps he realized that he would not regain custody of Robert. Or perhaps the official version of the story, as some believed, had holes in it. Some speculated that Rohm was about to surrender but overzealous state police officers gunned him down (a version preferred by many Rainbow Farm supporters).

Rohm's autopsy would throw light onto what occurred in his final minutes and provide physical evidence that would either support or contradict eyewitness statements. Like his lover, Rohm came to the morgue dressed in camouflage fatigues. Inside his pants pocket was a cigarette lighter shattered into fragments—an eerie symbol of Rainbow Farm's fiery ending. There were a number of small cuts and abrasions on his left upper thigh that at first sight appeared incongruous to a death by gunshot wound, but the minor mystery of these marks would become clear.

Rohm sustained two gunshot wounds. The fatal bullet struck him just below the left clavicle and tore through the innominate artery, the trachea, and the upper portion of the right lung before exiting in the upper right portion of his back. The bullet entry wound contained no soot or gunpowder residue. If fired from a close distance, execution style, the .308 the sniper used would have left gunpowder residue around the entrance site. The lack of gunpowder indicated that the sniper fired his weapon from a significant distance as reported. This bullet traveled from front to back, from left to right, and from above downward, indicating that the shooter fired at Rohm from in front of him and from an elevated point to his left. In short, the wound supports a scenario in which Rohm was crouched or even lying on the ground when shot in the chest.

A second bullet like the first, fired from a distance as evident from a lack of gunpowder residue around the entrance site, struck Rohm in the left thigh and traveled upward, exiting just below his belly button. This bullet passed through his pants pocket and shattered the cigarette lighter, spiking his upper thigh with shards and causing the irregular pattern of cuts and abrasions on the upper thigh. Like the fatal bullet that passed through his chest, this bullet also struck him in the front and passed from left to right. This bullet, however, traveled upward, indicating that he received the wound while falling backward or that the bullet's trajectory was altered when it struck and subsequently shattered the cigarette lighter.

Like that cigarette lighter, to the south, Crosslin's and Rohm's utopia lay in fragments. And from the pieces left by this tragedy, friends, relatives, and law enforcement would try to assemble some meaning.

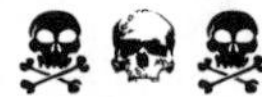

Grover "Tom" Crosslin's funeral took place on September 8 in Elkhart, Indiana. Popular even in death, Crosslin's last festival—his wake—was attended by an audience of five hundred people.

While friends and loved ones mourned the departed, thirty miles to the north, authorities occupied Crosslin's former cloud to study what had happened. They sifted through the remains of the ten buildings, now just burned shells. Even after Tom Crosslin died, the government would not leave Rainbow Farm alone. They surveyed a scene that would make a novelist jealous, a scene loaded with symbolism of Crosslin's life and death and the utopia he attempted to create: the blackened shell of a Volkswagen Beetle rested next to the charred remains of "The Joint"; the faded statement "Let Freedom Ring" painted on the basement wall of the house; protesters a few miles from the site, carrying handmade signs. One read, "They killed him."

In the subsequent months, protesters added to the symbolism by placing various emblems on the land in memory of their fallen comrades: an upside-down American flag and a sign that read, "Wake Up—Who's Next? You?"

The Rainbow Farm story might have received national media attention and become another Waco or Ruby Ridge, but three days after Tom Crosslin's funeral, an even bigger news story trumped all others: the tragedy of September 11, 2001. A surge of patriotism followed in the wake of the terrorist strike on the World Trade Center, and people wanted to rally around the flag, not burn it. In one day antigovernment protests became suddenly very unpopular.

In the following months, the Michigan state police, the US Justice Department, and the Cass County prosecutor reviewed the deaths of Crosslin and Rohm. After a lengthy study of the case, Teter pronounced that the shootings were legally justified homicide. Crosslin pointed his loaded weapon at the FBI agent, who fired in self-defense.

By pointing his rifle at the armed vehicle approaching him, Rohm threatened the two partially exposed officers. The state police sniper who shot him did so to protect them, thus Rohm's death was legally justified under Michigan law. In "defense of others," a killing is legally justified if the shooter reasonably believes that he faces imminent and life-threatening danger and that the killing is necessary to prevent the death of an innocent person.

The Michigan state attorney's office seconded Teter's exoneration of the officers. Despite the official pronunciations, the jury in the court of public opinion remains gridlocked in debate. For many, especially those who already hold a negative opinion of the government and its various entities, these findings came from sources prone to overlook discrepancies and errors. The justifiable homicide explanation did not explain why the two men had to die. The government "murdered" the two otherwise peaceful men, some said, then covered it up.

The two men committed "suicide by police," said others. They chose the manner of their deaths like one might write his own epitaph. They wanted to be left alone, and if the government would not cooperate, they were willing to die on their land, protecting it from what they saw as an invasion. Yet, the drug use at Rainbow Farm posed a threat to the community, both morally and literally, some maintained, citing reports of underage drinking and the tragic death of the seventeen-year-old killed in the collision with a school bus.

These arguments had been reincarnated from similar standoffs in which the government came under heavy fire from critical citizens who believed it overstepped its jurisdiction. Indeed, the deaths of Crosslin and Rohm created a line, and people chose sides.

The legal battle continues as well. Rollie Rohm's parents have filed a wrongful death suit in federal court, claiming that the killing of their twenty-eight-year-old son was anything but justified. The case is pending.

Despite the controversy that still surrounds the deaths of Crosslin and Rohm, one thing remains undisputed: they fought the law and the law won. Perhaps Crosslin and Rohm have now found a new cloud . . . one that no one can invade.

## Notes

1. Bob Fitrakis, "Siege at Rainbow Farm Leaves Two Dead," *Free Press*, October 1, 2001, http://www.freepress.org/journal.php?strFunc=display&strID=96&strJournal=14 (accessed July 20, 2007).

2. Quoted in Dean Kuipers, "Siege at Rainbow Farm," *Playboy*, October 2003. Kuipers's true-crime work, *Burning Rainbow Farm*, provides an exhaustive account of the case. Interested readers who want to know more about the case should consult Kuipers's book.

3. Ibid.

4. Ibid.

# 4. malice domestic

*What, my dear Lady Disdain! Are you yet living?*
—William Shakespeare, *Much Ado about Nothing*

Benedick and Beatrice in Shakespeare's *Much Ado about Nothing* despise each other. They throw verbal darts at each other, move closer, and throw verbal punches. They hate each other. By act five, they have fallen in love with each other. Their verbal sparring matches, though, provide some of the play's most humorous moments.

The feuding couple is an occurrence so common, it has become a staple of the sitcom since the inception of television. Ricky and Lucy Ricardo. Ethel and Fred Mertz. Archie and Edith Bunker. George and Louise Jefferson (the Bunkers' former neighbors before they moved "on up to a deluxe apartment in the sky"). Al and Peg Bundy. Fred and Wilma Flintstone. The Lockhorns (an apropos name for a feuding couple). The contentious relationships of these couples have entertained audiences for years. Audiences roar with laughter as they watch the couples engage in verbal sparring matches. The television reflects reality, often their reality, because like their fictional counterparts, they, too, at one time or another gave to *and* received from their loved ones the verbal equivalents of right hooks and uppercuts. So they know Petruchio and Katharina, Benedick and Beatrice, Archie and Edith Bunker.

Anyone who has enjoyed a romantic relationship understands the frustration that can result from a disagreement, a "honey-do" list, or any number of catalysts to a good whopper of a fight. For some couples, their animosity never escalates beyond extremely loud voices and a few expletives that result in nothing more than a few bruises to the psyche. For others, a good row turns physical, and someone ends up with a black eye. For still others, the dispute turns deadly.

The four cases that follow, each of which contains a unique forensic twist, demonstrate what can happen when someone in a relationship snaps, when verbal blows (real or perceived) turn into physical ones and tragedy results.

## Obsession

Many victims who have sustained massive and fatal head injuries never knew what hit them. Unfortunately, Linda Teeter knew what hit her, although she apparently didn't have time enough to react; her assailant struck so quickly, she apparently never even screamed, silenced by the shock of what was about to happen.

She was lying in bed, watching television when he rushed into the room. She knew him, lived with him, to a certain extent was controlled by him, and she feared him. This evening, her fears became reality, personified in the man standing over her with a baseball bat.

He raised the baseball bat, and with as much force as he could, swung the bat at her head. She held up her hand as if to shield herself from the bat, but the attempt was futile. The bat struck her head with a thud and fractured her skull. He raised the bat again and struck another blow, which sent drops of blood like an inverse rain against the bedroom ceiling, and another blow, while the television drama, oblivious to the real-life tragedy occurring at 220 Susan

Street, continued in the background. Though Linda Teeter lay unconscious and dying on the blood-soaked bedsheets, her killer had not yet finished . . .

The manager of the Meyer Service Station must have received quite a shock when he peered into the Ford Escort parked at the back of the lot and spotted Linda Teeter's body. A 911 call sent police to the scene.

Steven Bauder, Teeter's boyfriend and roommate, became a natural suspect. Bauder had been convicted of criminal sexual conduct against his daughter in the late 1980s and had completed a fifteen-year prison sentence. Five hours after the discovery of Teeter's body, police had taken him into custody.

During an interview, he confessed to murdering Linda Teeter. "Something happened to set me off," he recounted. "Everything just builds up. I was overwhelmed. I don't remember what I did."[1] He told investigators that he struck Teeter with a baseball bat, although he didn't remember if the bat was already in the bedroom or if he carried it into the bedroom (the latter would suggest a degree of premeditation), and he didn't know how many times he'd hit her.

At the trial, Teeter's son, William Shobway, would testify that he had last seen his mother around 9:30 p.m., and about two hours later, at around 11:30 p.m., he heard two "thuds." At the trial, a crime scene investigator would testify that the killer struck Linda Teeter at least three times; in his confession, Steven Bauder stated that he believed he struck Teeter two or possibly three times in a fit of rage motivated by a passion that would become clear only during the testimony of Teeter's friends and coworkers at the trial. Steven Bauder, according to the story he told investigators, had snapped.

The room in which Linda Teeter died provided vital clues about her last moments of life. Crime scene investigators discovered blood spatter evidence on the ceiling. Sergeant Chad Spence, a member of the major crime task force who studied the crime scene, testified at Bauder's trial that blood spatter on the ceiling, which he characterized as "impact stains," occur only after a second hit. The first strike, he explained in court, opens the head, while the second splatters the blood. Sergeant Spence also identified a "cast-off" stain in the blood spatter pattern, which occurs when the assailant draws back the weapon after impact. The blood spatter indicated that Bauder struck Teeter at least twice, and possibly a third time; the "cast-off" stain could have occurred when he drew back the baseball bat for another strike.

Linda Teeter's wounds bled profusely; this was evident in the way blood saturated the mattress, forming small pools that remained at the scene despite the fact that Steven Bauder replaced the blood-soaked linen with clean linen. The mattress contained two separate areas of blood. If Teeter's fatal injuries resulted from the blows of a baseball bat, what created the second area of staining?

While the forensic evidence allowed investigators to reconstruct the first half of the sequence of events that occurred that night, in his confession Bauder completed the second half of the sequence. After he killed Teeter, Bauder carried her body from the bedroom to her Ford Escort and placed it in the backseat. He cleaned the room, removed the blood-soaked bed linen and baseball bat, and left to dispose of the evidence. He discarded the linen in a Dumpster at McDonald's, the baseball bat in another waste receptacle, and left Teeter's body in the backseat of the car that he deposited in the weeds at the back of the Meyer parking lot. He returned to the bedroom in which he murdered Teeter, placed clean sheets over the blood-saturated mattress, and went to sleep. Bauder admitted to his interrogators that he was jealous of Teeter's ex-husband. Teeter apparently wanted to leave Bauder and reconcile with her ex, so the murder may have been Bauder's way of preventing this.

Investigators retrieved the bloody linen from the waste receptacle at the local McDonald's. After a painstaking, two-hour search through a garbage truck, investigators found a baseball bat they believed to be the murder weapon and also a used condom they found in waste near the bat. While tests revealed no DNA on the bat, testing confirmed the presence of Bauder's DNA inside the condom and both Bauder's and Teeter's DNA on its outside.

Yet in his confession, Steven Bauder left out one vital scene in the sequence of events—an action that would explain the second area of blood staining on the mattress—leaving a gap in the scenario that would be explained by anatomical evidence uncovered by the autopsy.

While the crime scene investigators gathered forensic evidence at Linda Teeter's residence, the autopsy being conducted at the Kent County Morgue revealed anatomical evidence of the violent, horrific end to her life. Linda Teeter arrived at the morgue in the state she was discovered in the backseat of her car: in a blood-soaked T-shirt, with her panties rolled down between her legs. Bruises on her hand—a defensive injury in this context—suggested that she held up her hand as if to shield herself from her attacker's baseball bat, which left her skull in pieces. The extent of the fracturing indicated that a tremendous force struck her head; similar damage occurs in pedestrians hit by cars. In fact, the head injuries occurred with such force that skull fragments, driven inward by the force of the blows, bruised and cut her brain, which exhibited bruising on the opposite side. She died as a result of these massive head injuries, the cause of death being craniocerebral trauma.

Another injury suggested the frenzied state of mind of her killer. Her vagina was torn from overstretching; her killer had raped her with some blunt object, the injury consistent with the handle of a baseball bat. The hemorrhaging in the area indicated that Linda Teeter, while unconscious and possibly brain-dead, suffered the injuries to her vagina while still clinically alive. The two distinct areas of bloodstains on the mattress indicate that she bled heavily from the injuries to both her head and vagina—evidence suggesting that she sustained both injuries while alive. This forensic evidence created an ugly picture of what occurred in the bedroom. In a frenzied rage, Linda Teeter's killer battered her with at least two blows from the baseball bat, slid her underwear down, opened her legs, and then raped her with a blunt object, possibly the same bat. Had she been conscious, this would have been an excruciatingly painful injury.

Just over a year later, one of the voices that would help convict Teeter's killer would come from the victim herself, who would testify through a series of statements admitted as evidence and recounted by her friends and coworkers. This testimony portrayed Steven Bauder as a sexual machine with an insatiable appetite and a handful of strange fetishes, such as an obsession with women's panties and feminine hygiene products, and a fierce jealousy of Teeter's ex-husband, with whom Teeter wanted to reconcile after leaving Bauder.

The testimony provided a chronicle of an abusive relationship that ultimately led to the final act of abuse in the bedroom that night. Teeter appeared the ultimate victim of domestic abuse, and Bauder emerged from the testimony as more than a jilted or cuckolded lover who lost his temper in the heat of an impassioned argument; he was a pervert whose sexual obsession with Linda Teeter led to a deadly climax.

Those who knew the couple alleged that Bauder treated Teeter as a sort of sex ATM machine, expecting her to give him sex upon demand, "24–7" as one witness characterized it.[2] If she didn't consent, he forced her.

In the days before Teeter's death, a friend explained during testimony, she appeared frightened and jumpy, like she anticipated that something bad might happen to her: "Any little noise, a car driving by, she would jump out of her skin."[3] According to this witness, Linda Teeter had told her that Bauder would kill her ex-husband if she even talked to him, and that Bauder had threatened her: if he could not have her, no one would. Neither she nor her son, Teeter apparently believed, were safe from Steven Bauder.

A coworker's testimony supported the notion of Bauder's sexual obsession. Linda Teeter went straight home from work because Bauder expected sex the minute she entered the door.

"'If I don't show up, call 911.'" This was one friend's account of what Linda Teeter told her—testimony that underlined the threat the victim perceived from Steven Bauder.[4] This statement, allegedly made by Linda Teeter and relayed after her death by a friend during trial testimony, provided the prosecution with a powerful and convincing piece of rhetoric, so powerful, in fact, that St. Joseph County prosecutor Doug Fisher repeated it during the prosecution's closing argument.

Through these statements, the potential motives underlying the horrific murder of Linda Teeter came into focus. Had she refused to submit to Bauder's demands for sex that night? Or did she tell him that she planned on leaving him and reconciling with her ex-husband, or had he found out some other way and made good on the threat that if he could not have her, no one would?

Emotions at the trial boiled and bubbled over, spilling into and flooding the courtroom. At one point during the trial, Teeter's brother snapped. The forty-five-year-old, David Meints, burst into the courtroom: "Where is that bastard?" he yelled.[5] Courtroom security prevented Meints from approaching Bauder. The jury exited the courtroom in one direction—retreating to the jury room—while Bauder exited in another direction, collapsing as officers escorted him. The scene proved too much for Bauder's elderly mother, who left for a local hospital and returned to the trial later that afternoon.

Meints's outburst would cost him a year in jail, but the cost of the outburst could have been much higher. Defense attorney Paul Stutesman requested a mistrial, but questioning of the jury about the effect of the incident convinced Judge James Noecker that the incident would not prejudice their deliberations or decisions, so he denied the motion. The trial would continue. The incident, though, would become an issue at an appeal of Bauder's conviction.

Bauder's defense admitted he was obsessed with Linda Teeter and had killed her, but that he did not premeditate or plan the murder in advance; instead, he snapped. The prosecution argued that Steven Bauder's actions suggested otherwise: he planned to kill Linda Teeter. He struck her not just once, but at least twice, and then inflicted an injury difficult to explain as a heat-of-the-moment action: he violated her with the baseball bat. He also disposed of evidence: the blood-soaked bed linen, the baseball bat, Teeter's body. And he returned to the bedroom and went to sleep in the same bed on which he murdered her. A remorseful killer who lost his temper and snapped, Fisher noted to the jury in his closing argument, would most likely have struck just once and at some point realized what he had done and called 911.

After eleven hours of deliberation, the jury returned their verdict: guilty on all counts charged, including second-degree murder, felony murder, and first-degree criminal sexual conduct. The trial court dismissed the second-degree murder conviction and sentenced Bauder to life in prison for the felony murder charge. It looked like Steven Bauder would spend the rest of his life in a cell.

Then came his appeal, which he based on two items he felt prevented him from receiving a fair trial: the outburst from Linda Teeter's brother, and the hearsay statements of Linda Teeter as recounted in court by her friends and acquaintances. Like the voice of a spirit at a séance, Linda Teeter had spoken at her own murder trial through her friends and coworkers, it appeared, because she could speak in no other way. Yet without Linda Teeter to confirm or answer for these statements, did they have any evidentiary value? Or worse, did they prejudice the jury and taint its decision, denying Steven Bauder a fair trial, as he claimed in his appeal?

A voice from the victim presented at trial is not a unique occurrence. In *Cause of Death: Forensic Files of a Medical Examiner*, we discussed the case of Sandra Duyst. Her death initially appeared to be a suicide, but when upon autopsy two entrance wounds were discovered, the police investigated it as a murder. During the investigation, a note (which testing confirmed as authentic) written by Sandra Duyst more than a year before her murder stated, "If anything has happened to me look first to David Duyst, Sr. . . . He could be my killer. I would never commit suicide. He may have killed me."[6] A jury convicted her husband, David Duyst, of her murder. While David Duyst maintains that Sandra's suicide and the note created an intentional frame and placed his picture, as a murderer, inside of it, the note provided a key piece of evidence that helped to convince the jury of his guilt.

The trial court had addressed the issue of Teeter's hearsay evidence. Before the murder trial began, the court ruled that the value of the hearsay statements outweighed any possible prejudice they potentially caused. The State of Michigan Court of Appeals agreed with the trial court's decision. The trial court admitted the hearsay statements "for the proper purposes of proving the victim's state of mind, specifically showing domestic discord, and, indirectly, for evidence of motive for murder."[7] The appeals court decision reads like a succinct summary of the case: "She had said she was fearful of defendant, that defendant had threatened to kill her, her son, and her ex-husband, that she was tired of defendant's incessant demands for all kinds of sex and defendant's forcing sex if she refused, that she wanted to end her relationship with defendant and reconcile with her ex-husband, that defendant was jealous of her ex-husband, and that defendant stalked and beat her."[8]

The statements about Bauder's sexual fetishes, the appeals court decided, did not create an unfair trial because they did not alter or affect the outcome. Too much other evidence proved beyond a reasonable doubt that Steven Bauder murdered Linda Teeter. And the court also rejected the appeal that Meints's outburst prejudiced the jury and created an unfair trial.

Steven Bauder will spend the rest of his life in prison, convicted in part by the statements his victim made in the year before her murder. Perhaps he will be haunted by that moment when his obsession turned homicidal; perhaps his mind will replay those final moments in Linda Teeter's life: the expression on her face . . . the look in her eyes . . . the sound of the bat striking her . . .

. . . or perhaps *he* will become someone's obsession . . .

. . . and justice will be hers.

## Notes

1. Quoted in Corky Emrick, "Outburst Lands Victim's Brother in Jail; Jury Hears Taped Confession," *Sturgis Journal*, March 19, 2004, http://www.sturgisjournal.com/print.asp?ArticleID=15857&SectionID=2&SubSectionID=65 (accessed May 11, 2006).

2. Ibid., "Victim's Friends Testify," *Sturgis Journal*, March 18, 2004, http://www.sturgisjournal.com/print.asp?ArticleID=15844&SectionID=2&SubSectionID=65 (accessed May 11, 2006).

3. Quoted in ibid.

4. Quoted in ibid., "Jury Deliberation Begins," *Sturgis Journal*, March 25, 2004, http://www.sturgisjournal.com/print.asp?ArticleID=15891&Section ID=2&SubSectionID=65 (accessed May 11, 2006).

5. Quoted in Emrick, "Outburst Lands Victim's Brother in Jail."

6. Quoted in Doug Guthrie, "'My Life Is Over,' Shooting Victim's Message Says; Jurors Hear Sandra Duyst's Voice Mail Message, Telling Her Husband to 'Enjoy Your Life,'" *Grand Rapids Press*, March 9, 2001. For a detailed discussion of the Duyst case, interested readers should consult *Cause of Death: Forensic Files of a Medical Examiner*, by Stephen D. Cohle and Tobin T. Buhk (Amherst, NY: Prometheus Books, 2007).

7. *People v. Bauder*, 269 Mich. App. 174 (2005).

8. Ibid.

## "It's Not a Weapon; It's a Tea Mug!"

At his trial, Charles Lange did not deny that he repeatedly struck his wife on the head with a glass mug. He did not deny that he caused the head injuries that led to his wife's death. He maintained, however, that when his wife informed him of her alleged marital infidelity, she provoked a passion in him that forced his actions. In short, he believed, he was guilty of voluntary manslaughter and not second-degree murder. And as surprising as it may seem, he did not believe, in the context of his attack on his wife and in the context of Michigan's sentencing guidelines, that the glass mug constituted a weapon. At the appeal he also raised the question of whether medical malpractice may have ended his wife's life.

On August 20, 1999, Charles Lange struck Georgia Lange a fatal blow with a glass mug, then made a phone call. Actually, he struck her six times, his attack leaving her skull shattered. Unlike Steven Bauder, who hid evidence by discarding it, Lange called 911 twice and alerted authorities, who arrived at the Lange residence a few minutes later. Charles Lange admitted to striking his wife in the head with a glass object.

At the scene, they found Georgia Lange in a coma and the apparent murder weapon—a bloodstained glass mug. She appeared to be the victim of a frenzied attack and was battered beyond recognition.

Mrs. Lange was transported to Spectrum Hospital in Grand Rapids, where, after periods of periodic consciousness, she would die two weeks later, on September 3, 1999. Georgia Lange: deceased at forty-nine years old.

Charles Lange alleged that the incident occurred after his wife told him that she had been involved in an extramarital affair. According to Lange, he snapped and attacked his wife, beating her and slamming the glass mug into her head, causing extensive injuries evident in the autopsy conducted in the Kent County Morgue.

If she had told him of a marital infidelity—an accusation that remains without substantiation—the admission would have just ignited a fire that had been stoking for some time. By the time of Georgia Lange's death, the Lange's once happy marriage of thirty years had all but dissolved. More likely, the conversation that turned fatal for Georgia centered on an impending separation.

Charles Lange, though, apparently could not accept the split. The physical blows that ended his wife's life represented the latest manifestation of what seemed to be a growing hostility. Testimony at the subsequent trial revealed that following an argument, while Georgia was at work, Lange left her a surprise and perhaps a message. He glued dishes together. He cut up her clothes. He slashed her couch with a knife. He even flushed her jewelry down the toilet.[1]

Some men eager to reconcile with their lost loves attempt to purchase forgiveness with dozens of roses. Others, designer clothes or accessories like Gucci handbags. Still others, expensive jewelry, such as a diamond "upgrade." And some just apologize. Perhaps Lange tried all of these. Perhaps he tried none of them.

Whatever the case, some element of their conversation ignited the fire and burned Georgia Lange—perhaps it was the realization that a reconciliation would not occur, that the marriage, to which Charles had contributed for thirty years, was bankrupt. The victim's head showed evidence of the ferocity of Charles Lange's attack. Georgia Lange sustained no fewer than three skull fractures that resulted from six blows with a blunt, heavy object: the glass mug.

Two blows to the top of the head resulted in depressed skull fractures, or fractures that occur when portions of the skull are driven inward by the tremendous force of a heavy object brought down with all the strength an adult can muster. Georgia Lange also sustained other fractures that indicated the frenzied nature of the attack: a comminuted (pulverized) nasal fracture and a fracture to the right orbit (eye socket), as well as cuts on her inner lips and chin. The attack occurred with enough force to crack Mrs. Lange's upper dentures, loosen three of her teeth, and knock out one of them, which was found in her stomach—she had swallowed it.

Charles Lange would have faced an attempted murder charge, but Georgia Lange succumbed to the wounds her husband had inflicted on her. Just after arriving at the courthouse for the preliminary hearing on the attempted murder charge pending against him, Charles Lange learned that his wife had died. Now, he faced murder charges. He admitted to striking Georgia with a glass object, and if her death resulted from the blows to her head, he had caused her death.

At the subsequent trial, the prosecution depicted Lange as a man obsessed with his soon-to-be ex. Georgia Lange, the object of her estranged husband's obsession, paid the ultimate cost.

Charles Lange's defense depicted him as a wounded man who would do anything, anything, to reconcile with his wife. Clearly, the impending doom of a failed marriage had bothered Charles Lange, who tried to end his life with a handful of prescription pain pills while living with a daughter in Virginia a few weeks before the attack. He appeared desperate to save the marriage, and even attempted to use his children as marriage counselors; he asked them to call their mother and plead his case. When the attack occurred, Lange told one of his children, he was visiting his wife in one last attempt to save the marriage.[2] When Georgia told him, as his defense alleged, that she had been cheating on him, he just snapped, just lost it, and in an uncontrollable fit of rage grabbed a glass mug filled with tea and hammered at the thing he loved most.

The forensic evidence, the prosecution argued, did not jibe with the "he just snapped" defense that Lange gave in to an uncontrollable rage. Georgia Lange's injuries did not suggest a lack of control. He did not grab her arm and throw her across the room after sinking his fist into her stomach. He did not slap her repeatedly before throttling her with his belt. He struck Georgia six times, all on her head. The prosecution argued that the lack of randomness in her injuries suggested *controlled* rage.

Lange's defense also argued that the second-degree murder charge did not fit the elements of the crime. According to Lange, his wife admitted to having an affair; his wife's admission of marital infidelity was like pouring gasoline on a fire that had already begun with their conversation and ignited a rage that led to the murder. In other words, the admission provoked his response.

For a second-degree murder under Michigan law to have occurred, evidence of four criteria must exist: "(1) a death, (2) caused by an act of the defendant, (3) with malice, and (4) without justification or excuse."[3] If Georgia Lange's alleged admission provoked Lange, the defense argued, the proper charge would be manslaughter, not murder, and a much shorter sentence.

In fact, of these four elements, the only one not challenged during the trial and subsequent appeals was that Georgia Lange's death occurred.

As for cause of death, some evidence did exist to suggest that accumulated secretions in her airway could have led to asphyxia and death. This cause of death would have resulted from negligence at the hospital and not from Charles Lange. This possibility raised an interesting question: did Mrs. Lange's death result from gross medical negligence? The evidence of massive blunt force trauma to her head, though, indicated that Mrs. Lange most likely died as a direct result of the blows to her head, blows Charles Lange by his own admission inflicted on his unsuspecting wife. And the defense offered no evidence or arguments regarding gross medical negligence other than to raise the possibility of this cause of death. In fact, in both the opening and closing arguments, the defense admitted that Lange was guilty of voluntary manslaughter. Therefore, the first two criteria of Michigan's legal definition for second-degree murder applied.

As for the third criterion, the additional injuries, such as the fractures to her nose and eye socket, indicate the presence of malice. The jury, then, had to determine if the prosecution proved criterion number four. During the trial, Lange's defense admitted that his attack on his wife was not accidental but argued that he had justification: her alleged admission of an affair provoked the attack.

The jury did not buy this excuse. The defense could not substantiate this alleged affair, and even if it could, the mention of an affair would not justify murder. Nothing would. The jury found him guilty of second-degree murder. After listening to Lange's daughter, who requested that her father be given a maximum sentence, the trial judge initially sentenced Lange to between fourteen and thirty years in prison for the murder of his wife. After correcting an error in calculation, the judge reduced Lange's sentence to twelve to thirty years.

Lange appealed to the State of Michigan Court of Appeals, which reviewed the case and delivered its decision on May 10, 2002. Lange argued that the prosecution failed to prove the elements necessary for second-degree murder, but the court rejected this argument.

Lange also argued that the trial court made a sentencing error based on the notion of "weapon." Michigan common law establishes sentencing guidelines. The more points scored, the longer the sentence issued.

> (1) Offense variable 1 is aggravated use of a weapon. Score offense variable 1 by determining which of the following apply and by assigning the number of points attributable to the one that has the highest number of points:
>
> (a) A firearm was discharged at or toward a human being or a victim was cut or stabbed with a knife or other cutting or stabbing weapon . . . 25 points

(b) A firearm was pointed at or toward a victim or the victim had a reasonable apprehension of an immediate battery when threatened with a knife or other cutting or stabbing weapon . . . 15 points

(c) The victim was touched by any other type of weapon . . . 10 points

(d) A weapon was displayed or implied . . . 5 points

(e) No aggravated use of a weapon occurred . . . 0 points[4]

Lange argued that while he used the glass mug as a weapon, no evidence existed to indicate that he planned to use the mug as a weapon, therefore the trial court erred when it assessed him ten points.

The appeals court also rejected this argument. A person can convert just about anything into a weapon with the use of deadly force. Everyday household objects—a screwdriver, a lamp, a dinner plate, even a shoe—can become weapons despite the fact that they were never intended to be used as such. While he may never have intended to murder his wife that morning, that glass mug became as deadly a weapon as a .44-Magnum or a hunting knife. Its use as a weapon earned Charles Lange twelve to thirty in prison.

Yet with that glass mug, Charles Lange delivered his wife's death sentence.

## Notes

1. Jennifer Ackerman-Haywood, "Wife Dies, and Now the Charge Is Murder," *Grand Rapids Press*, September 4, 1999; Tanda Gmiter, "Husband Found Guilty of Beating Wife to Death," *Grand Rapids Press*, January 28, 2000.

2. Tanda Gmiter, "Husband Found Guilty of Beating Wife to Death," *Grand Rapids Press*, January 28, 2000.

3. *People v. Lange*, 251 Mich. App. 247; 650 N.W. 2d 691 (2002).

4. Quoted in ibid.

## A Slap in the Face

Like Charles Lange, Greg Datema most likely never intended to kill his wife, Pamela. Like Lange, something, some piece of conversation triggered a reaction; he snapped and delivered an inadvertent death-blow to his wife. The comparison, though, ends here. Lange's attack on his wife, a frenzied barrage of blows with a weapon in the form of a glass mug, indicates that while perhaps he did not intend to kill his wife—that her death resulted from a frenzied attack that went too far—he did intend to harm his wife with significant bodily injury . . . in short, with malice.

Greg Datema didn't attack his wife in a frenzy; he didn't jab her in the chest with a screwdriver, or batter her with a baseball bat, or smash a beer bottle over her head. He slapped her. Once. Just once, but once with all the force needed to kill her. Her death resulted, oddly, in the form of a slap in the face . . .

December in Michigan is a cold month characterized by overcast skies and periodic outbursts of freezing rain, sleet, ice, and snow. Under the gray skies, families color the holidays with blinking lights running along roof awnings and around evergreen pine trees and presents are stacked under Christmas trees. A Currier and Ives image on a postcard.

On December 21, 1988, three days from Christmas, desperate shoppers descended on the area's shops and malls to procure last-minute presents, while others huddled inside to celebrate the holidays and recharge before facing months of frigid temperatures and rain frozen into various forms. It is a time for families and friends to mingle.

The Datema residence seemed the picture of domestic bliss from the outside. Thirty-one-year-old Pamela had four children—two from a previous marriage and two with her present husband, Greg. The blinking lights on a Christmas tree in the front window of their duplex signaled the approaching holidays, although a warm spell would leave the area uncovered by snow. Yet inside this home, the image of tranquility that characterizes the early morning hours would be shattered with the sound of a slap.

The Datemas's and a few friends' revels extended into the early morning hours of December 22, their socializing lubricated with alcohol and marijuana. With their inhibitions removed, conversation turned to a topic that lovers often wonder about but rarely discuss: past romantic liaisons. The Datemas's conversation took on a form of verbal sparring. The figurative temperature grew with each statement until the cauldron of passions spilled over to physical violence.

Pamela Datema leveled a devastating verbal blow: she told Greg that she had slept with other men in front of Greg's children. With this verbal slap, Greg Datema reeled back, his face stinging. As Pamela began to rise from her chair, he returned her figurative slap with a literal one. The openhanded blow knocked Pamela Datema back; she slumped back into the leather chair and yelled at her husband, telling him that she wished he would leave and not return. She then slid from the chair to the floor, unconscious.

The three eyewitnesses present believed that Pamela had simply consumed too much alcohol and passed out. After five or ten minutes, they tried to revive her, but she would not awaken. An ambulance would arrive shortly after their call, but Pamela Datema would never come to. When they arrived at the duplex, police would find her on the floor where she fell at approximately 4:30 a.m., and a little over an hour later, she would be pronounced dead.

What force or forces killed Pamela Datema? As the others present would report, Greg slapped her and nothing more. Perhaps she had consumed one drink too many and died of an ethanol overdose. At the time of this writing, the legal blood-alcohol limit for driving a car is 0.08 percent, or 80 milligrams per deciliter. In a person of approximately 154 pounds or 79 kilograms, a mixed drink or a beer would raise the blood-alcohol level by 15 milligrams per deciliter, so five to six drinks would make a person mildly intoxicated.

At the time of her death, Pamela Datema's blood-alcohol level was 0.03 to 0.05 percent—not enough to prohibit her from driving a car and not enough to have killed her. As a forensic rule of thumb, a blood-alcohol level of 400 milligrams per deciliter is needed for an ethanol overdose to occur. She also consumed marijuana the night she died, but the combination of alcohol and marijuana did not lead to her death, either. So the question remained: what killed Pamela Datema?

The autopsy would reveal a shocking revelation: she died as a result of a torn artery in her brain. Although those present would later testify that Greg Datema delivered the deathblow with an open hand and without a maximum amount of force, in order for him to hit her hard enough to burst a blood vessel, the hit must have been powerful. Such an injury would likely occur only as the result of a blow administered with all of one's might.

Another factor may have led to the tear in the artery: the consumption of alcohol and marijuana. When struck, a person's reflexes usually lead to a stiffening of the neck muscles—a reaction that lessens the possibility of serious injury. The consumption of substances like alcohol and marijuana relaxes the reflexes. When struck, a person under the influence of these substances might not react as quickly, and a hit, in this case a slap, could lead to a torn artery.

The physical dynamic would occur something like this: the slap to the face led to a violent turning of the head to one side, which led to the stretching and tearing of one of the paired arteries arising from the cord traveling through the cervical spine to the brain stem.

Such a cause of death, however, is as rare as a blue diamond. Rarer. Every day of the week, people receive harder blows than the one that killed Pamela Datema and escape without injury.

In fact, Greg Datema had allegedly administered blows harder than the slap. At some point, Pamela Datema had had enough. Six years after their marriage, she filed for divorce. The court records establish a chronicle of alleged abuse that began years before Pamela's untimely death. The documents state that Datema's violent temper would lead to incidents in which he punched and kicked his wife.

One severe beating allegedly occurred just short of a year before Pamela's death, in February 1987. During the incident, Pamela claimed, Greg punched her in the face before throwing her to the ground and trouncing her in the head with the heel of his boot. The incident led to facial contusions and the need for stitches. When Pamela's daughter from her previous marriage yelled at Greg to stop, he allegedly chased her upstairs and punched her.[1] This, according to Pamela Datema, was not a singular instance.

A few years earlier, the court documents allege, in separate incidents Greg broke Pamela's nose and in a rage set their apartment on fire.[2] The allegations in the court documents portray Greg Datema as a man prone to violent outbursts, prone to snap occasionally. The volatile couple, though, had apparently reconciled and planned to spend the holidays together. Now, ironically, he would face a jury for an incident less violent than those his wife had previously accused him of and for which he escaped punishment.

A jury convicted Greg Datema of involuntary manslaughter, but his prison stay would not be a short one. A previous felony for malicious destruction of property would extend his sentence: he received seven to twenty-two and a half years in prison. For a slap . . .

Datema would argue in his appeal that the slap he delivered that morning lacked gross negligence or recklessness and therefore did not fall into the category of involuntary manslaughter. His appeal would reach the State of Michigan Court of Appeals, but they would not agree. The forensic evidence suggested that Greg Datema struck his wife with all of his force, and when such a blow leads to a person's death, the court reasoned, the proper charge is manslaughter and not assault.

With this finding, the court delivered a slap of its own, the sting of which Greg Datema would feel for a long time.

For seven to twenty-two and a half years, to be precise.

## Notes

1. John Hogan, "History of Abuse Preceded Killing; Husband Sought," *Grand Rapids Press*, December 23, 1988.

2. Ibid.

## Punch Drunk

When she arrived at the Kent County Morgue six days after she died, Debra Barth looked like she went twelve rounds with a heavyweight . . . or like something else had happened.

Barth was last seen alive on September 14, 2000, during a night of partying with her live-in boyfriend. Supposedly everyone knows everyone's business in a small town, and if this is indeed true, then the notion that Debra Barth left town and all of the strings that tied her to the tiny rural community of Frankfurt, Michigan, including two children, without anyone noticing would seem strange indeed. She would have informed friends and relatives, or someone would have seen her packing.

Michael Salagovich, a friend of the couple, became concerned when he had not seen Barth for several days after September 14, when both she and her boyfriend, Brian Slade, had been drunk at his residence. Concerned, five days after he last saw her alive, Salagovich notified police about the disappearance. Members of Barth's family, who could not reach her by telephone to tell her of her older brother's death (he died the day after her disappearance), also notified authorities.

Salagovich had good reason for concern. He testified that when he last saw Barth and Slade together, Slade had become rather "physical with Debbie," repeatedly poking her in her head.[1] He also heard Barth state, according to Salagovich's recollection in court, "Get your hands off my neck and leave me alone, keep your hands off me."[2] This exchange characterized their relationship, which tended to be violent. Salagovich had witnessed fights between the contentious couple and, as he would later testify, even called the police about fights between them. Perhaps Barth did leave town, finally breaking with Slade. Earlier on the fourteenth, according to Salagovich, she told him that she had packed her possessions. She was ready to leave.[3]

No one, though, knew where Barth had gone.

No one had seen Brian Slade, either, although as the last person to see Debra Barth alive, Slade could perhaps provide vital information as to her whereabouts. But his disappearance led to suspicion.

Another factor caused suspicion to fall on Brian Slade and motivated investigators to find and question him about the night of the fourteenth and his missing lover: a history of arrests and convictions including a prison term for domestic violence. Slade's résumé of legal troubles began at the age of eighteen with a conviction for assault and battery and continued in 1984 with the first of three drunk driving convictions, followed by three more convictions for driving with a suspended license and an additional conviction for possession of marijuana.

In January 1996, Slade was convicted for assaulting his girlfriend (the mother of his two children) and spent three months in jail. As part of his sentence, Slade had to attend a counseling program for men hosted by the Women's Resource Center—a program teaching men how to avoid violent conflict.

Slade didn't take notes apparently, as he would return to the program two more times as a result of two more convictions: another conviction for assaulting his girlfriend (in September 1996), and a third conviction for stalking. Charged with aggravated stalking, Slade faced up to five years in prison but avoided that fate by pleading guilty to misdemeanor stalking, which would send him to jail for a year.

The year did not cool Slade's hot temper; his troubles would continue in 1997 with a charge of fourth-degree child abuse for allegedly striking his son with enough force to cause extensive bruising on his face and body. The police report details the particulars of the case, including the son's statement that Slade slapped him several times for crying. Slade offered the police a different version: he admitted to slapping the boy only after the boy bit his sister. The bruises? The result of rough play.

The rough play, though, would continue. Court documents chronicle a terrifying incident. In violation of a personal protection order that forbade Slade from calling or visiting his now ex-girlfriend, he allegedly called her several times one morning, demanding to see his children. In addition, Slade allegedly threatened to kill her. He waited at her house until she returned with her children and refused to leave. When police arrived, he jumped out a window and ran away.

In fact, local police were well acquainted with Slade and the volatile nature of his relationship with Barth. They visited Barth's home on two separate occasions a year before her death. After one particularly nasty squabble between Barth and Slade, they arrested both of them and Barth's adult daughter. Police photographs show various bruises and bite marks on Slade's face and neck indicating that their squabble had escalated to physical violence. No charges, though, followed these incidents.

Benzie County sheriff's deputies arrived at Barth's home with a search warrant and discovered evidence in the form of blood spatter in the kitchen and bedroom that indicated something awful had occurred to the home's missing occupant. They did not, however, find Debra Barth. The next morning, crime scene investigators from the Michigan state police arrived to process evidence at the scene and discovered, buried under boxes and insulation in the basement, Debra Barth's body.

The external damage done to her body gave mute testimony to a frenzied physical struggle that had occurred before her death. Numerous scrapes and bruises covered her body like faded purple polka dots and indicated that her demise came after a violent struggle. She sustained blunt force trauma to the right side of her head. In some autopsies, the cause of death lies hidden, like a marble that rolls to the back of the closet, only to become evident after a toxicology screen or a close examination of tissue under a microscope. Not in this case. Barth's cause of death would present itself after the first cut of the autopsy procedure.

The Y-incision would reveal the massive internal injuries that accompanied the external ones and establish just how violent a struggle Barth experienced before she gasped her last breath. Her ribs had been broken in thirty places, and all of her ribs except one had been fractured in the front and on both sides. This damage to her ribs occurred while she was alive—the result of repeated instances of blunt force trauma.

Such extensive rib injuries sometimes occur in accidents

involving sudden and massive force, like car accidents, but seldom appear as the result of murders. To have inflicted these injuries, Barth's attacker would have to have generated a tremendous amount of force. While these injuries could have resulted from punches, the assailant would have had to punch with the force of a professional boxer to inflict the rib injuries that led to Barth's death. More likely, her assailant kicked or trounced her while she lay on the ground. Either case would lead to the same result: the fractured ribs, several of which punctured her lungs, impeded her breathing, and she suffocated—a horrifically painful death.

The forensic evidence played a key role in determining the fate of Barth's killer, who would face a second-degree murder charge and possible life in prison instead of a manslaughter charge of ten to fifteen years.

Two days after discovering Barth's body, police tracked down Brian Slade and arrested him in a convenience store. He told two stories about Debra Barth's disappearance. First he told police that he drove her to Traverse City, from where she would travel to a powwow held in Michigan's Upper Peninsula (Barth was a member of the Chippewa Indian Tribe of Sault St. Marie). During the interview, Brian Slade began to cry, which left police doubting his first version of the story. During subsequent questioning, he told a much different version.

According to this version of the story, after a round of arguing with Barth, he went to sleep, and when he awoke around 4 a.m., he found himself in bed next to Barth, who was dead. He told his interrogators that he knew nothing of Barth's death, but after attempting to resuscitate her with CPR, he panicked. Fearing that police would blame him for her death, he dragged her to the basement where he concealed her body. In a later interview, he would amend this story. The night before Barth's death, he obtained the narcotic Stadol—a painkiller—from a friend. He had consumed a combination of Stadol and alcohol that night. He and Barth argued, and he fell into a drug- and alcohol-induced stupor. The drugs and alcohol made him so drunk, he didn't know or remember what had happened before he came to.

So why didn't you call for help? one of the officers asked. Slade said that he thought the phone in the house had been disconnected. He left the residence and traveled to a nearby store, where he used Barth's checking account to purchase cigarettes. In the period between the morning he discovered his girlfriend's body and his arrest, Slade drove to various places in Barth's car, including Detroit. One witness at the murder trial testified that Slade appeared at her cottage on the morning of September 15 and that she noticed bruises on his arms.

The presence of the bruises suggested that at some recent time, Slade was involved in a physical altercation. While one could pair these injuries with the scuffs on Barth's body and conclude they came from the struggle that resulted in Debra Barth's murder, the conclusion would be premature, given the violence that characterized their relationship.

Approximately a year after Debra Barth disappeared, Brian Slade would face a jury on second-degree murder charges. During the trial, a parade of witnesses for both the prosecution and the defense would testify about the volatile, often violent nature of the couple's relationship. Both, it appeared, would fall into the category of mean drunks—people who, under the influence of alcohol, tend to become violent, flying into bursts of rage that result in arguments that escalate from arguing to shouting to striking.

Debra Barth, it appeared, had a bit of a Jekyll and Hyde personality, and drinking brought out the Hyde, as witnesses for the defense testified. One witness after another told stories of Barth's penchant for violent outbursts and excessive use of alcohol. Slade's sister Tawny testified that Barth drank "constantly" and she witnessed Barth hit her brother. Another witness—a neighbor—corroborated with an anecdote: once when Brian Slade complimented Barth's daughter on her singing ability, Barth without provocation punched him.[4]

Fellow victims of Barth's wrath also testified. An ex-boyfriend told of an incident when she hit him on the head with an iron skillet. Her former husband explained that during their seven-year marriage, he witnessed her become violent after imbibing. He recounted an incident when, during a heated argument, Barth cut his back with a knife.

**NOTE TO THE READER: Michigan law prevents the display of autopsy photographs identifying specific victims by name or by physical features. In accordance with law and in the interest of good taste, the authors selected photographs that illustrate the types of injuries described in the text but that are not necessarily from the victims discussed in the text.**

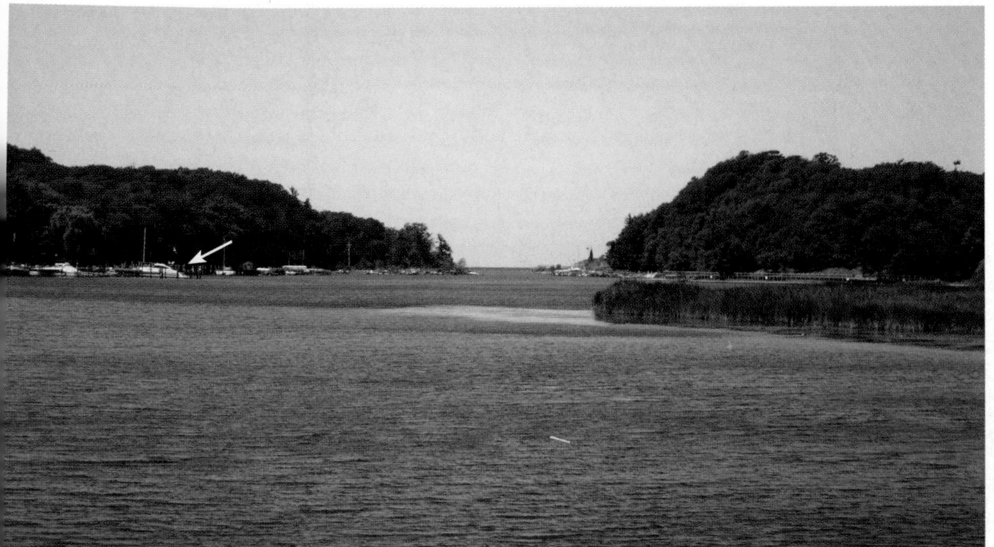

Pigeon Lake, looking west toward Lake Michigan. How did "Jane" get into this lake? Arrow represents approximate location where Jane Doe's body was found. The channel leading to Lake Michigan appears in the center of the photograph. The Consumers Energy plant is to the right, across Pigeon Lake from where the body was discovered (see "The Sea Shall Give Up Her Dead"). *Image courtesy of Tobin T. Buhk.*

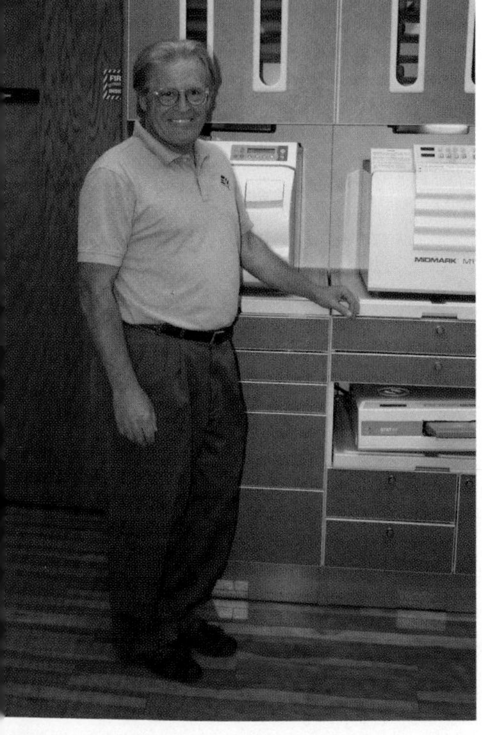


Forensic dental consultant Dr. Roger Erbaugh in his dental laboratory. Forensic dentists play a vital role in identifying victims (see "The Sea Shall Give Up Her Dead"). *Image courtesy of Tobin T. Buhk.*

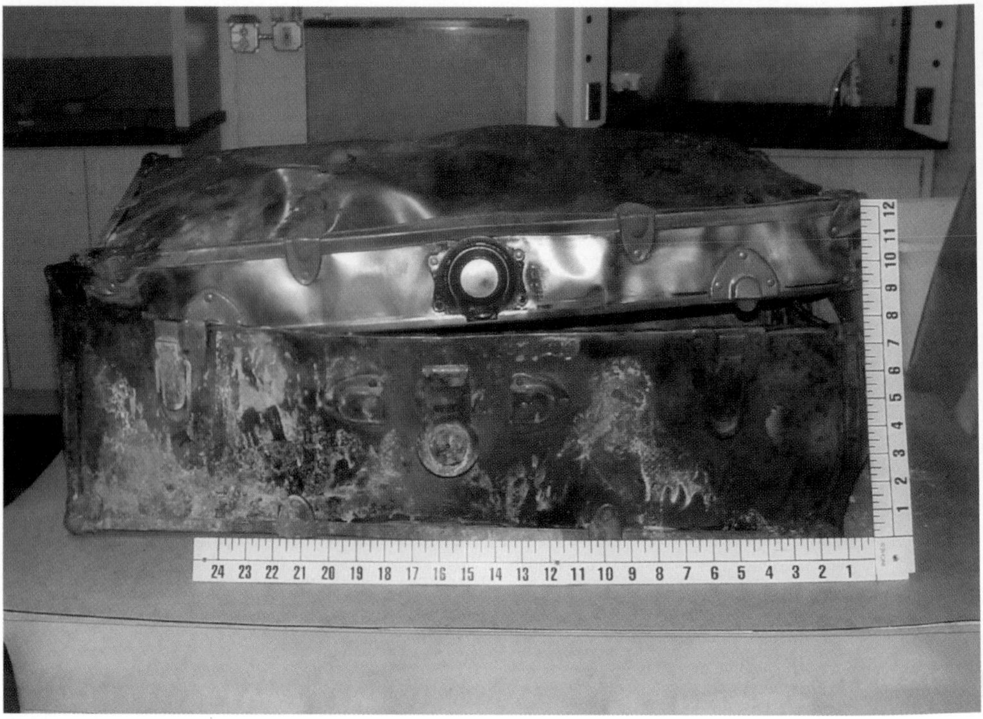

The box from the "Jack in the Box" case. Investigators would find the charred remains of "Jack" inside (see "No Tombstone for 'Jack': An Untitled Story in Five Acts"). *Image courtesy of Ottawa County Sheriff's Office.*

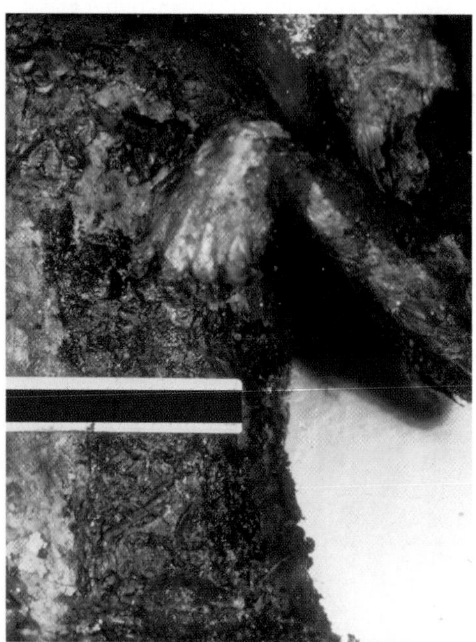

The charred remains of a victim whose killer tried to conceal his crime with fire. Note the victim's posture: when a body burns, the muscles of the arms shorten and contract, creating a pose reminiscent of a boxer. *Image courtesy of Stephen D. Cohle, MD.*

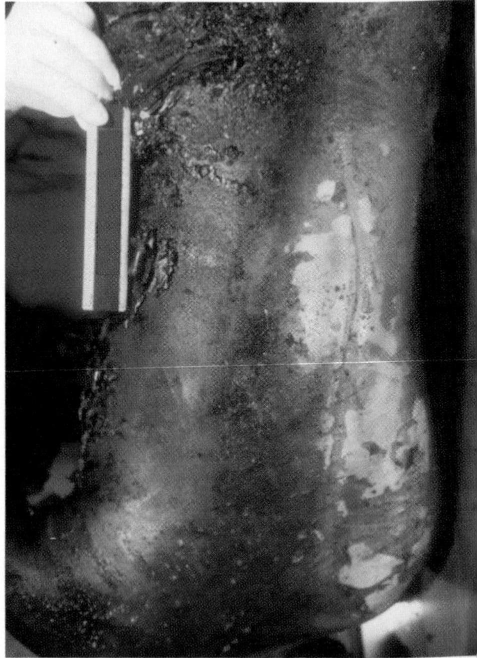

Back of a victim whose body was burned postmortem. Less severe burning indicates the victim was lying on his back when burned. *Image courtesy of Stephen D. Cohle, MD.*

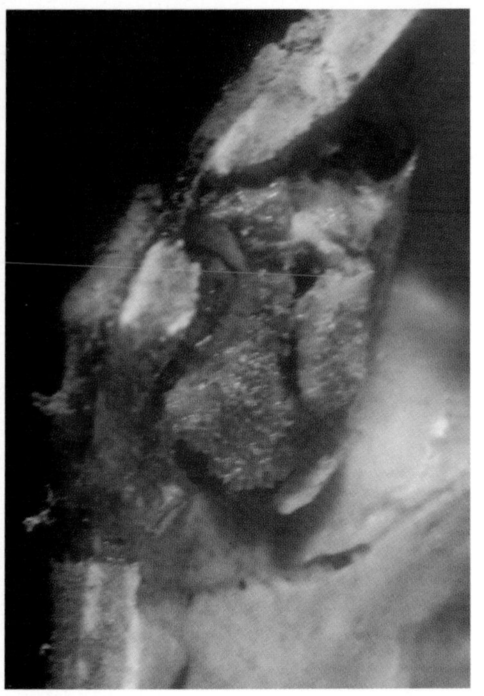

Close-up of a depressed fracture in the skull (see "No Tombstone for 'Jack'"). *Image courtesy of Stephen D. Cohle, MD.*

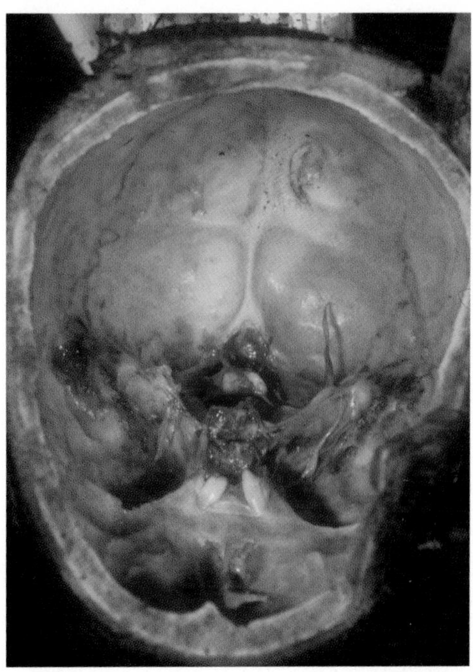

Interior view of the skull from a victim killed with a hammer (see "No Tombstone for 'Jack'"). *Image courtesy of Stephen D. Cohle, MD.*

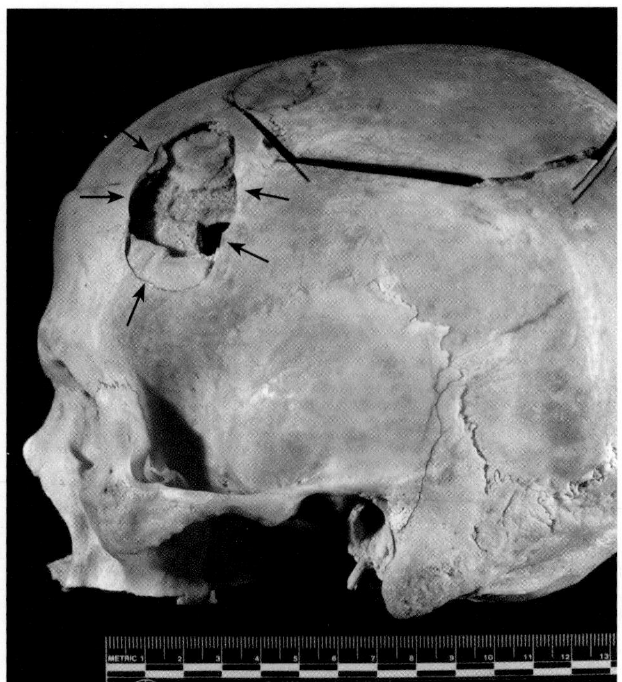


Skull showing depressed fractures. This damage is consistent with a hammer blow *(see next page, top left). Image courtesy of Michigan State University's Department of Anthropology.*

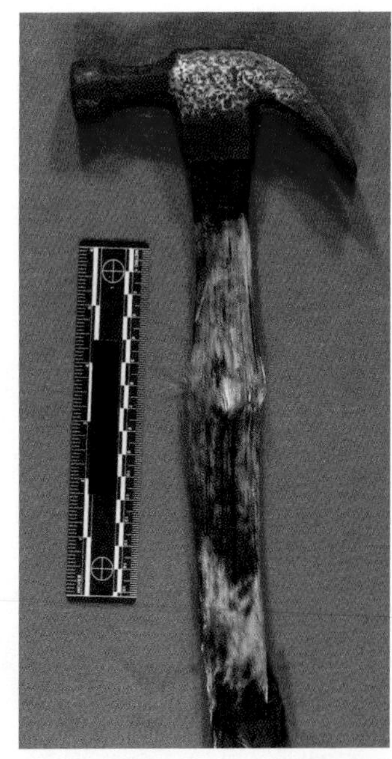

The murder weapon in the "Jack" case: a claw hammer with a fiberglass handle. *Image courtesy of Michigan State University's Department of Anthropology.*

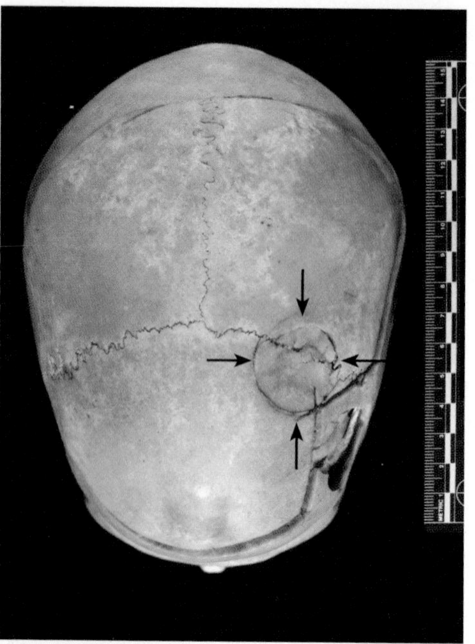

Skull showing a depressed fracture. The shape of the fracture leaves little doubt about the weapon this victim's killer used (see "No Tombstone for 'Jack'"). *Image courtesy of Michigan State University's Department of Anthropology.*

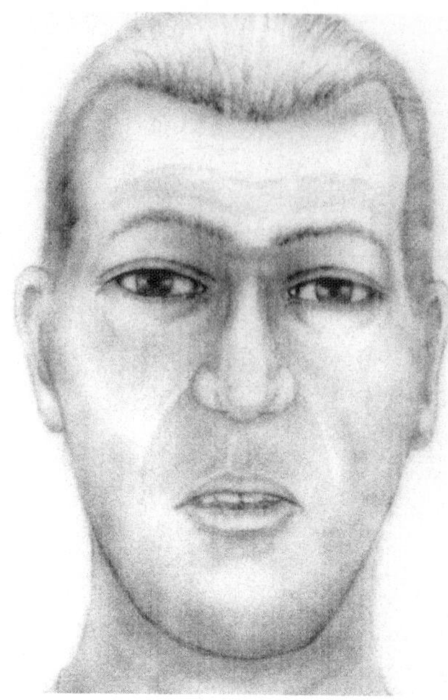

Michigan State forensic artist (retired) Fernando Martinez's sketch of "Jack." If you know this man or have any information that may lead to the identification of him, please contact the Ottawa County Sheriff's Office. *Image courtesy of Ottawa County Sheriff's Office.*

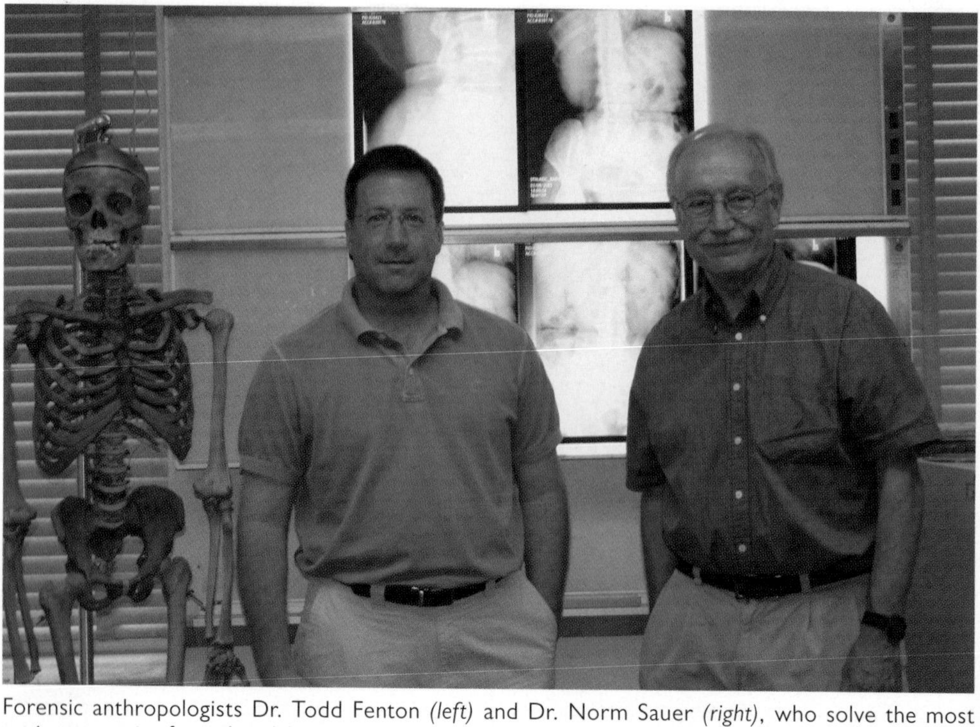

Forensic anthropologists Dr. Todd Fenton *(left)* and Dr. Norm Sauer *(right)*, who solve the most vexing mysteries from their laboratory at Michigan State University in East Lansing. *Image courtesy of Tobin T. Buhk.*

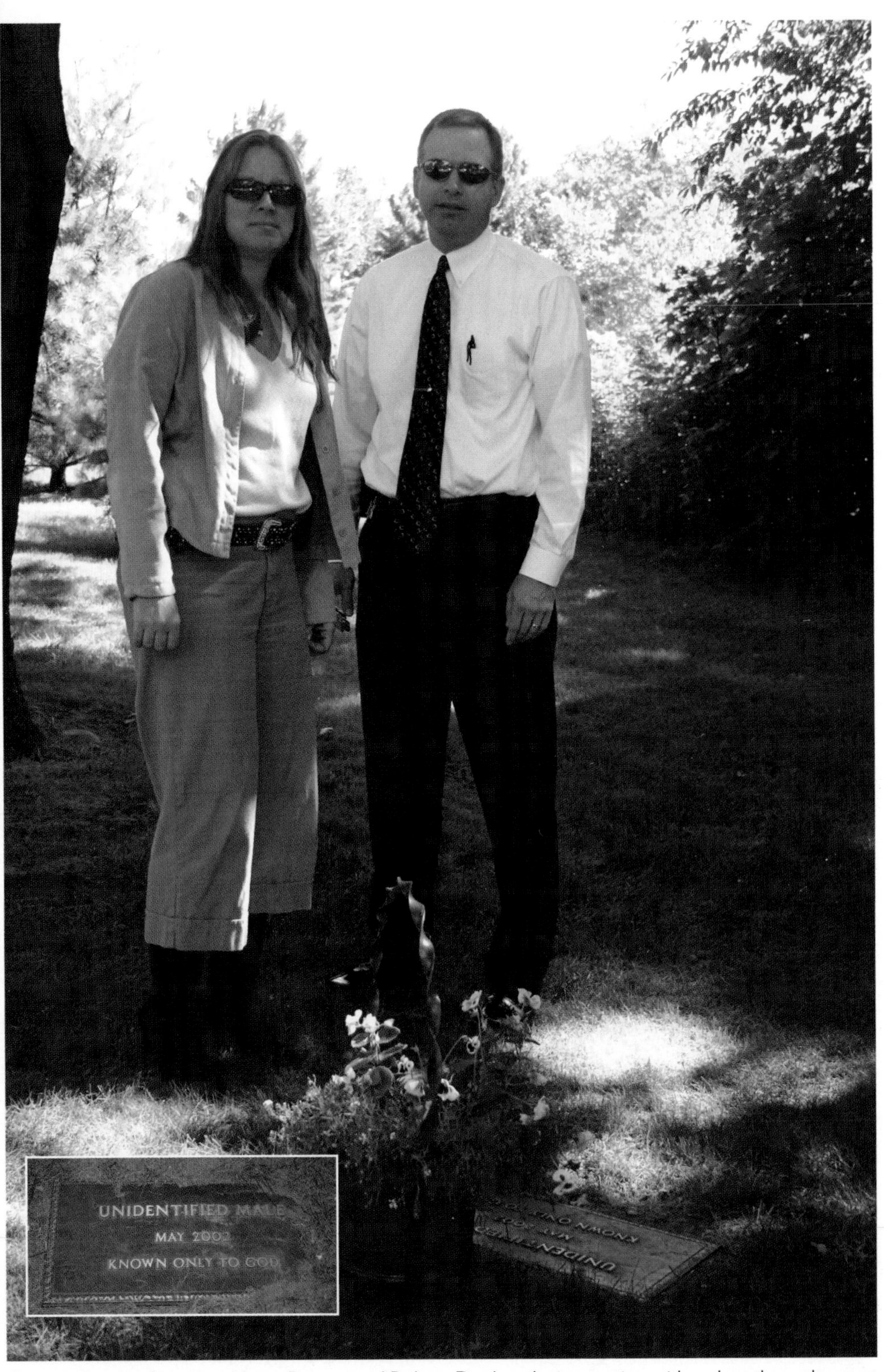


Ottawa County detectives Venus Repper and Robert Donker. An interesting aside: when the author met with the detectives at "Jack's" grave, someone had placed this floral arrangement there. *Inset:* Memorial bronze plaque that serves as "Jack's" headstone in Lakeshore Cemetery. *Images courtesy of Tobin T. Buhk.*

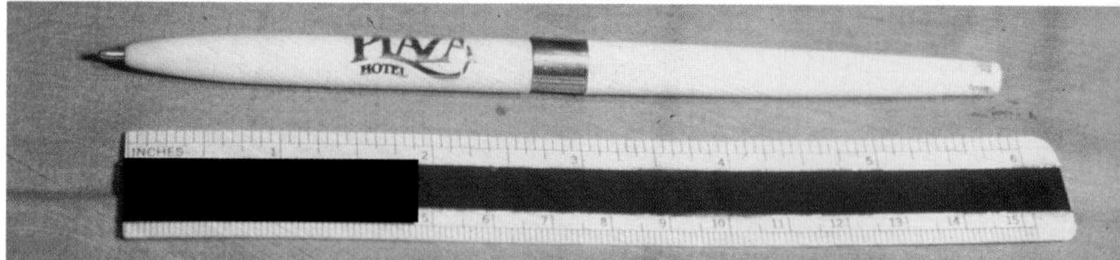


A key piece of evidence tying two Michigan victims to the Amway Grand Plaza Hotel in downtown Grand Rapids, Michigan. Randy Kraft stayed at this hotel when the two men went missing. The entire length of the pen was inserted into the victim's penis and shoved into the pelvis area, where it was discovered during the autopsy (see "Scorecard"). *Image courtesy of Stephen D. Cohle, MD.*

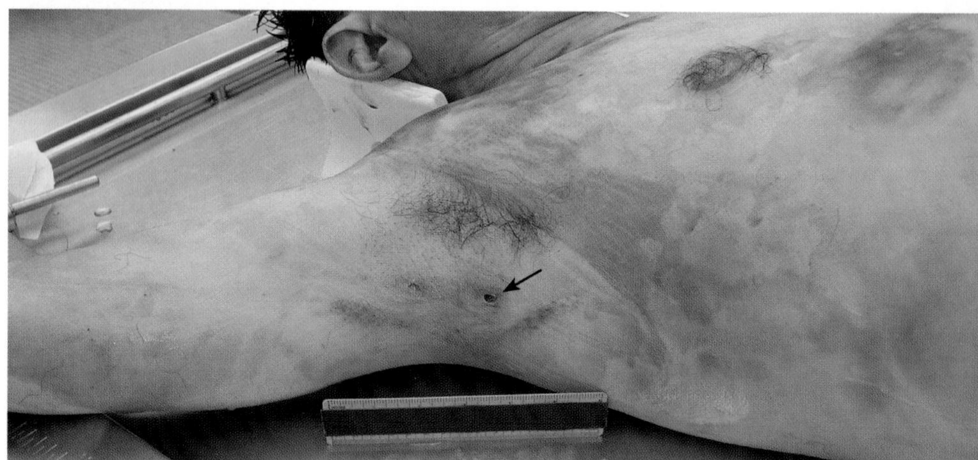

Victim of a gunshot homicide. Note the bullet entry wound under the armpit. The placement of this wound suggests a defensive posture, as if the victim threw up his arm to shield himself. Such forensic evidence can help an ME reconstruct the shooting, and thus confirm or refute eyewitness accounts of a shooting, or prove or disprove a defendant's story (see "I Fought the Law and the Law Won"). *Image courtesy of Stephen D. Cohle, MD.*

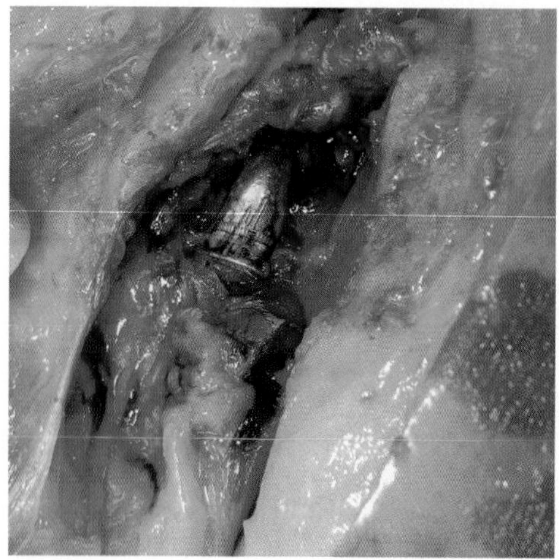

Bullet from an assault rifle inside a wound track (see "I Fought the Law and the Law Won"). *Image courtesy of Stephen D. Cohle, MD.*

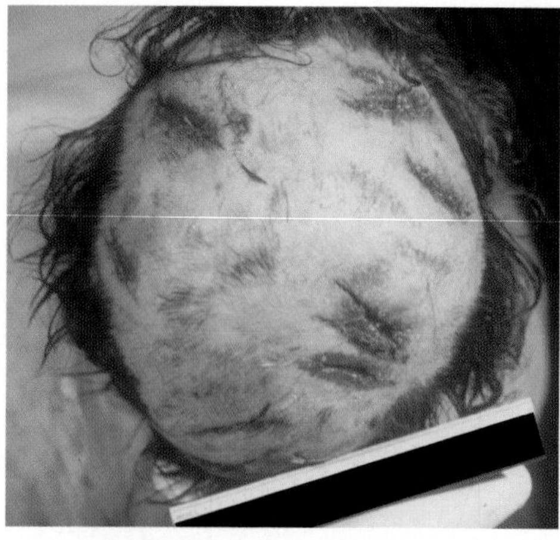

Injuries caused by repeated blows from a blunt object. Such injuries typically indicate that the ME will find skull fractures under the surface. *Image courtesy of Stephen D. Cohle, MD.*

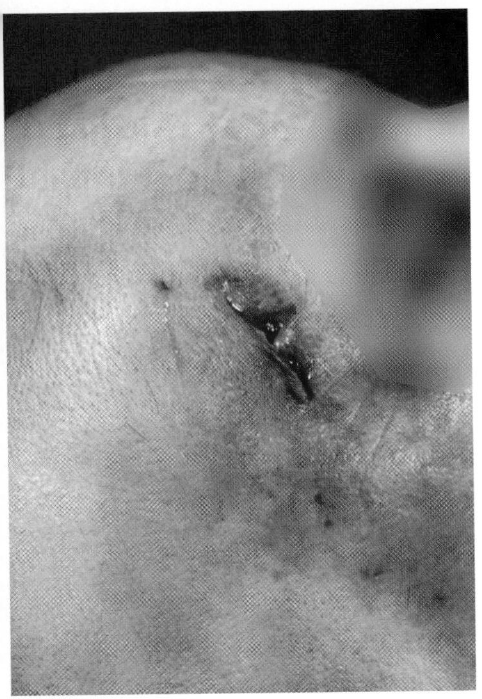

Skin laceration over a skull fracture caused by a blunt object such as a baseball bat, a board, or a steel pipe. *Image courtesy of Stephen D. Cohle, MD.*

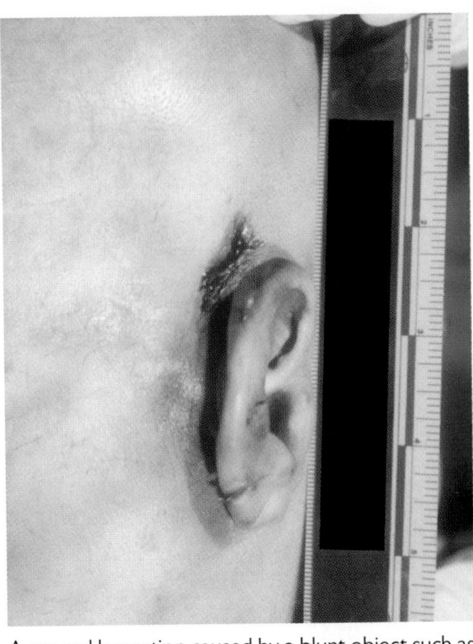


A second laceration caused by a blunt object such as a baseball bat or a steel pipe. This wound suggests that after the initial blow, the killer brought the blunt object back for a second strike, which could create a cast-off blood spatter stain at the scene. *Image courtesy of Stephen D. Cohle, MD.*

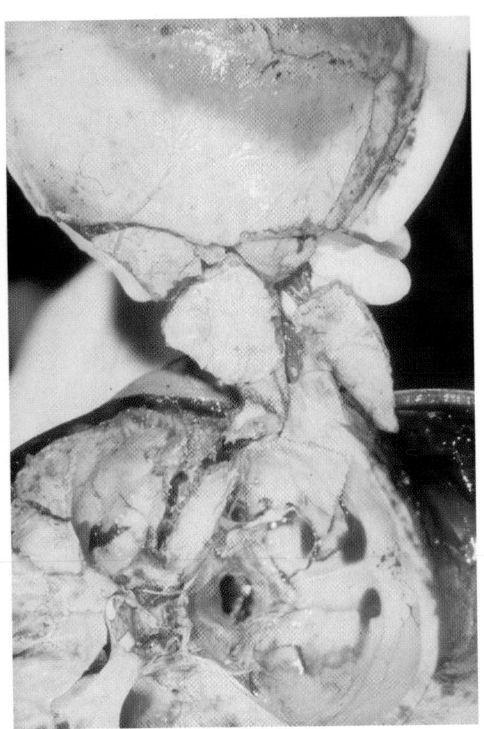

A skull shattered by a blunt object. *Image courtesy of Stephen D. Cohle, MD.*

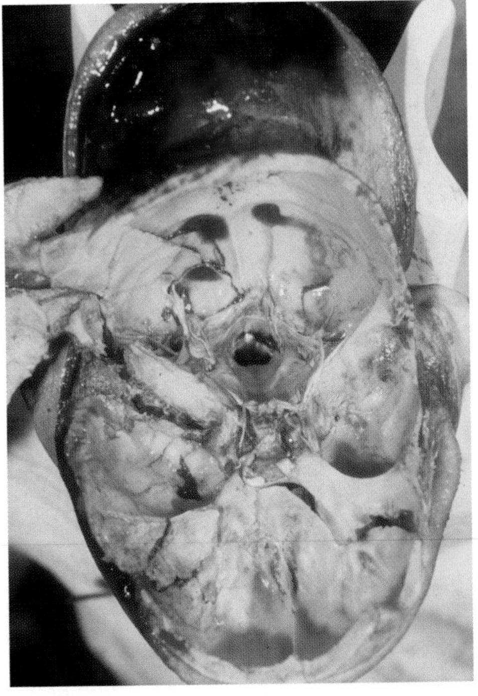

Interior of a skull showing evidence of blunt force trauma: multiple fractures in the bottom of the skull. *Image courtesy of Stephen D. Cohle, MD.*

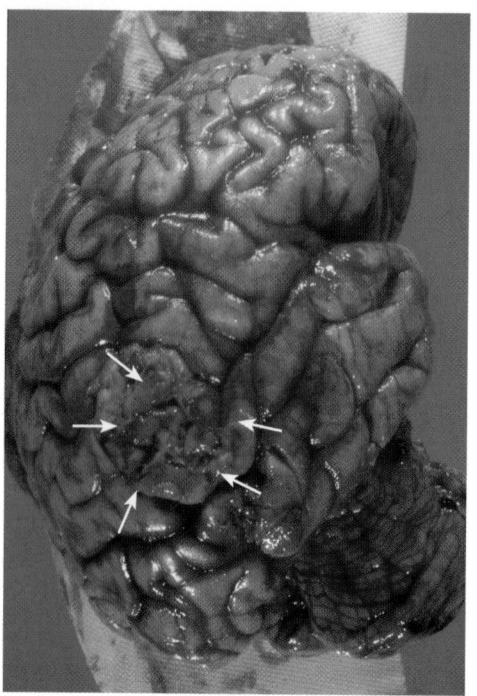

A brain showing contusions (bruises marked by arrows) from blunt force trauma. *Image courtesy of Stephen D. Cohle, MD.*

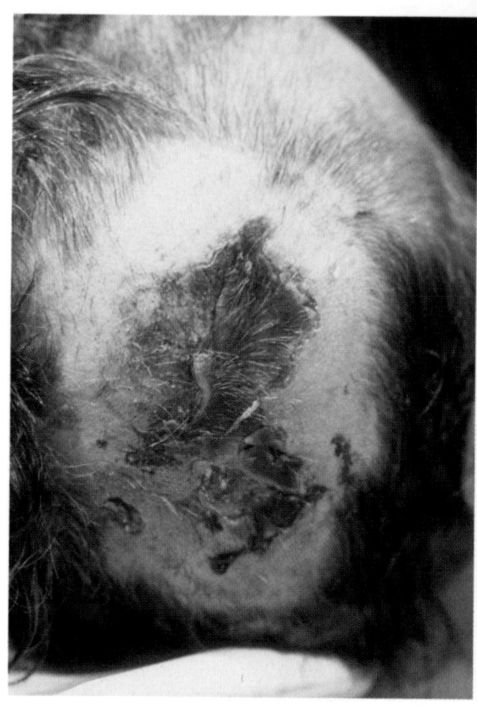

This victim was struck by a forceful blow to the head with a blunt object, leaving scalp lacerations. *Image courtesy of Stephen D. Cohle, MD.*

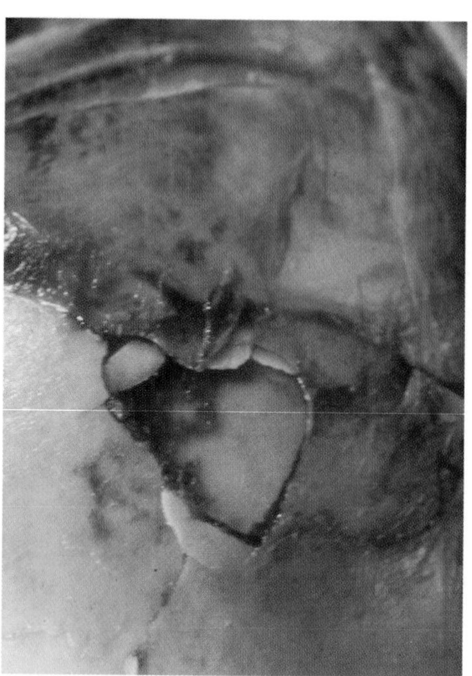

Depressed skull fracture from a blunt object. The massive skull damage indicates that the killer struck his victim with full strength. *Image courtesy of Stephen D. Cohle, MD.*

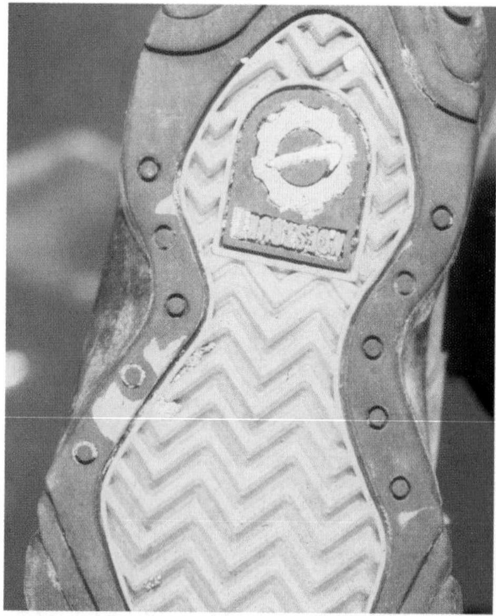

Murder weapons come in all shapes and sizes, from a glass tea mug (see "It's Not a Weapon; It's a Tea Mug!") to a tennis shoe (see "Head Case"). Each weapon leaves telltale forensic evidence, from depressed fractures to patterned abrasions tattooed onto a victim's skin. *Image courtesy of Stephen D. Cohle, MD.*

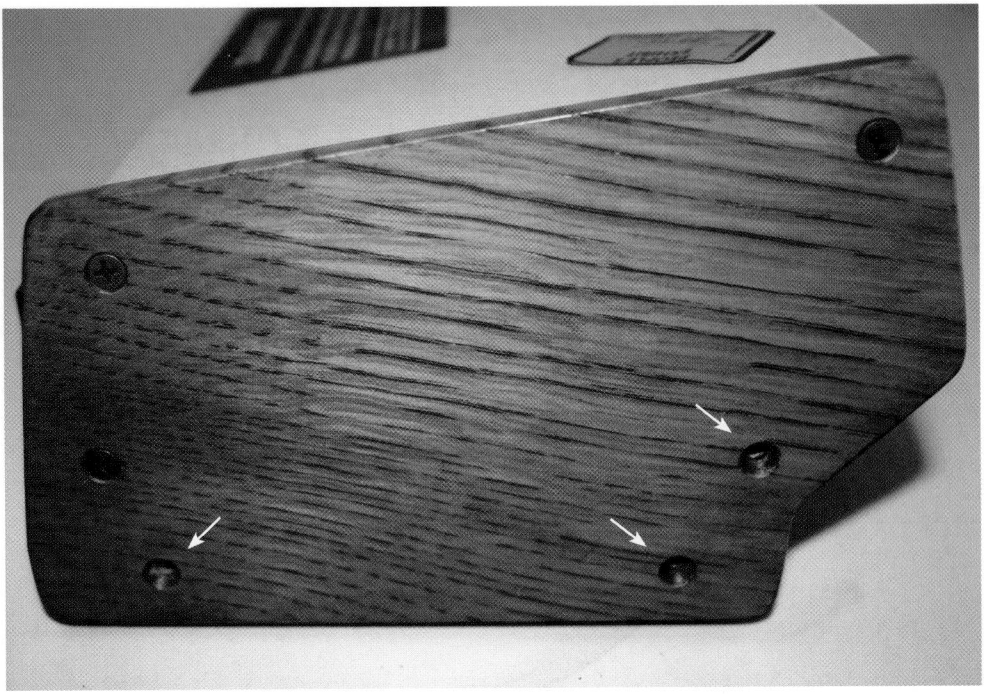

Right side of a fetal monitor showing three missing screws—evidence that someone had tampered with the device. Two screws were missing from the left side as well (see "Loved Him to Death"). *Image courtesy of Tobin T. Buhk. Evidence provided by Dan Miller, Chief of Public Safety, City of Wayland.*

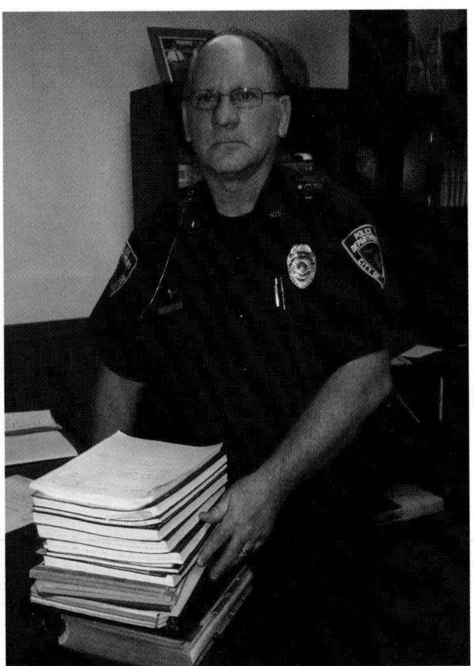

Dan Miller, City of Wayland Chief of Public Safety, standing next to the case files and trial transcripts from the Spencer case (see "Loved Him to Death"). *Image courtesy of Tobin T. Buhk.*

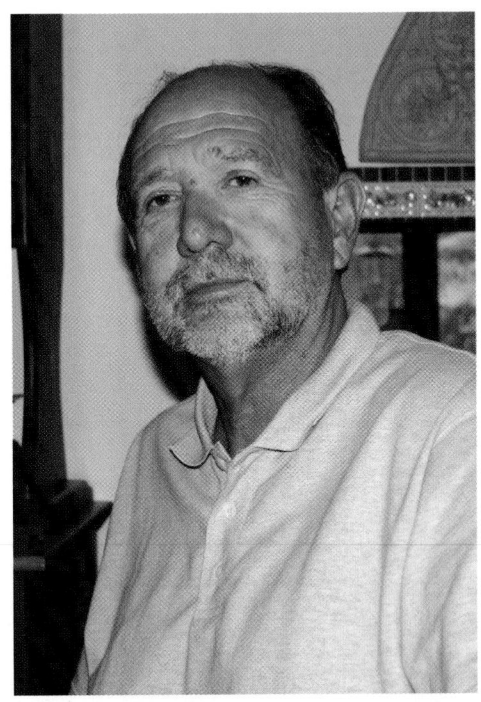

Michigan State Police Detective Sergeant (retired) Ron Neil (see "The Hand That Feeds"; "Loved Him to Death"). *Image courtesy of Tobin T. Buhk.*

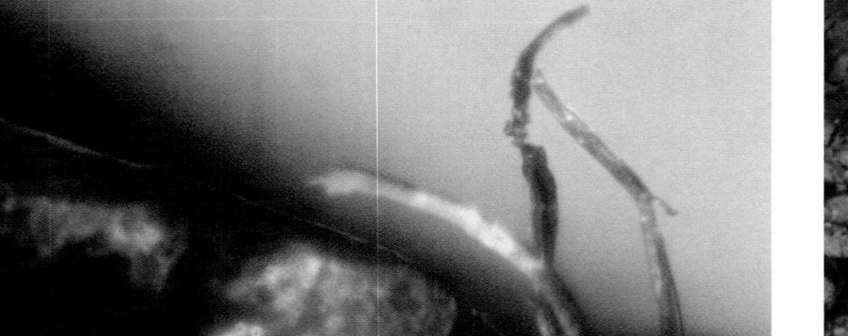

Tiny metal fibers found in the head wounds of a victim bludgeoned to death with a metal object like a steel pipe or a tire iron. These fibers linked the killer to the murder weapon (see "The Hand That Feeds"). *Image courtesy of Stephen D. Cohle, MD.*

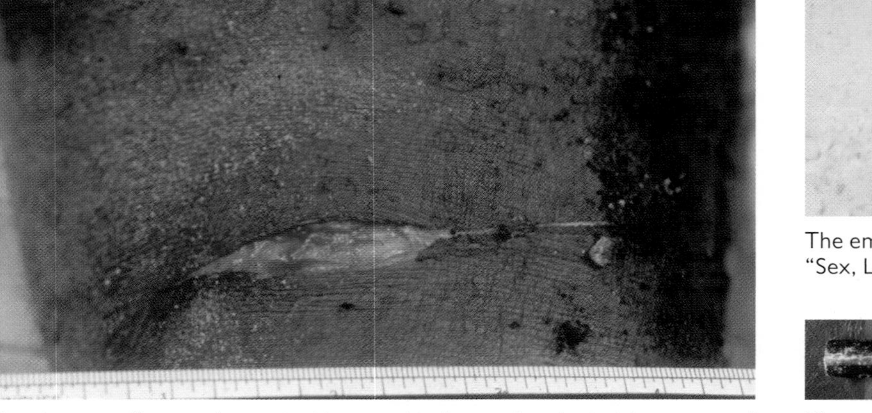

The absence of hemorrhaging in this wound indicates that the incision occurred postmortem. *Image courtesy of Stephen D. Cohle, MD.*

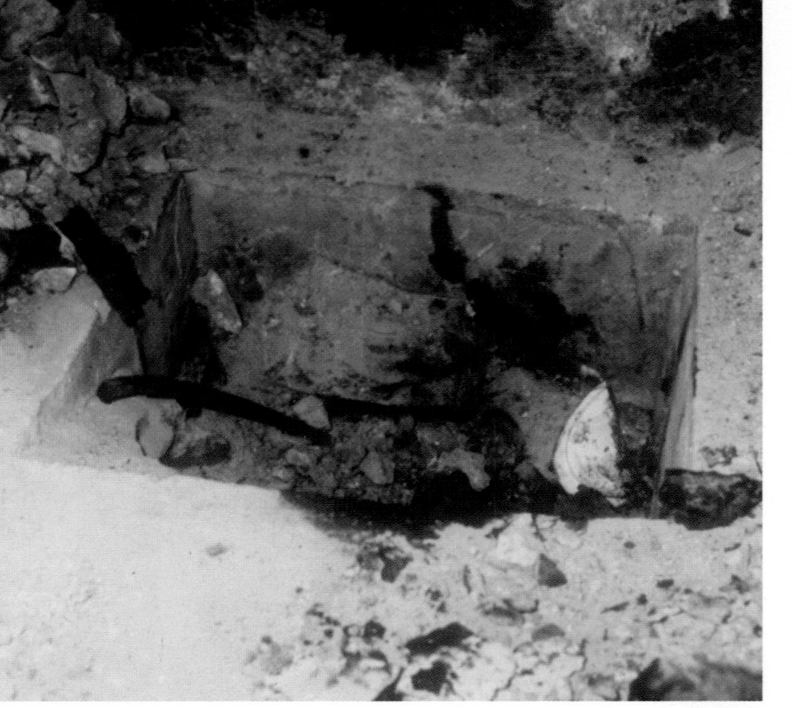

The empty crypt after investigators managed to remove the victim's body (see "Sex, Lies, and Cement"). *Image courtesy of Stephen D. Cohle, MD.*

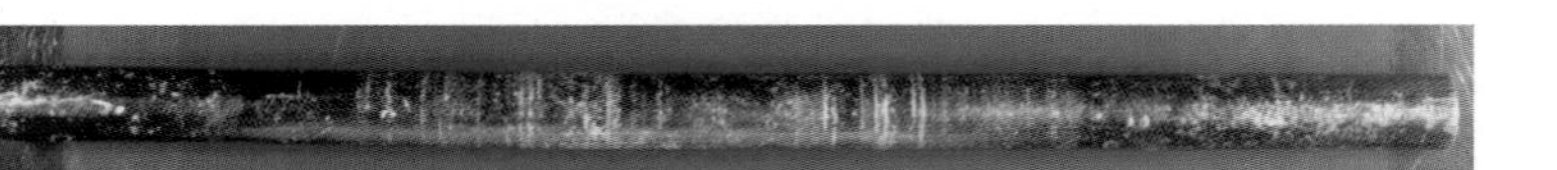

The type of weapon Keith Prong used to murder his two elderly victims (see "The Hand That Feeds"). *Image courtesy of Stephen D. Cohle, MD.*

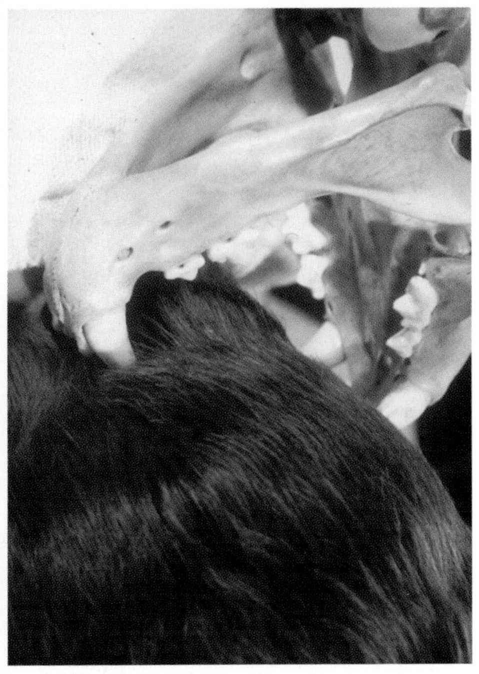

A jaguar skull placed on a hospital volunteer to confirm that Naudi inflicted the deadly wounds on a zoo employee (see "Big Cats"). *Image courtesy of Stephen D. Cohle, MD.*

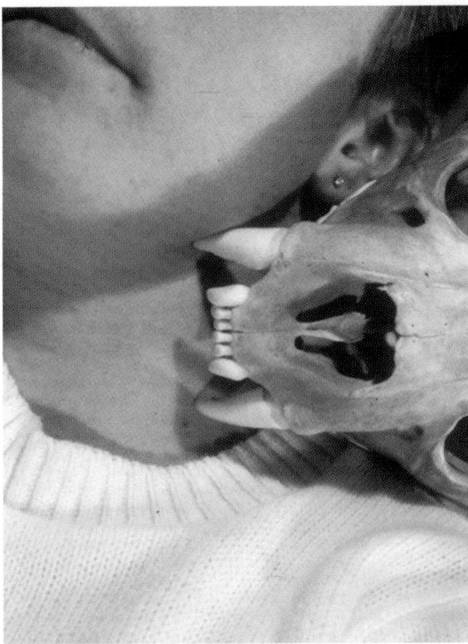

This image illustrates the manner in which Naudi killed the zoo employee: his canine teeth punctured her left carotid artery and jugular vein, and she bled to death (see "Big Cats"). *Image courtesy of* American Journal of Forensic Medicine and Pathology.

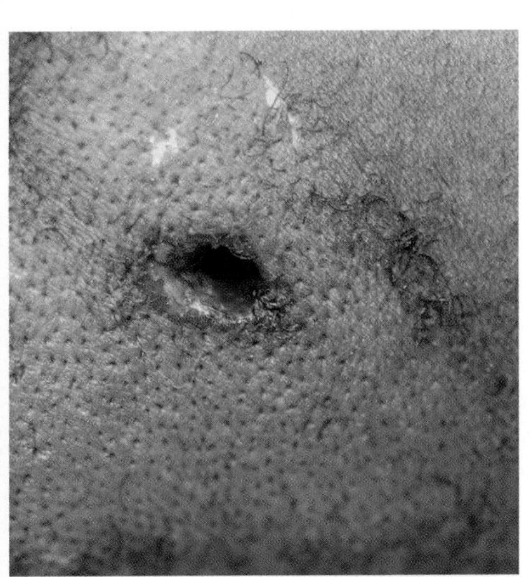

(Picture 1 in a sequence) The characteristics of a bullet entrance wound can provide vital information about a shooting, such as the type of weapon used and the angle/range from which the gun was fired. This information can help confirm or disprove eyewitness accounts of a shooting, or in cases without witnesses, help re-create the event (see "I Fought the Law, and the Law Won"; "Things Ain't Always What They Seem"). *Image courtesy of Stephen D. Cohle, MD.*

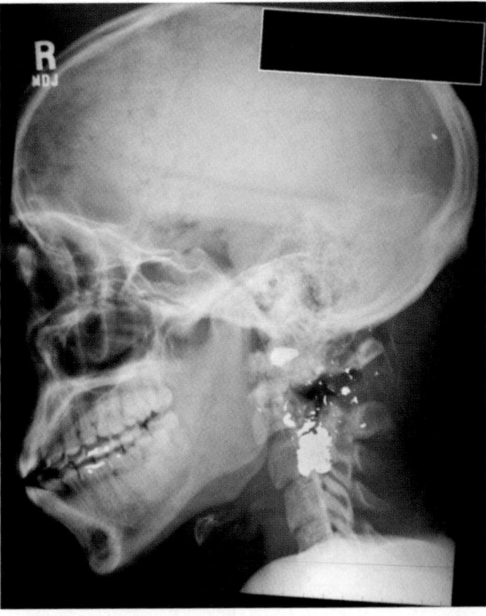


(Picture 2) The x-ray showing the bullet still in the victim's neck. "Jacketed" bullets often separate into two pieces. This can sometimes create a red herring for the ME, since the core of a jacketed bullet often exits, creating an exit wound while the jacket remains inside the victim. *Image courtesy of Stephen D. Cohle, MD.*

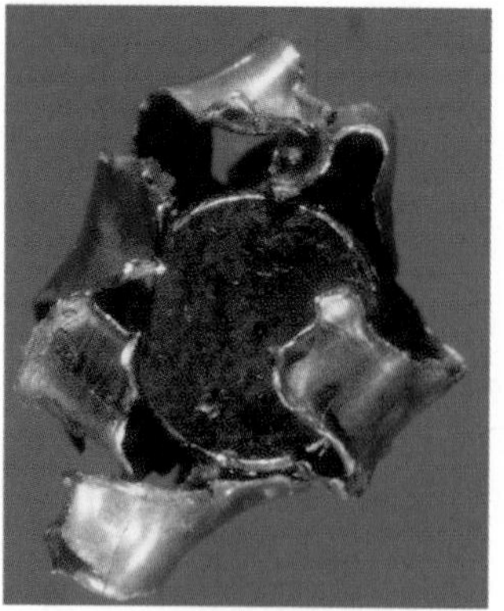

(Picture 3 in a sequence) The jacket from a jacketed bullet. *Image courtesy of Stephen D. Cohle, MD.*

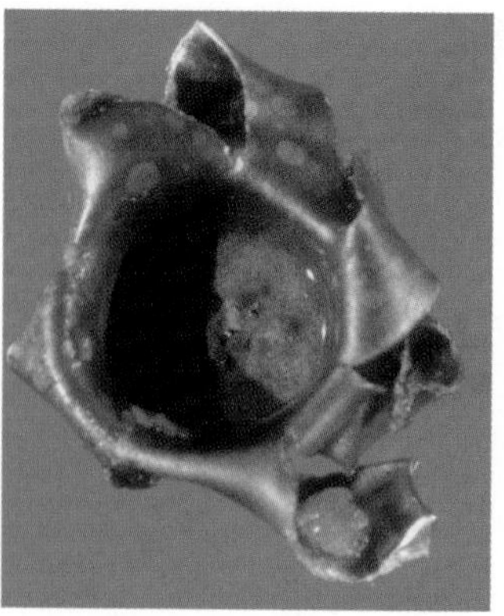

(Picture 4) Another view of the jacket without the core. Police do not use such ammunition because while the jacket often remains inside a victim, the core can pass through and strike a bystander. *Image courtesy of Stephen D. Cohle, MD.*

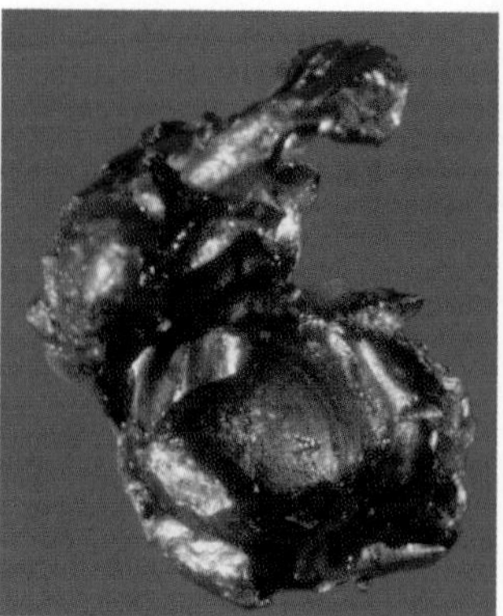

(Picture 5) Bullets can often fragment upon impact and create separate wound tracks. *Image courtesy of Stephen D. Cohle, MD.*

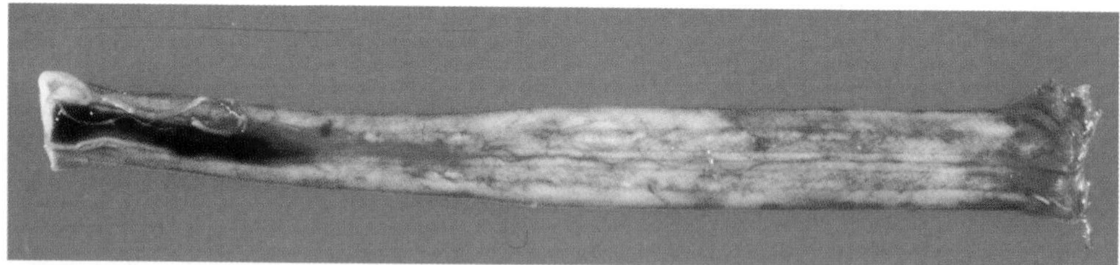

(Picture 6) The severed spinal cord of a victim shot by the jacketed bullet. The severed end is at the right. *Image courtesy of Stephen D. Cohle, MD.*

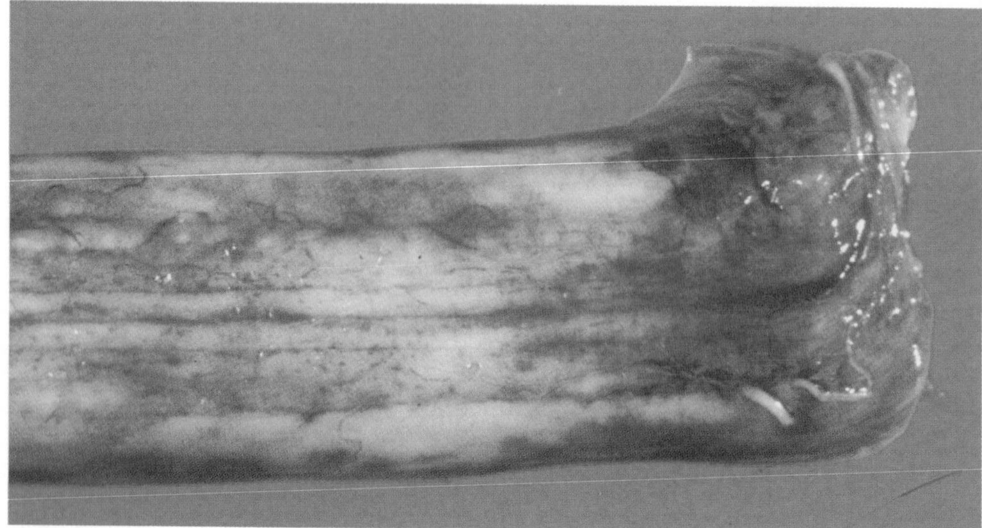

(Picture 7) Close-up of the damage to the victim's spinal cord. *Image courtesy of Stephen D. Cohle, MD.*

At the hospital, they spun the tale that the injury occurred when he fell off a ladder.[5]

Slade's defense attempted to cast doubt on what appeared to be cold-blooded murder: the pair had taken drugs and consumed a copious amount of alcohol that night, the two argued . . . Slade woke up to find Barth dead. He panicked and hid the body. Since Slade didn't remember what occurred in the time period represented by the ellipsis in the previous sentence—during the interval between the argument and his waking up next to his deceased lover—perhaps testimony about Barth's violent behavior would help the jury to fill the missing hours with the image of Debra Barth's Hyde attacking Brian Slade. As he testified that he did not recall what occurred, however, Slade could present no real evidence of self-defense. The prosecution countered by describing his actions after he concealed the body: after the murder, the prosecution alleged, Slade partied—a week-long bender that ended with his arrest.

No matter who threw the first punch, though, the forensic evidence suggests that Barth's killer did more than just defend himself; he did more than just assault her; he beat her to death with the force of a professional boxer.

Almost a year from the date police arrested Brian Slade, the jury would discuss what they heard in court. They found him guilty as charged, and a month later, a judge sentenced him to life in prison.

Slade did appeal his conviction partly on the basis that a reference to a polygraph test during testimony unfairly prejudiced the jury. During the trial, the prosecution played a portion of an audiotape that contained a reference to a polygraph test. On the tape, one of the investigators questioning Slade suggested that he had the opportunity to take a lie detector test, and when the prosecutor played the tape, the jury heard the reference. Polygraphs are not considered accurate enough for use in court, so the reference on the audiotape, according to defense attorney John Dougherty, could leave the jury wondering if Slade took a lie detector test and if he did, if he passed or failed.

Dougherty immediately moved for a mistrial, but the trial judge denied the motion. The State of Michigan Court of Appeals reviewed the appeal but affirmed the trial court's decision that the inadvertent reference did not call for a mistrial.

The tie that bound together Brian Slade and Debra Barth was a rubber band. Occasionally, the rubber band stretched, sending the two hurtling toward each other.

On one late summer night, the rubber band stretched too far, Brian Slade snapped, and a vicious murder resulted. The thirty-eight-year-old was arrested on the first official day of fall; the arrest represented the beginning of the final season of Slade's life, which he will spend in prison.

## Notes

1. Quoted in *People v. Slade*, Mich. App. 238129 (2003), unpublished opinion, http://courtofappeals.mijud.net (accessed April 3, 2007).

2. Ibid.

3. Additional details about Salagovich's testimony from Stacey Smith, "Witness: Barth Intended to End Ties with Slade," *Traverse City Record-Eagle*, September 15, 2001, http://www.record-eagle.com/2001/sep/15sladet.htm (accessed April 3, 2007).

4. Stacey Smith, "Jurors Deliberate Slade Verdict," *Traverse City Record-Eagle*, September 21, 2001, http://www.record-eagle.com/2001/sep/21slade.htm (accessed April 3, 2007).

5. Ibid.

# Ghosts of Arcadia

> *"Singularity is almost invariably a clue. The more featureless and commonplace a crime is, the more difficult is it to bring it home."*
>
> —Sherlock Holmes, "The Boscombe Valley Mystery," *The Adventures of Sherlock Holmes* (1891)

The justice system dragged Mark Unger, kicking and screaming, to the edge of the lake and threw him in, drowning his screams of innocence.

Because, a jury believed, that is just what he did to his wife, Florence, except she was unconscious. He committed a crime and attempted to cover it up as a commonplace accident. And, as Sherlock Holmes suggested in "The Boscombe Valley Mystery," it was difficult for the prosecution to "bring it home." Unger had motive and opportunity, but the forensic evidence—in this case the difference between guilt and innocence—hinged on a few feet. A few feet: the distance from the cement slab to the shallow water in which Florence Unger was found dead. "A few feet" also applied to the figurative ledge on which Mark Unger stood: a few feet between safety and the abyss of prison. These few feet raised an interesting question: how did Florence Unger's unconscious body move the few feet from the concrete slab on which she fell into the water of Lower Herring Lake?

This question raised another question posed for the jurors at the subsequent trial, a question that for some remains unanswered and a matter for further debate in court: was Florence Unger's death the result of a relatively commonplace accident, or did Mark Unger murder her and attempt to make her death appear to be an accident?

The ugly incident occurred in the middle of one of Michigan's most beautiful areas—an area some consider paradise.

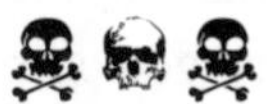

With its scenic overlooks and quaint fishing villages, Highway M22 is Michigan's version of California's Pacific Coast Highway; it runs up the northwest coast of Michigan. Those making the scenic drive may feel like they are riding a roller coaster, following the undulating route as it crests to the highest point in Michigan's lower peninsula at the top of a gigantic sand dune before plunging to the quaint lakeside villages of Elberta, Onekama, and the aptly named Arcadia. In Greek myth, Arcadia was a wooded paradise somewhere west of the Pillars of Hercules (the Strait of Gibraltar).

In the nineteenth century, the area hosted fishing villages and port cities born from and raised by the logging industry. Today, these same cities have become a tourist mecca for hikers who explore the forests and rivers of the Manistee National Forest and water sport enthusiasts who play on the surfaces of the area's numerous inland lakes or the Big Lake.

Like the area's many villages, the Watervale Resort, six miles from Arcadia, has been reborn as a resort. The Leo Hale Lumber Company built the village of Watervale in 1892. The village contained a lumber mill, a post office, a general store, and accommodations to house the company personnel: eight cottages for married employees and a boarding house for single employees.

The village had a short life, though, because after the Panic of 1893, the company folded and the village became a ghost town. Almost a quarter of a century later, in 1917, a Chicago physician purchased the complex and converted it into a resort for his seven brothers and sisters. The Watervale Resort opened in 1918 and, still owned and operated by the family of the physician who purchased it, continues to delight tourists with its charming Victorian structures furnished with period antiques. With a hotel (the boarding house) and over a dozen houses or cottages (seven of the original loggers' cabins) nestled on the southern edge of Lower Herring Lake, the resort provides visitors with access to the inland lake as well as a mile of Lake Michigan shoreline.

In late October, the leaves on the deciduous trees throughout northern Michigan begin to change colors, creating a vibrant canvas of crimson, scarlet, and orange. A period of unseasonable warmth, an Indian Summer, mixes with the bitter cold—a harbinger of the winter to come—to create unpredictable weather mood swings. One could call it Mother Nature's version of (a meteorological) manic depression. This was the setting for the horrific drama that began as a family getaway.

Mark and Florence Unger visited the Inn at Watervale Resort each year, and despite a failing marriage, they would make their annual jaunt in 2003. With their two boys, the couple traveled across the state from their suburban Detroit community of Huntington Woods to the idyllic peacefulness of Watervale.

The couple ended the evening of October 24 on the deck of a boat dock, twelve feet above a concrete slab that served as a boat launch into Lower Herring Lake. Huddled in blue comforters among chaise lounge chairs, perhaps the couple reminisced about better times. At some point, their discussion may have turned to their impending divorce, perhaps the division of assets, or the most sensitive issue of all, the custody of their two boys.

At approximately 7:38 the next morning, the innkeepers, Linn and Maggie Duncan, who lived in a cottage on the premises, received a call. On the other end of the line, Mark Unger informed them that his wife, Florence, had apparently gone missing. He had last seen her on the boat deck the night before, but he had returned to the cottage without her and she never returned. The Duncans, co-owners of the Watervale, left their cottage to search for the missing woman.

The Duncans began a search of the resort, but they didn't need to look far. They found Florence Unger floating facedown a few feet from the edge of Lower Herring Lake in five inches of water. Fractured wooden railings on the boat dock suggested that Mrs. Unger had had a horrific accident, falling over the railing to the cement slab twelve feet below. A bloodstain marked the spot where it appeared she landed. Candles and shards of broken glass were sprinkled across the cement surface. Somehow she wound up in the lake; some force, perhaps the momentum from the fall, carried her body into the water.

Police forensic experts studied the scene and found some curious, even suspicious elements at the scene. A large, diluted pool of blood indicated that Mrs. Unger lay on the pavement for an interval of time bleeding profusely from her head wound. Yet no streaks of blood appeared on the few feet of pavement between the point of impact and the lake's edge. This anomaly raised disturbing questions: if the momentum of the fall carried Florence Unger into Lower Herring Lake, how did the pool of blood, which indicated she lay in that same area for some time, occur? And why did no streaks of blood appear on the pavement marking her path into the lake?

Although the distance between the point of impact and the lake's edge was only a few feet, the scene suggested that Florence Unger did not roll into the lake. But if she didn't, how did she get into the water? One possibility seemed to answer the inconsistencies: someone carried her body into the water. Perhaps an autopsy would reveal information that would solve the riddle presented by the scene.

Certain counties, such as Benzie County, that do not have a forensic pathologist contract the Kent County medical examiner team to conduct autopsies for suspicious deaths. Benzie County medical examiner Matthew Houghton turned to the Kent County ME, and Florence Unger traveled to Grand Rapids, where her autopsy was performed. Although the death may have appeared to be an accident, the evidence uncovered at the autopsy suggested that a more sinister scenario occurred that late October night.

Florence Unger had suffered a massive head injury—cranial-cerebral trauma; when she landed headfirst on the concrete, the impact cracked her skull. The severity of the head injury also caused her to aspirate blood. This finding suggested that she lay, likely unconscious, on the concrete for perhaps twenty or thirty minutes, during which she breathed in the blood. The amount of blood on the concrete also suggested that she may have lain on the slab for some time before moving. The fall also fractured her hip. If conscious, an unlikely but nonetheless possible scenario, she could only have moved with excruciating pain.

Yet her body was found in Lower Herring Lake. So, if she lay on the concrete for twenty to thirty minutes, likely unconscious from the fall, with a fractured hip that would have rendered any movement painful and thus unlikely, how did she get into Lower Herring Lake? Did she at some time regain consciousness and, in absolute agony, walk into the water, only to lose consciousness and die? While possible, this is a very unlikely scenario. Rather, the forensic evidence suggests that someone had to move her into the water. Manner of death: homicide, not accident.

Yet a vital question remained: did the head injury *kill* Florence Unger? If she died from the head injury, she could have accidentally fallen onto the concrete and died. If someone then moved her body into the lake, it was possible that her "killer" didn't kill her but simply moved her dead body: not murder. The blunt head trauma would have eventually killed Florence Unger, but did drowning replace this eventual fate? The position and disposition of her body—floating facedown in Lower Herring Lake—raised the possibility that she drowned. If someone moved her body into the lake and she drowned, then her death became a murder, not an accident.

Drowning, however, leaves no conclusive forensic or physical evidence that the medical examiner can find during an autopsy. Therefore, the autopsy of a victim suspected of drowning becomes an autopsy of exclusion. Only after all other possible causes of death have been *excluded*—and only if the context of the incident warrants such a conclusion—can a medical examiner rule drowning as the cause of death. Discovery of fluid in the victim's lungs may suggest a death by drowning, but pulmonary edema can occur secondary to head injury, narcotic overdose, and heart failure, to name a few other causes.

Thus, while Florence Unger likely died from the head injury she sustained when she fell onto the concrete slab, the possibility that she drowned could not be eliminated. This raised a very important question that forensic experts would debate in court; the possibility that Florence Unger drowned spurred a forensic chicken-egg debate. Either process could have led to her death, but which one occurred first: death by drowning or death by cranial-cerebral trauma?

L. J. Dragovic, the Oakland County (Detroit area) medical examiner consulted by authorities during the investigation, opined that the forensic evidence indicated Florence Unger drowned and was thus alive when moved into the water.[1] Although she would have eventually succumbed to the cranial-cerebral trauma, he believed the drowning trumped the head injury. Florence Unger, according to Dragovic, died when her lungs filled with water as she lay unconscious and facedown in inches of Lower Herring Lake.

Although Dragovic did not participate in the autopsy, he based his conclusions on the circumstances and the autopsy report. Her lungs contained fluid. Her brain lacked the degree of swelling one might expect for a person who died from a closed head injury. And the context supported such a conclusion: she was found floating facedown in a lake . . . it all added up to drowning. And if the pelvic fractures coupled with the cerebral trauma made movement unlikely, how did she get into the lake? Dragovic's conclusion indicated that someone moved Florence Unger's unconscious yet *living* body into the lake, where she drowned. This scenario created a murder rap for the person who moved her body into water.

And that person, investigators believed, was Mark Unger. Unger, police believed, had pushed his wife over the rail and dragged her unconscious body into the lake to make it look like an accidental death.

The lack of swelling in the brain, however, did not necessarily prove that she did not die of cranial-cerebral trauma. In some closed head injuries, the brain strikes the inside of the skull, which causes bleeding to occur under the protective membrane separating the skull from the brain (this area is called the dura). This bleeding, called subdural (beneath the dura) hematoma, creates pressure inside the skull that causes the brain to swell. The portion of the brain responsible for controlling respiration—the brain stem—is at the bottom of the brain and is surrounded by a portion of the skull called the foramen magnum. When the brain stem swells into the foramen magnum, it ceases to function, the heart stops beating, and death occurs. Physicians often must stop the swelling before this happens in a time frame known as "the golden hour." Treatment can involve removing the blood by drilling a hole in the skull or stopping the swelling through the use of drugs. Because of this dynamic, one could reasonably expect to find a swollen brain in a victim who died from blunt force trauma to the head. In some cases of massive head trauma, however, such as one might see in car accident victims, the damage to the brain may be so severe and death so rapid that the brain does not have time to swell.

The fluid in Florence Unger's lungs, while perhaps indicative of drowning, would also be consistent with a severe closed head injury.

Massive trauma to the brain impedes breathing, which in turn could cause a buildup of fluid in the lungs. The same signs that led L. J. Dragovic to conclude that Florence Unger drowned could also indicate that she died from a head injury.

Although the prosecution did find an eyewitness who saw the Ungers on the boat dock that night, there was no eyewitness to the incident, nor a confession. With L. J. Dragovic's conclusions, though, they had a smoking gun: if Florence Unger drowned and the hip injury immobilized her, how did she get into the lake?

The answer, authorities began to believe, could only be that Mark Unger pulled her into the lake, thus purposely ending her life. For a prosecutor to prove that Mark Unger committed first-degree murder, he must prove that he planned to kill her; in short, he premeditated the crime. According to criminal law, if Mark Unger did move her *living* body into the lake, this action would indicate that he intended to murder his wife. Under Michigan law, someone found guilty of premeditated murder receives a sentence of life in prison without the possibility of parole.

But what if Florence Unger had accidentally fallen over the railing and sustained a fatal head injury on the concrete slab twelve feet below? What if Mark Unger had for some reason or another left his wife on the deck—to check on his children, for example—only to return and find her body in a heap on the concrete, already dead? Perhaps afraid the police would finger him for throwing her off the deck, he dragged her *lifeless* body into the lake to make it appear that she died of an accident. This scenario would make him guilty . . . of moving a body: a relatively minor crime compared to first-degree murder. It would be a strange scenario indeed; if an accidental fall had killed Florence Unger, why would he need to move the body to make it appear that she drowned?

Perhaps he panicked. Yet, *if* the forensic evidence proved that Florence Unger drowned, as L. J. Dragovic concluded, someone would have moved her into the lake while she was still alive. This would destroy the viability of and possible legal defense that Unger moved his wife's lifeless body to stage an accidental death and made it appear that his wife drowned.

Thus, how Florence Unger died—the cause of death—became the key item of contention in this case. Dragovic's opinion, and whether he would have the chance to testify at the preliminary hearing, became the center of a legal battle. A recent Michigan law changed the way evidence can be presented in court proceedings. The law was created to prevent shoddy expert testimony and required experts to support their conclusions with legitimate scientific research. After opposing council wrangled over the legality, the presiding judge at the preliminary hearing allowed Dr. Dragovic's testimony. When asked by the defense to support his conclusions, he explained that no such support exists; the circumstances of Florence Unger's death were unique and thus without precedent.[2]

After Dragovic's testimony, Mark Unger was headed for trial. The prosecution had a strong case against him—a case rich with overwhelming yet circumstantial evidence accumulated over the eight-month interval between the incident and the preliminary hearing. If Dragovic was allowed to testify at the criminal trial, they would also have their smoking gun, and Unger's defense would have to explain how Florence Unger wound up in the lake.

The expert testimony, though, would also pose a problem for the prosecution; "competing" theories and well-respected medical examiners who do not agree about the victim's cause of death can leave a jury with reasonable doubt.

Dr. Cohle, who conducted the autopsy, testified that he believed Florence Unger died of a massive head injury, but he admitted she could have drowned. Under cross-examination, he also admitted that she could have regained consciousness, suffered a seizure, and fallen into the lake. Dragovic testified for the prosecution that she would have died from the head injury, but she drowned first. He also testified for the prosecution that the injuries on Florence Unger's body were consistent with a scenario in which someone pushed or kicked her off of the deck.

To remove any reasonable doubt that resulted from the differing forensic expert testimony, the prosecution needed to convince the jury that a jealous, vindictive Mark Unger murdered his wife because her death served his personal interests in their upcoming divorce, that he lured her to the boat deck where he pushed her over the railing and dragged her into Lower Herring Lake to finish the job and stage an accident.

A mountain of circumstantial evidence corroborated this scenario. The family trip to Watervale, investigators learned, was pregnant with subtext. To others at the resort, the family of four may have appeared as the perfect family, but when investigators began to open doors, they found skeletons rushing out at them. These skeletons came out in court as a parade of friends and acquaintances who testified for the prosecution about the couple's troubles. They collectively told a story of sex, drugs, deceit, and a powerful motive for murder.

Mark Unger had worked as a sportscaster and mortgage broker in the Detroit area, but then drug addiction and gambling gripped him tightly. Rehabilitation followed, but the lure of Vicodin, marijuana, and gambling had created a mountain of debt that Florence Unger felt was crushing her. In early 2003, Mark Unger received $10,000 a month in disability payments from policies he bought in preceding years, but according to a friend of Florence Unger, the money was not enough to support the family and pay a mountain of debt that apparently emanated from Mark Unger's gambling habit.[3] To pay the bills, Florence took a job as a mortgage broker.

Another friend testified that Florence wanted to leave Mark because of his addictions and financial troubles.[4] In fact, Florence Unger had filed for divorce two months before their trip to the Watervale Resort. And four days before her death, she and Mark attended a hearing during which her attorney presented Unger with divorce papers that asked questions about his substance abuse problems. Florence remained living with her husband and agreed to take the family jaunt to Watervale, but friends and her divorce attorney testified that she had no interest in reconciling. Their marriage had long ago dissolved; all that remained was a façade.

Mark Unger, however, did not want the divorce. And he did not want to lose custody of his children. (At a custody hearing prior to the trial, Mark Unger did lose custody of his two sons, ages seven and ten, due to his substance abuse and forthcoming murder trial.) According to the testimony of friends, the couple had been battling each other over the divorce in the week preceding the trip to Watervale.

Mark Unger also had a jealous streak. A friend of Florence told the jury an anecdote to illustrate this. During a dinner with this friend, Florence received several calls from someone the friend assumed to be her husband, Mark. It seemed to the friend that Florence was attempting to reassure the caller; she reiterated several times that she was having dinner with her friends and not some lover.[5]

Mark's suspicions and fears about marital infidelity were not just a figment of a paranoid imagination. At the preliminary hearing, Glenn Stark, a good friend of Mark Unger, shined a light on a skeleton dangling in his closet: he admitted to having an affair with Florence. In the two-year duration of their relationship, they sent each other intimate e-mails and had romantic liaisons on multiple occasions, the last time just a week before Florence's death.[6] Stark testified that Florence characterized her husband as a "Jekyll and Hyde" because of his "increasingly erratic" behavior.[7]

This was the subtext of the drama that may have played out on the boathouse deck the night Florence Unger died. Had Mark Unger had enough of marital disharmony and decided to end all of the debates and outmaneuver the divorce court by engineering an "accident" for his wife?

Another aspect of the incident raised questions about Mark Unger's role in his wife's "accident": he told two different versions of what occurred that night. He told the police that around 9 p.m., Florence asked him to return to the cabin to check on their children. When he returned to the deck, she had gone, he assumed, to visit with a friend at the resort.

According to his wife's hairdresser and former coworker, who testified for the prosecution, Mark Unger told her a different version of events that occurred the night his wife died. The hairdresser, unaware of the tragedy unfolding at the Watervale across the state, telephoned Florence at nine the next day. Mark Unger answered the phone. He told her what had occurred the previous night. He had left Florence on the deck and when he returned, he found her on the deck, alive and well, so he returned to the cabin. In her testimony, the hairdresser characterized Mark Unger as a habitual liar.[8] Did this slight alteration of his story suggest that it was a fiction conjured to hide a cold, calculated murder plot?

Were both of Mark Unger's versions merely variations of the same lie? Florence Unger's father, a witness for the prosecution, testified that his daughter was afraid of the dark. Friends who testified corroborated this idiosyncrasy; since childhood, she had an almost pathological fear of the dark and had not shaken it in adulthood. This fear of the dark made it unlikely that Florence wanted to be on the deck alone in the middle of the night, and called into question that element of Mark Unger's story.

And Unger's actions after the death of his wife were suspicious. When Linn Duncan told him that he found Florence Unger's body in Lower Herring Lake, Mark Unger, apparently wild with grief, ran to the exact spot in the lake where her body had been found. Duncan, however, had not shown Unger where he had found her body. And Unger, Duncan testified, could not have seen her body from the place where they stood when he broke the news. Had Mark Unger made an educated guess, or did he already know that his wife was in the lake? He also acted like a manic depressive, wailing one minute and calm the next. Were these emotions merely histrionics—a show to convince the police—or genuine grief?

Other crime scene evidence appeared to support the prosecution's scenario that Florence Unger's "accident" was no accident. The railings of the boat deck had been broken, but Linn Duncan testified that the day before Florence Unger's death, he had used the boat railings to lower over twenty pieces of furniture. They were stable. They held his weight.[9]

In addition, Michigan state police crime lab technicians found paint chips on the soles of both Mark's and Florence's shoes. Testing of paint chips cannot produce an exact match, but it can indicate if the chips came from a common source. Testing indicated that the paint was consistent with the paint used on the railings but not with the paint used for the boathouse walls. Had Mark Unger kicked the railing to damage it and thus make it appear that it gave way when his wife leaned on it?

If the defense team was to convince the jury that Florence Unger had had an accident, it would need a countermeasure to deflect the bomb of Dragovic's testimony; it needed to produce a reasonable explanation for how Florence Unger's body got into Lower Herring Lake—an explanation that would create a reasonable doubt about the prosecution's version of events. Defense attorneys called upon their own expert witnesses and posited a different scenario of what occurred that night on the boat deck.

The defense maintained that Florence Unger, alone on the boat deck, accidentally fell over the railing. The deck railings were in a state of disrepair. They were mottled with spots of growth, and the posts were cracked. And they were ten inches under code height. The railings were, in the words of a structural engineer who testified for the defense, an "accident waiting to happen."[10]

To contradict Dragovic's testimony, the defense called another Detroit area medical examiner, Dr. Carl Schmidt of Wayne County. Dragovic testified that Florence Unger's injuries indicated that someone had pushed or kicked her off the deck, but Schmidt testified that she could have received the same injuries if she fell through the railing by accident.[11] In other words, the medical evidence could not prove if the fall that created the head injury—the cranial-cerebral trauma that Cohle, who conducted the autopsy, and Benzie County ME Houghton believed killed Florence Unger—was an accident or a homicide.

So how did Florence Unger's body get into the lake? The defense posed a few possibilities: the momentum of the fall carried her the few feet into Lower Herring Lake; the edge of the lake is just a few feet from the place where the bloodstain indicated she landed from the fall. If, as Dr. Cohle opined, she lay on the concrete for a time—an opinion corroborated by the amount of blood on the cement—this explanation seemed unlikely.

Another possibility posed by the defense addressed this problem: she hit the pavement, lost consciousness, and lay on the cement, bleeding from the head wound. At some point, she regained consciousness, suffered a seizure caused by the head injury, and fell into the lake where she drowned—a possibility Dr. Cohle confirmed in earlier testimony.

The curious lack of blood on the pavement between where Florence hit the cement and the lake's edge seemed to support the prosecution's theory that she could not have rolled into the lake from the fall. This same curious fact also indicated that Mark Unger could not have dragged her body into the lake. The pool of blood indicated that her injury caused significant bleeding, yet crime scene investigators found no blood between the point of impact and the lake's edge. They didn't find blood or clothing fibers on the metal breakwater, either. Had Mark Unger dragged Florence over this area, certainly some blood would have appeared in this area. Unless he *carried* her body . . .

Although he did not take the stand and testify, Mark Unger maintained his innocence throughout the murder trial; he still does. Each side—the prosecution and the defense—posed a scenario to answer the question at the center of the forensic debate: how did Florence Unger's body get into Lower Herring Lake? After eights weeks of listening to two drastically different versions of Florence Unger's death and evidence to support them, the jury had to decide which version to believe. If the length of their deliberation was any indication, it was not an easy debate. After four days and twenty-six hours of deliberation, they returned their verdict. Mark Unger: guilty of first-degree murder—a verdict that led to an automatic sentence of life in prison without the possibility of parole.

Mark Unger has not yet submerged into the prison system; arms flailing, thrashing, through a series of appeals, he will fight against the rapids of the criminal justice system. For Mark Unger, the general maxim "innocent until proven guilty" has now become reversed: "guilty until proven innocent." His guilt or innocence aside, the central question posed by the forensic evidence will resurface: how did Florence Unger get into Lower Herring Lake?

The visitor to the Watervale Resort cannot help but feel a sense of nostalgia as he walks past the nineteenth-century structures that once housed exhausted lumberjacks. It can be said that the collective memory of a place is peopled by ghosts of its past. If that is true, Watervale has a new resident: a lovely, very sad brunette. In October 2003, the terrible death of Florence Unger added another chapter to the life of Watervale . . . another memory . . . and another ghost.

## Notes

1. Patrick Sullivan, "Examiners Don't Agree," *Traverse City Record-Eagle*, February 1, 2004, http://www.record-eagle.com/2004/feb/01unger.htm (accessed April 3, 2007).

2. Ibid., "Doctor: Death No Accident," *Traverse City Record-Eagle*, September 9, 2004, http://www.record-eagle.com/2004/sept/09unger.htm (accessed April 3, 2007).

3. Ibid., "Witnesses Recount Unger's Financial Woes," *Traverse City Record-Eagle*, May 11, 2006, http://www.record-eagle.com/2006/may/11unger .htm (accessed April 3, 2007).

4. Ibid.

5. Ibid.

6. Frank Witsil, "Unger Jury to Visit Site of Death Today," *Detroit Free Press*, May 3, 2006.

7. Quoted in Patrick Sullivan, "Suspicious Death: Preliminary Hearing for Mark Unger Begins," *Traverse City Record-Eagle*, July 7, 2004, http://www.record-eagle.com/2004/jul/07unger.htm (accessed April 3, 2007).

8. Jennie Miller, "Hairdresser Perceived Mark Unger as Habitual Liar," *Woodward Talk*, June 7, 2006, http://nl.newsbank.com/nlsearch/we/Archives?p_action=doc&p_docid=115DC52C34F6A3B8 (accessed August 6, 2007).

9. Mike Martindale, "MI Husband Behaved Oddly at Wife's Drowning Scene," *Detroit News*, May 5, 2006.

10. Quoted in "Examiners Disagree over Cause of Death," *Traverse City Record-Eagle*, June 2, 2006, http://www.record-eagle.com/2006/jun/02unger.htm (accessed April 3, 2007).

11. Ibid.

# 5. by reason of insanity?

In Ken Kesey's *One Flew over the Cuckoo's Nest*, Randle McMurphy attempts to scam the criminal justice system. Yet he soon learns the truth in the cliché "what comes around goes around." His girlfriend lied to him about her age, and a conviction for statutory rape follows. Like many savvy criminals, he knows that he can ameliorate his situation if he can serve his time in a psychiatric ward. With a little acting, McMurphy manages to convince prison guards that he needs psychiatric help. And off he goes to what he thinks is a vast improvement over the prison cellblock.

Kesey peoples his hospital with many fascinating characters who seem to drive McMurphy to figurative insanity, but what could be better? Cons know that guilty by reason of insanity can be a get out of jail card. Consider a hypothetical: two men are accused of the identical crime of engineering their wives' murders. One receives a first-degree murder conviction and is taken, kicking and screaming, to a maximum-security prison to serve a life sentence without parole or worse. He will languish for years in a jungle of gang warfare.

The other, who suffers from schizophrenia, is judged to be not guilty by reason of insanity. He will travel to a psychiatric hospital for incarceration and treatment. While his future freedom depends on his condition and the subjective opinion of his physicians, he could one day emerge from the hospital a free man.

The same crime. One in prison forever, in a hell straight from Dante's *Inferno*. A vast, criminal society replete with illicit drugs, homemade alcohol, rape, and brutality.

The other, in a relatively quiet hospital ward, while still incarcerated, can look out the window and see the trees of the forest just beyond, reasonably assured that he will not wake up with a shank in his chest because he wore the wrong colors.

To those accused of crimes, this juxtaposition is evident, as it was to the fictional Randle McMurphy, who managed to trade hard labor for afternoons playing poker.

Then he meets the custodian of the ward—Nurse Ratched—who is harder than the hardest prison warden. She is Machiavellian, oppressive, dictatorial, tyrannical; she is made of the same clay used to form third-world, ironfisted dictators. McMurphy's scam goes bad and ends up being worse than a life sentence when he receives a lobotomy after his protracted feud with Ratched. He traded his cellblock for Ratched's ward and consequently traded a short prison stint for a life sentence.

McMurphy's real-life parallels will do anything, including feign mental illness, to avoid prison. They will create "demons" that plague them, personalities who inhabit them, and strange compulsions that drive them to commit crimes. The legion of criminals attempting to whittle a life sentence down to a stint in a psychiatric hospital have, for some, made the phrase "not guilty by reason of insanity" synonymous with "scam." Exposing the scam is like catching a fish with bare hands: it takes a strong hand and a steady eye.

Some, on the other hand, are not faking their symptoms and really do need help. They do hear the voices of demons. Some must split time between multiple personalities. And some are driven by compulsions and cannot help themselves.

Demons, real and imagined, have contributed many skeletons to the medical examiner's closet. While the ME and forensic pathologist determine cause of death, attorneys and mental health professionals argue about mental pathology, because as the following stories illustrate, legal sanity and actual sanity are not the same thing.

## "I Did It, but *I* Didn't Do It"

Every city has a back pocket in which its underground commerce is conducted. Until the recent attempts to revitalize the inner city transformed old factories and hotels into first-class apartments and condominium developments in Grand Rapids, the underground sex and drug industries were centered in a territory bisected by North Division Street. This was a frontier of sorts, a boundary between the legal and decent and the illegal and indecent. Human life could be cheap along this frontier, the cost driven down by desperation caused by poverty or addiction. For the price of a bottle of cognac, or less, a woman could be purchased for an hour or two.

Part of the aptly named Commerce Avenue runs through this territory. Legitimate businesses line the streets of this area and conduct their affairs alongside of illegitimate businesses such as prostitution and drug peddling. It is on Commerce Avenue that an illicit business transaction turned into a murder case.

On the evening of April 19, 1988, as she left work at approximately 5:45 p.m., Margaret Gillis witnessed a curious scene: two people—a woman and a man—who appeared to be talking in the front seat of a burgundy-colored car parked on the side of the road. Thinking nothing of it, Gillis started toward her own car when she heard a bang, like the sound of a car backfiring.

A few seconds later, when she reached her car, Gillis heard another bang. When she turned to find the source of the noise, she saw a strange sight: the car in which the two people had been conversing was rolling backward down the street toward her, its passenger door open and now with only one occupant—a man on the driver's side. The woman—a blonde wearing a black leather jacket—had disappeared.

As the car rolled closer, she glimpsed a grisly scene. The man was slumped forward, leaning over the steering wheel with lines of blood running down his face. The car rolled by, then stopped when it ran into a telephone pole. Gillis raced back into her workplace and placed a 911 call.

When the victim, thirty-seven-year-old Raphael Alverado, stepped into the car with this woman, he may have thought he would be with Bambi; he couldn't have realized that instead he would face Lucy—a smoldering cauldron of rage.

The rage that ended with Alverado's murder began earlier that evening. It was an unseasonably cold day; the mercury topped out at 44 degrees Fahrenheit—14 degrees cooler than average, and inside Levata Stewart's apartment, a fire had begun to smolder.

That night Rosemarie McSwain, a twenty-year-old streetwalking prostitute and mother of two, brought her john—a man matching the description of the victim—to Stewart's apartment so they could use one of her rooms. The pair disappeared behind the door of the bedroom; fifteen or twenty minutes later, they emerged, McSwain enraged by something that had happened behind the closed bedroom door. Stewart's testimony at the trial suggested that the argument centered on money; Rosemarie McSwain demanded that he pay her for wasting her time; the man claimed he didn't have any money. Stewart further testified that McSwain reached into her purse, pulled out a handgun, pressed it against the man's penis, and declared that "she was going to blow his nuts off."[1]

Stewart took the gun from McSwain and put it back in her purse.

McSwain's threats escalated. As McSwain and the john left the apartment, Stewart testified that she heard McSwain threaten the man again: McSwain stated that "she was going to blow his head off."[2] At the time, Levata Stewart, according to her testimony at the subsequent trial, considered the statement a joke because she never knew Rosemarie McSwain as a violent person. A fire, though, had begun to burn inside the young prostitute.

An autopsy confirmed that the sound of a car backfiring came from a small-caliber handgun used to send two slugs into Alverado. One bullet entered above the victim's right eyelid. Stippling or gunpowder at the entrance wound suggested that the perpetrator fired the handgun from a distance of between six and twelve inches. If the perpetrator had pressed the gun against the victim's head, gas following the bullet discharge, with no place to escape, would follow the bullet and explode under the scalp, creating a stellate shape to the entrance wound. If the gun had been closer than six inches, the soot would surround the hole where the bullet entered the skull.

Of course, one could argue that the victim committed suicide, although the forensic evidence seems to suggest otherwise. Most suicide victims would not hold the gun so far from the head in case they were to miss, although one cannot dismiss the possibility as strange as it might seem. R. E. Kohlmeier et al. conducted a study of 1,704 suicides by firearm.[3] Some of the study's results are predictable; for example, the largest number (50 percent) used handguns to shoot themselves in the right temple (the majority being right-handed). The study, though, also produced some odd statistics: 3.6 percent used handguns to shoot themselves in the *back of the head* (3.8 percent used rifles and 1.2 percent used shotguns in the same manner)! And some (1.4 percent) even used handguns to shoot themselves in the stomach.

The fact that this victim did not appear to have held the gun tightly against his head does not dismiss suicide as a possibility. The second shot, though, makes suicide an unbelievable scenario. The second shot struck the victim in his right arm; the bullet moved through the arm, into his chest, and was found in the victim's aorta. Unless he shot himself in the arm before shooting himself in the head (it couldn't work the other way around), someone else pulled the trigger.

Because an eyewitness saw two people in the vehicle, heard the shots, then saw the car and its victim roll past, homicide seemed to be a foregone conclusion—a "date" between a prostitute and her john that turned murderous. Someone murdered Raphael Alverado.

That someone was Rosemarie McSwain. Or so it *appeared.*

Indeed, the alleged killer admitted her role in the murder. At one point during their date, McSwain took the handgun from her purse and shot her victim twice—a fact that she confirmed through confessions and partial confessions made to her cellmates in the Kent County Jail as she awaited trial. One cellmate heard her first deny her role in the murder, then state that "she didn't mean to do it"—a statement that both admits culpability for the crime and suggests she felt remorse.[4]

The defense invoked an argument of mistaken identity, but prosecutors had no shortage of evidence to prove that the murder resulted from premeditation inspired by the victim's failure to pay for services rendered. Levata Stewart, whose apartment the pair used for their first liaison of the evening at approximately 5 p.m. (forty-five minutes before the murder), testified that although she knew McSwain as a brunette, the night of the incident at the apartment, McSwain had blonde hair and wore a black leather jacket. Her description of McSwain matched the one provided by Margaret Gillis, who saw the two in Alverado's burgundy car just before hearing the gunshots.

McSwain's defense produced an alibi: her half sister picked up McSwain and her boyfriend from a nearby corner and drove them to a house about two miles from the murder scene, where they spent several hours together. This story, however, actually helped the case against McSwain. The alibi indicated that she had been in the area of the shooting and could have walked the distance from the scene to the corner where she supposedly met her half sister.

The prosecution argued a different scenario: Alverado picked up McSwain at approximately 5 p.m. The pair traveled to Stewart's apartment, where behind closed doors an argument erupted regarding payment for McSwain's services. They returned to the corner where Alverado had initially picked up McSwain, and the argument continued, this time ending in his murder.

The trial was what a prosecutor might call a slam dunk, or an open-and-shut case. The eight-day trial concluded with a verdict of guilty and a life sentence for premeditated murder and the possession of a firearm in commission of a felony.

This case appeared to be over. But appearances can be deceiving. A strange twist led to a reexamination of the murder trial that sent McSwain to prison for life without the possibility of parole.

During the next eleven years of her incarceration, Rosemarie McSwain exhibited what many fellow inmates considered strange and inconsistent behavior. On one hot summer day, she wore an extravagant ball gown; on another occasion, she awoke in the middle of the night and began to color with crayons on paper and even on the walls of her cell.

Her mannerisms would vacillate from childlike to authoritarian. Even though McSwain referred to herself by different names—variations of Rosemarie such as "Rose," "Marie" and "Maria," as well as other names such as "Passion"—acquaintances in prison knew her by her street name, "Bambi." But when they came across Rosemarie McSwain, they never knew which Rosemarie McSwain they would see: the shy, reserved, childlike Jekyll or the aggressive, brazen Hyde. Who would they see, they wondered? They didn't realize that they may have met not only Rosemarie McSwain but also several others who inhabited the same body.

Someone else, though, did realize this bizarre possibility.

Dr. Steven Miller examined Rosemarie McSwain in March 1997—almost nine years after the crime that sent her to prison for the rest of her life—to determine if she suffered from a legally defined mental illness. After more than seven hours during which he examined and tested McSwain, he concluded "very little doubt" existed that she suffered from an illness known as dissociative identity disorder (DID), more commonly known as multipersonality or split personality.[5]

Many psychologists, psychiatrists, and others who have studied the human mind believe that DID can result from some traumatic event. The human mind is like a pane of glass. A horrific, traumatizing event, such as a gang rape or a violent crime, can, like a hammer, shatter the pane of glass, fragmenting it into several distinct personalities.

For Rosemarie McSwain, the hammer may have fallen as the result of horrific sexual abuse by her stepfather. In her testimony at the appeal, Rosemarie McSwain described the alleged abuse she suffered as a young girl. According to McSwain, the alleged abuse began when she was about ten, when her stepfather tied her up in a shed and forced her to have sex with him, including oral, anal, and vaginal. In one instance, she alleged, he raped her vaginally with a glass bottle. She recounted another incident when he hanged her upside down, and stated in court that he often burned her legs with smoldering cigarette butts; she showed the scars from this alleged abuse at her appeal hearing. This brutal treatment would explain the existence of a street-wise personality that acted as the guardian of the group: Lucy.

The alleged abuse may have begun at an earlier age, but by age twelve, Rosemarie McSwain began a downward spiral; an initial hospitalization at a psychiatric facility at age twelve would be followed by several more in her teen years for drug use and depression. She testified that she became involved in several abusive relationships with men, including her stepfather, and eventually turned to prostitution.

Dr. Miller believed that Rosemarie McSwain's personality split occurred at about the age of three to three and a half, when she developed the personality of "Baby Rose" (perhaps the personality who colored on her cell walls). She developed a "core" personality as a teenager. Others appeared later: the prostitute "Bambi"; "Passion"—an entity Dr. Miller characterized as a "sexual person"; and "Lucy"—a streetwise personality and the protector of the whole clan.[6] When the other personalities needed protection if they felt threatened, they turned to Lucy.

A second expert, Dr. Greeley Gregory Miklashek, who interviewed Rosemarie McSwain for a little over an hour in September 2000, also concluded that she suffered from DID. According to Rosemarie McSwain, no fewer than eight personalities inhabited her person, ranging in age from three to the late forties. These personalities included (their ages in parentheses) "Baby Rose" (three); "Rosemarie" (sixteen); "Maria" (seventeen); "Passion" (eighteen); "Bambi" (nineteen); "Gemini Light" (nineteen); "Lucy" (forty-three); "Gemini Dark" (forty-seven). "Lucy," like an older sibling or even a parent figure, played the role of protector for "Rose," "Rosemarie," and "Gemini Light." Like Dr. Miller, Dr. Miklashek believed that the split likely dated from an early incident of abuse, most likely one that occurred when she was around the age of three.[7]

During the interview with Dr. Miklashek, McSwain expressed her remorse for the death of her victim, but offered an explanation not forwarded at her 1988 trial: Lucy committed the murder to protect Bambi, whom she apparently felt was in harm's way.

So why didn't McSwain present this as a defense at her 1988 trial? During her interview with Dr. Miklashek, she stated that "we didn't correspond and share the way we do now."[8] According to his testimony at the appeal hearing, Dr. Miklashek witnessed a switch as Lucy took over, accompanied by a drastic change in facial expression.

The possibility that Rosemarie McSwain suffered from DID in 1988 created an interesting legal question: who killed Raphael Alverado on the night of April 19, 1988? Perhaps Bambi stepped into the car that evening, but it appears that Lucy emerged. One can imagine the scene of a john assaulting or perhaps raping a prostitute—a defense invoked by Florida's serial killer Aileen Wuornos. If Bambi felt at all at risk, Lucy would have appeared to protect her, and she did: with two bullets from a handgun. Dr. Miller opined that to protect the other personalities, Lucy committed the murder.[9]

A motion for relief from judgment followed, based on the notion that in 1988, Rosemarie McSwain was not competent to stand trial. The court did not revisit her guilt or innocence in the murder; at no time did Rosemarie McSwain deny involvement. In fact, she continued to express her remorse that Lucy shot the man and caused so much trouble.

At the behest of the trial court, a third doctor interviewed Rosemarie McSwain, Dr. Arthur Marroquin. Unlike the other experts, Dr. Marroquin also studied the original trial transcripts as part of his examination. In his three interviews with Rosemarie McSwain, he witnessed nothing—no sudden changes in demeanor, voice tone or inflection, or facial expression—to suggest the presence or even existence of alter egos. McSwain signed prison forms with the name "Rosemarie

McSwain," which seemed to belie the idea of a fragmented psyche. In short, Dr. Marroquin opined that the evidence suggested she was competent to stand trial both in the present and at her 1988 murder trial.[10] The voices of the other experts, though, would drown out this dissenting voice.

In August 2001, after hearing from a parade of convincing witnesses including Drs. Miller and Miklashek, the court granted Rosemarie McSwain's motion; she would have a second day in court and the opportunity to present a new defense based on her alleged DID. A portion of their reasoning, quoted in the opinion of the state appeals court, bears reproducing here:

> This court is extremely reluctant to open up once again a murder case that was tried before a jury some eleven years ago. The court fully recognizes the need for finality. Similarly, the court is of the opinion that medical evidence involving psychiatric conditions is not always as objectively reliable as other types of medical testimony. Furthermore, given the offense for which defendant was convicted, and the life sentence with no possibility of parole necessarily imposed following trial, defendant has nothing to lose by bringing this motion, and everything to gain. Defendant could well be scamming the court and the system.
>
> On the other hand, defendant through very competent and diligent counsel presented a compelling case that she had and continues to have several distinct personalities. Until hearing the evidence presented, this court would have been very much inclined to dismiss as psycho-babble the claims presented by defendant. In the end, justice and fairness is every bit as important to the system as is finality and convenience. If defendant is scamming the court, she is doing so only after convincing two attorneys, four mental health professionals, and a close friend that she has a mental illness (DID), and that such illness made her incompetent and criminally not responsible at time of the offense and trial in question.[11]

Three possibilities exist: (1) Rosemarie McSwain suffered from DID in 1988, but her condition was unrecognized, and one of her other personalities committed the 1988 murder; (2) her personality split was the result of some event that occurred after 1988, perhaps something that happened to her in prison; or (3) she does not suffer from DID. In its opinion, the court acknowledged the possibility of (3) and that she could be "scamming the court and the system"—a possibility diminished under the weight of the experts who testified that they believed she did suffer from DID.

Not surprisingly, the matter wound up in front of the State of Michigan Court of Appeals, which reviewed the trial court's decision to grant the motion for relief. After deliberation, the court of appeals overturned the trial court's decision; McSwain would not have a second day in court after all. Even if Rosemarie McSwain suffered from DID, the court reasoned, no evidence was presented during her appeal to indicate that she suffered from DID in 1988, or that she was not competent to stand trial, or that a jury would rule any differently than it did in 1988. In fact, Dr. Marroquin, who studied the original trial transcripts, testified that he believed her competent to stand trial in 1988.[12]

Rosemarie McSwain and all of her alleged alter egos returned to prison to serve her sentence for premeditated murder, where she (they) will spend the rest of her (their) life (lives) in prison. At least, if she does suffer from DID, she won't be lonely.

The plot of the William Diehl novel *Primal Fear*, the basis for the 1996 film of the same name starring Richard Gere and Edward Norton, provides an interesting comment on the issue of DID and criminal responsibility. An altar boy, Aaron Stampler, played by Edward Norton, is accused of murdering Archbishop Richard Rushman, who sexually abused his charges. Attorney Martin Vail (Richard Gere in the cinematic version) takes the case. In the course of his preparation, Vail discovers that Aaron suffers from DID.

In the end, though (humble apologies if you have not yet read the book or seen the movie) Martin Vail discovers that Stampler is a superb actor who is faking it.

Despite claims of multiple personality disorder, one certainty remains: Raphael Alverado died in his car on Commerce Avenue.

The argument that precipitated his murder was over $50. Life can indeed be cheap on the street.

## Notes

1. *People v. McSwain*, 259 Mich. App. 654 (2003).
2. Ibid.
3. R. E. Kohlmeier et al., "Suicide by Firearms," *American Journal of Forensic Medical Pathology* 22 (2001): 337–40.
4. *People v. McSwain*, 259 Mich. App. 654 (2003).
5. Ibid.
6. Ibid.
7. Ibid.
8. Ibid.
9. Ibid.
10. Ibid.
11. Ibid.
12. Ibid.

## Loved Him to Death

The pile of manila files stands several feet high on top of the desk in Wayland chief of police Dan Miller's office. It consists of various reports, trial transcripts, and several long pieces of graph paper, which, pieced together, form a chronicle of murder that occurred almost seventeen years ago. The files detail the most complicated and disturbing case any cop could encounter in his career, a case Chief Miller, a thirty-year veteran of the Wayland police department, remembers well. How could he forget?

Miller points to the window of his office. It all happened about two blocks from the station.

In fact, the evidence room at the back of the Wayland police station still contains vital items from the city's highest-profile and most shocking case to date: the perpetrator's personal Bible, the clothes she wore when arrested, a stack of journals completed during stints in drug rehab, and the most important piece of evidenced: an electronic monitor about the size of a shoebox.

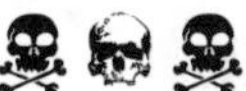

The City of Wayland police department is a small-town station. It doesn't even contain a holding cell. It doesn't need one. If the need arises, and it rarely does, an officer must drive the prisoner twenty miles to another town.

Wayland is a living remnant of small-town America. It's a place where residents can leave their cars unlocked in their driveways. And some do. A place where residents can leave their homes unlocked without fear of becoming a violent crime statistic. And some do that, too.

It is a place where residents walk down the streets and give a thankful nod to a passing police officer, where they know Dan Miller as a neighbor and friend as well as chief of police.

It is a peaceful place.

One fall night almost twenty years ago, that peace was shattered by the sound of a mother's screams . . .

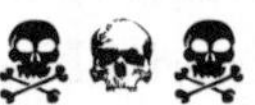

A 911 call from a desperate mother brought paramedics to the Wayland home in the middle of the night of September 25, 1990. The mother, Diane Spencer, reported that her six-month-old son, Aaron, had stopped breathing.

This serious problem had occurred in the past. One state trooper had been to the home a few months earlier on a similar call. And on three previous occasions in the last few months, Spencer had brought the child to a Grand Rapids hospital and reported to physicians that Aaron had trouble breathing and that his breathing had even stopped. A pediatrician had even prescribed a sleep monitor to warn of trouble.

As the emergency personnel arrived, they heard screaming. Inside the house, they found the mother—twenty-two-year-old Diane Spencer—leaning over her son's unconscious body, performing CPR on the infant. She told them that she had discovered him unconscious and not breathing.

But had she? The scene, although horrific, contained a few oddities that raised suspicions despite the boy's medical history. Aaron Spencer was not wearing the sleep apnea monitor his pediatrician prescribed and he was blue, as if he had died some time before they arrived, raising the possibility that some time had elapsed between the baby's death and the 911 call.

But why would she wait?

Perhaps she found her son dead but desperation caused her to attempt resuscitation.

Or a more sinister possibility: perhaps the scene was staged . . .

The paramedics rushed Aaron to a downtown Grand Rapids hospital about twenty-five miles away, but he arrived too late. The child would never see his first birthday party, never enjoy his first Christmas.

His body was sent to the Kent County Morgue to find out what had caused his untimely death. Aaron Spencer's death appeared to be caused by SIDS, or sudden infant death syndrome—a killer as frightening to parents as the worst serial killers. An autopsy is typical for cases in which SIDS appears to have reached out its hand and pulled another helpless infant into an early grave.

Many questions remain unanswered about SIDS, sometimes called "crib death," in which some force or forces cause a child to stop breathing. One possible scenario that leads to a SIDS death: an infant rolls onto his stomach and, unable to roll over again, suffocates, as his head becomes buried in soft bedding, a sheet, or even a plush toy. The infant does not necessarily suffocate from a lack of oxygen; rather, the infant inhales his own exhalation. The carbon dioxide–rich gas paralyzes the brain stem, which controls breathing. The infant dies of asphyxia.

SIDS has no clear cause of death, but SIDS deaths sometimes do leave forensic clues for the ME to find. One piece of forensic evidence appears in about half of SIDS cases: tiny red spots called petechial hemorrhages will dot the thymus (a fan-shaped organ that produces T lymphocytes; by adulthood, the gland has atrophied to the point of virtual nonexistence) and the lungs. Aaron Spencer's lungs did contain such petechiae, or pinpoint hemorrhages, which look like red pepper sprinkled on a deep purple surface.

Yet curiously, the autopsy revealed no anatomical cause for Aaron's alleged breathing problems—the same breathing problems that caused his mother to call 911. A few other circumstances raised the suspicion of foul play and with it the seemingly unbelievable, horrific possibility that someone had murdered the six-month-old infant. Too many factors suggested murder: what appeared to be a significant time lapse between when Aaron died and his mother called 911; the fact that when he stopped breathing, Aaron was not wearing his prescribed sleep apnea monitor; and a medical history of cardiopulmonary problems with no clear cause. A criminal investigation followed, and the trail led to Aaron's pediatrician and the fascinating story of the sleep apnea monitor . . .

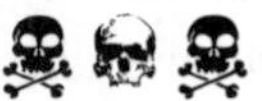

Like a good mystery novel, this story begins in *medias res*—in the middle of things; Aaron's death represents only the opening scene. This story had a significant back story that would begin to materialize as investigators probed Diane Spencer's background. The investigation began simply enough with a phone call.

Suspicious circumstances led Dr. Cohle to contact Wayland chief of police Dan Miller. Miller recalls the exact moment his investigation began, when he received the fateful call from the Kent County ME suggesting he probe the premature death of Aaron Spencer. He was sipping coffee at his brother's Phillips 66 gas station. Miller had known about the case before the call, because state police officers at the scene had discussed it with him. And Miller had known of Diane Spencer from a pending check forgery accusation. Now, on the other end of the phone was the Kent County ME, calling from twenty miles north. Several aspects of the case were suspicious. "Things just didn't add up," Miller recalls.[1]

Miller's investigation had begun. He traveled north to the ME's office to study the autopsy reports. It was there that he first heard about a strange mental condition called Munchausen by proxy syndrome. And it was there that he learned about the apnea monitor.

Miller followed the trail to hospital personnel who had treated Aaron for numerous ailments, one of which was sleep apnea. The trip to the hospital the night he died was *not* the first time Aaron Spencer had visited; his mother had sought help for the child because, she claimed, he had moments when he experienced trouble breathing or cessation of breathing (apnea) and he suffered from seizures. Consequently, Aaron had made several visits to the hospital. One of those visits occurred in early September 1990.

During this visit, hospital personnel observed some strange, inexplicable behavior from Aaron's mother, including an incident when Diane Spencer disconnected a monitor connected to Aaron by unplugging it from the wall. She got in the way while they treated Aaron. She was told to do one thing, and she did the opposite. She became so intrusive, she was warned that if she didn't stop interfering, steps would be taken to keep her from visiting Aaron while in the hospital.

After a thorough examination and a battery of tests, physicians could find nothing wrong: no congenital heart abnormalities, no abnormal heart rhythm, nothing to explain how or why the child had episodes during which he stopped breathing or had seizures. Nothing could explain the boy's problems. The absence of a medical cause for the boy's breathing troubles led to some speculation.

*Did* Aaron Spencer have trouble breathing, or was the boy's affliction a figment of his mother's imagination? The presentation of illness with no clear cause led to speculation that Aaron's Spencer's illness may have begun in his mother's mind.

Perhaps his mother imagined her son's difficulties.

Perhaps she misread some symptom, real or imagined, and as all parents do on occasion, made a diagnosis but an incorrect one.

Perhaps the paranoia of an overzealous and worried parent led to a perceived medical condition.

Or perhaps something else occurred, perhaps another, more sinister possibility had brought Aaron to the hospital. Perhaps Diane Spencer created a fictional medical illness for her son and forced him to live through it.

Perhaps Diane Spencer suffered from a mental condition known as Munchausen by proxy syndrome—an extremely rare disorder. (In fact, this possibility was raised to Spencer during her son's early September hospitalization, and she was offered counseling, but she refused.) The condition is so rare, in fact, that many practicing clinical psychologists can complete their careers without ever treating a patient who suffers from it. For psychologists, Munchausen by proxy syndrome is the psychological world's version of a blue diamond . . . or perhaps uraninite makes for a better analogy. This rare, radioactive metal is found in tiny amounts in other rock. And a prolonged exposure to a significant quantity can lead to sickness and even death.

It is an appropriate analogy, because people who suffer from Munchausen by proxy syndrome can be very dangerous to those around them. They can be deadly. Especially to children like Aaron Spencer.

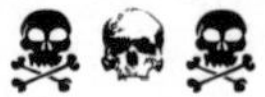

The disorder takes its name from an eighteenth-century German baron named Karl Friedrich Hieronymus, Freiherr von Münchhausen.[2] Münchhausen served with the Russian military and saw action against the Ottoman Empire on two separate occasions, eventually achieving the rank of cavalry captain. Like his name, Münchhausen was a larger-than-life character, or at least he presented himself that way; in his retirement, he earned a reputation for telling wildly embellished stories of his past.

Before Münchhausen died, an anonymous author wrote a book that supposedly represented a collection of Münchhausen's stories and semifictitious experiences; the book, which reappeared in various editions for years, took many of the stories from other sources. The tall tales became wondrous examples of exaggeration.

For example, the first English version published in 1785 depicts the baron as visiting the moon and riding on a cannonball. In one adventure, he spots and shoots down a balloon, only to find a French philosopher dangling from it! In another adventure, he protects himself from a wolf by wondrously turning the wolf inside out. Ironically, in chapter 20, the baron expounds the virtues of veracity, or truthfulness! The baron, it appeared, had become larger than life in print, larger than the larger-than-life character he presented to friends through his stories. Much larger . . .

The book's publication damaged the baron's reputation. While the actual baron told embellished stories to entertain and charm his company and not to further his reputation, the exploits of his fictional counterpart gave Münchhausen a reputation as one of the world's great prevaricators. His name became synonymous with the tall tale and those who delight in creating and telling such stories.

Unfortunately and perhaps unfairly, his name has subsequently been linked with a very dangerous mental condition—a fact that no doubt would have bothered the gregarious German baron, who never used his stories to harm others, unlike those who suffer from the condition that carries his name.

Like the fictional Baron Münchhausen, those suffering from Munchausen syndrome—a mental condition that falls into a category called factitious disorder—tell tall tales. They compulsively fake medical conditions. It goes beyond malingering. A malingerer fakes illness for a specific purpose; for example, a high school student may fake an illness to miss a test.

For those suffering from Munchausen syndrome, the medical care is the purpose of the fictitious illnesses. These people crave the attention that such feigned illnesses bring; the symptoms of illness do not lead to suffering but to the attention they desire. The treatment by a physician may represent the love they perceive as missing in their lives (people who suffer from such factitious disorders often had a cold, loveless parent who neglected them). And their desperation for such affection from doctors and hospital staff leads them to some desperate measures to feign illness, including self-mutilation.

An extremely rare variant of this factitious illness is called Munchausen by proxy syndrome and it represents one of the worst forms of child abuse. A parent, almost always the mother, will fake an illness in a child or worse create an actual illness, which can lead to physical harm or even death. The parent presents the child to a physician for treatment and thrives on the attention that results. The parent often causes real illness or injuries for the physician to treat, and misadventure or miscalculation may lead to the death of the child. Likewise, the physician may actually unwittingly harm or injure the child when attempting to treat for an illness that does not exist.

The child, often an infant, does not understand the fictional web in which he has become entangled and is powerless to alter the situation. The child is the pawn in the parent's deadly game. And the parent is usually a very accomplished game player. She becomes extremely adept at fooling medical professionals; her medical knowledge is usually very detailed and extensive, because to fool a doctor, it would need to be. She's so convincing that often practitioners question themselves rather than her. And she typically has had practice by the time her ruse is discovered, practice that sometimes has ended in tragedy: in some cases, an older sibling has died of mysterious and undiagnosed causes.

In most cases of Munchausen by proxy syndrome, the mother appears to care for the child, while behind the curtain she is the cause of injury and potentially even death. When her lie becomes exposed, most associated with her cannot believe her capable of perpetrating such horrific injuries on her child. And some of the injuries can be extreme: she may induce in her child seizures or diarrhea or an infection . . .

. . . or trouble breathing? Aaron Spencer's doctor could find no medical explanation for a breathing problem, which raised the suspicion that the mother and not the child was the source of the problem: that she possibly suffered from Munchausen by proxy, that she faked the symptoms of Aaron's pseudomedical condition, that her son had become her pawn in a game that could and did turn deadly.

Through a follow-up interview with Diane Spencer, investigators also learned that, while a resident of Pennsylvania, she had lost another child to SIDS—a medical rarity bordering on an aberration. And investigators subsequently learned that she had lost yet another to SIDS. Aaron would have made a third SIDS death. This raised the level of suspicion even higher. SIDS, although the most common cause of death of children less than a year old, very rarely is the cause of death of more than one child in a family. A second instance of SIDS striking the same family occurs with the frequency of lightning striking the same place twice. In humans, the cause of a second "strike" could be an inherited mutation or an environmental factor, such as a faulty furnace producing carbon dioxide. As his pediatrician discovered, however, Aaron Spencer had no heart disease or other inherited diseases. Something else went wrong to cause his death, something like homicide.

But if Aaron's troubles really originated in his mother's mind—a conclusion that fit the absence of any real medical problems but seemed incongruous with the loving mother's personality—the apnea monitor would not or could not protect little Aaron Spencer. It would, however, provide vital evidence if the boy's heart stopped and would indicate what occurred during the event. Ultimately, Diane Spencer would be trapped in the web by the sleep apnea monitor—a web she created when she repeatedly complained about Aaron's breathing trouble.

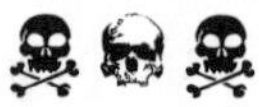

Aaron left the hospital, but this time with some protection. During his investigation, Chief Miller discovered that on September 10—a few weeks before Aaron's death—Diane Spencer had obtained a sleep apnea monitor from a medical equipment supplier—White and White.

A pediatrician prescribed the monitor to protect Aaron from an untimely death at the hands of the fiendish SIDS and also because he suspected that Diane Spencer feigned her son's problems. The sleep apnea monitor—a device the size of small shoe box and weighing about four pounds—was designed to measure an infant's breathing. The little box contains a few dials and four leads with suction cups that adhere to the baby's body. A green light indicates proper functioning; a red light indicates that an "event" (apnea, meaning a cessation of breathing) has occurred, and an alarm sounds to wake up the baby and/or alert the parents that the child has stopped breathing. It is an alarm that screams trouble loud enough to wake a sleeping parent. It was designed that way. It was designed to be loud enough to wake the dead.

Yet Diane complained that the monitor didn't function properly. She also reported that Aaron had continued to experience seizure and apnea episodes, so once again Aaron was hospitalized. When he was released, another apnea monitor was prescribed and subsequently placed in the home on September 14. This time, however, the monitor had a memory chip. Spencer had asked the technician who delivered the device what the memory chip recorded, but it appeared that she didn't entirely understand its function. Just over a week and a half later, Aaron was dead.

Chief Miller did not know about the apnea monitor chip until three days after Aaron's death, when he interviewed hospital personnel who had treated Aaron. By this point, Spencer had returned the monitor to the medical supplier. Now, Miller needed to know what the monitor remembered about that night in late September. He needed to locate the monitor's memory chip and get a printout that could provide information about Aaron Spencer's last night. So Miller visited the medical supplier and obtained the apnea monitor and the printed downloads from the monitor's chip.

It was clear that someone had tampered with the monitor. Five screws were missing from the ends of the device (three from the left side and two from the right). But it was the memory chip that contained the evidence that something other than SIDS had taken Aaron Spencer's life.

The printout provided a chronicle of the minutes during which Aaron died:

| | |
|---|---|
| 0449 | monitor turned off |
| 0525:21 | monitor turned on; five-second alarm sounded |
| 0525:26 | monitor turned off |
| 0526:42 | monitor turned on |
| 0526:53 | monitor turned off |
| 0529:04 | monitor turned on for a duration of three seconds then turned off permanently[3] |

State police detective Ron Neil (see "The Hand That Feeds"), who was attached to the Wayland post and had joined the investigation, recalls seeing the printouts. "It was shocking," he recalls. "We were able to pinpoint time of death."[4] The printout also showed that someone had manually shut off the apnea monitor at 4:49. The alarm had not gone off; it was turned off. Thirty-six minutes later—at 0525:21—the printout shows that the monitor was turned back on, and all the vital signs monitored and recorded were "flatlined"—Aaron had died. The printout also indicated that once again the monitor was shut off briefly and then turned on again a few times: strange events in the chronicle.

The printout provided investigators with a horrific scenario and one that presented a sharp contrast to the story Spencer told them. Spencer's story: the apnea alarm went off, she went in to check on Aaron, awakened him, placed the monitor back on him; it seemed to be functioning properly. A period of time elapsed, and it went off again. She went back in and found him not breathing.

The scenario suggested by the apnea monitor's printout: someone shut off the monitor and, in the thirty-six minutes not recorded by the monitor, murdered Aaron, probably by pressing something soft like a pillow or a towel over his face. That someone replaced the monitor on Aaron's dead body, which explains the flatline. This time line raised a few questions: why did that someone wait for an extended period after the flatline—perhaps an hour—before alerting authorities? And why did that someone turn the monitor off again and then on after the flatline? Detective Neil speculated that that someone turned the monitor off and then on because it was one way to see if Aaron was dead.[5]

That someone, investigators believed, was Diane Spencer.

Chief Miller did some investigative legwork. He probed Diane Spencer's biography. Spencer, he learned, had lived for a time in Pennsylvania. And in Pennsylvania, she had lost not one, but *two* other children to SIDS. "Now I knew that something was up," Miller recalls.[6] This last piece of information left little doubt. The day after Thanksgiving 1990, he traveled to Pennsylvania to gather information.

Aaron Spencer's "SIDS" had begun to look more like a homicide, and the murder investigation focused on the one suspect in the case. Chief Miller and Michigan state police detective Ron Neil went to interview Diane Spencer, but they could not find her. They eventually managed to track her down: she had checked herself into a drug rehab center in Grand Rapids, technically "off-limits" for investigators, so they waited. Meanwhile, Chief Miller obtained an arrest warrant for uttering and publishing (a felony): Spencer had allegedly taken checks from her mother without permission and forged her mother's name.

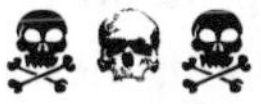

Spencer's presence in the drug rehabilitation center represented the next step in a cycle that characterized her life from the late teenage years until the present. Diane Spencer's biography would read like a season of episodes from a soap opera: melodrama ending with tragedy.

Diane Spencer's life story is replete with abuse and addiction. She claimed to have been a victim of sexual abuse as a child.[7] At a very early age, she heard the siren's song and, unable to resist temptation, began abusing substances including alcohol, cocaine, marijuana, methamphetamine, and speed. In one of the journals she completed as part of a drug rehabilitation program, she explains that she first got drunk at age twelve on sloe gin. She became so sick, she swore she would never drink again.

She got drunk the next weekend.

Her substance abuse escalated. By age fourteen, she notes in another journal entry, she drank five days a week, smoked marijuana every day, took "drop speed" almost every day, and experimented with LSD and hash. She ran away from home on several occasions and eventually found her way into a youth home.

She also had trouble with relationships. Beginning in her teen years and extending into adulthood, she became entwined in a series of disastrous relationships resulting in three children sired from three different men.

At fifteen, Diane left the youth home and began a two-year trek hitchhiking. During this nomadic period, she fell back into habitual drug use. Her last ride, it appeared, came from a truck driver who became her lover and fathered her first child. Although she did not wed the truck driver, Diane settled in Pennsylvania and at sixteen gave birth to Joyce Anne Denochick in August 1983. The pair broke up after the birth of their daughter. Six weeks later, Joyce Anne died, presumably a SIDS victim. After the death of her daughter, Diane once again fell under the spell of drugs.

This time Diane wound up in jail facing drug-trafficking charges; there she met her future husband, the father of her second child. For Diane, however, history would repeat itself. She gave birth to Autumn Dawn in August 1987, but for a second time, SIDS took her child. She was seventeen days old. In the wake of Dawn's untimely passing, the relationship dissolved, although the couple would never divorce. Diane Spencer, it appeared, was a modern version of Tantalus, for whom domestic bliss remained just out of reach.

She moved to Michigan to spend time with her mother. Diane left

Pennsylvania, it appeared, to come home (she was raised in a suburb west of Grand Rapids), to start over, because in her wake she left tragedy. Her friends and acquaintances initially believed that Diane's two daughters died as a result of a horrific coincidence.

Despite the change in setting, Diane Spencer could not flee the siren's song, although she tried. It was at a Narcotics Anonymous meeting that she would meet the future father of her third child. A six-month romance followed, but the relationship ended before the birth of their child, Aaron, in March 1990. Aaron would follow his older sisters to an early grave and die before he reached his first birthday. And Diane would once again start using, which led her to check into a rehabilitation center.

Outside, investigators waited for her to leave. They wanted to discuss the night Aaron Spencer died and the possibility that Aaron's SIDS death was one more of his mother's fabrications.

Diane Spencer, in addition to a recurring substance abuse problem, also had a penchant for lying. She told wild stories to gain attention, according to a former roommate with whom Spencer lived while pregnant with Aaron.[8] When she came home on crutches and sporting several abrasions, she told her roommate that she was hit by a car. Later, when confronting her disbelieving roommate, she changed the story: a drug dealer beat her for the five hundred dollars she owed. During this period, Spencer wrote letters to her husband. The letters, which perhaps represent a life she desired but never obtained, contain more lies: she tells him that she completed an engineering degree, for example. No one, though, seemed willing to believe that Spencer, who appeared to care very deeply for Aaron, could have perpetrated so horrific a crime as murdering her own child.

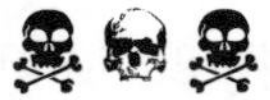

When she left the drug rehabilitation center in downtown Grand Rapids in December 1990, Chief Miller and Detective Neil arrested her. They took her to Lansing, where a state police polygraph examiner waited to administer a polygraph test. Spencer signed a waiver indicating that she understood her Miranda rights and that she was willing to talk with investigators. About six hours of intense interviewing followed—from about 8 p.m. to 2 a.m. the following morning—during which Spencer never asked for an attorney.

The process began when Michigan state police detective sergeant John Palmatier administered three polygraph tests, which clearly indicated she was lying about events that occurred that night.

When confronted with the results of the polygraph tests and the possibility that she murdered her son, Diane Spencer flatly denied it. She claimed that even though she knew she shouldn't have, she took Aaron off the apnea monitor and fell asleep on the couch with Aaron in her arms. When she awoke later, he was dead. She tried desperately to revive him, but her efforts were in vain.

Yet Spencer sprinkled into her conversation with Palmatier a few suspicious statements: she said that she was going to prison and at one point asked Palmatier if she was going to prison for the rest of her life. Despite these cracks in her façade, she maintained her story of how Aaron died.

After a cigarette break, the conversation shifted to the deaths of her two children in Pennsylvania. Again, she laced the conversation with strange statements about going to prison. When once again confronted with the idea that she killed her children, her façade crumbled. She began to cry. She admitted to murdering Joyce—her first child—by placing a towel over the child's mouth. She then admitted to murdering Autumn—her second child—in the same manner. She murdered the two children, but she didn't know why.

Then the conversation returned to her third child—Aaron. At first, she stuck with the story she initially told investigators, but after a few minutes, she said that she was going to prison and would likely be killed there because of what she did. She then admitted to murdering Aaron by pressing a pillow over his face and suffocating him. Several times throughout her confession, she noted how much she loved Aaron.

Now Spencer agreed to repeat the confession to Detective Neil, who waited in another room with Chief Miller and watched Palmatier's discussion with Spencer.

"'You know, he really knows what's going on in my fucking head,'" Miller recalls Spencer saying of Palmatier.[9]

She repeated her confession.

She told Neil that she placed a towel over Joyce's face with the intent to kill the six-and-a-half-week-old infant. When asked to show how she did it, she demonstrated by placing her open hand over her own mouth and nose. Joyce didn't die, though, so she called an ambulance. The infant lived on life support for a few days at the hospital before it was removed.

She loved Joyce, she told Neil, but she intended to murder the child by suffocating her. She just didn't know why.

She killed fifteen-day-old Autumn in the same manner, but this time she smothered the baby with a blanket. Diane admitted that she intended to kill the baby, but again, she told Neil, who found the lack of motive frustrating, she didn't know why.

Aaron, who was the final victim in this ghastly series of murders, suffered the same fate as his sisters. Diane lay down with him on the couch and pressed a pillow over his face until he stopped breathing. She did this with the intent to kill him, but once again, she did not know why. After he stopped breathing, she tried to resuscitate him. She turned the monitor on several times to see if he was alive or dead, which explains the bizarre sequence of events recorded on the apnea monitor's memory chip. She told Neil, however, that she never tampered with the monitor. When she failed to revive Aaron, she called for help.

She acknowledged that some of Aaron's ailments for which she consulted a doctor were not real. She gave a detailed report on things she had done to Aaron so she could take him to the doctor. And she knew what symptoms Aaron needed in order to fit a certain diagnosis. According to Detective Neil, Diane Spencer had a wealth of knowledge of medical terms, a knowledge that became obvious from his interviews with her, a knowledge that transcended that of a layperson.

Subsequent investigation would also reveal that she had done the same thing to herself: she cut herself so she could go to the hospital.

Throughout her confession, she kept reiterating her love for the child. "She kept saying, 'You have no idea how much I loved him,'" Neil recalls.[10] She punctuated the interview by reiterating the truthfulness of her statements.

On the return trip to Grand Rapids, Diane Spencer, after the terrible truth about her son Aaron's death finally had been exposed to authorities, curled into a ball and remained in a fetal position the entire ninety-minute journey from the state's capital city.

Diane Spencer faced one count of first-degree murder and, if convicted, a life sentence without the possibility of parole. When the judge read the charge, Neil recounts, she collapsed onto the floor. She "crumbled."

By this time, Diane Spencer had come to trust and respect Detective Neil. As sometimes happens between investigators and the accused, a relationship of trust develops and the investigator becomes the confidante of the accused. Yet, as a law enforcement agent, he could act on information of a criminal nature she told him in confidence, so initially Spencer's attorney barred communication between the two.

Spencer, though, had become attached to her confidante, so an agreement was reached between the prosecution and the defense: Detective Neil could visit her in jail, but anything that transpired was privileged.

"I honestly believe that it resulted because I had treated her fairly decently," Neil explains.[11] Many visits followed, during which she described in great detail the Pennsylvania murders. The legal agreement only covered Spencer's Michigan murder, so Neil passed the information to Pennsylvania state police who by then had opened an investigation. Like a nimbus cloud, Spencer's confession and the very real possibility that she murdered Aaron cast a dark shadow over the cause of death of the infants Joyce Anne Denochick and Autumn Dawn Spencer. So while Spencer faced a murder charge in Michigan, the Pennsylvania investigation created the real possibility that she could also face a double-murder charge there.

Before Spencer's shocking confession, Pennsylvania authorities believed that *both* children died of SIDS. One SIDS death is rare, but two? Joyce Anne was buried without an autopsy with the cause of death listed as SIDS, although a SIDS cause of death cannot and should not be established without an autopsy. An autopsy was conducted on the second victim, Autumn Dawn, but no signs of trauma were found, and the cause of death was subsequently listed as SIDS. Since an autopsy had been conducted upon Autumn Dawn's death, the Pennsylvania authorities did not exhume her body and did not change the manner of death to homicide. The absence of a word change on Autumn Dawn's death certificate would not prevent a murder charge, though, because Spencer had admitted to murdering the child.

Yet, a question remained about Spencer's first victim: did Joyce Anne die of SIDS, or did her mother, as she confessed to Michigan state police, smother the infant? Perhaps opening the casket and performing an autopsy on the infant's body would reveal the truth about what had happened. Perhaps an autopsy would uncover valuable corroboration of Spencer's confession and thus provide evidence that could lead to murder charges and that prosecutors in Pennsylvania could use in a future murder trial.

In December 1990, a Pennsylvania judge ordered the exhumation of Joyce Anne's body. The autopsy uncovered no signs of trauma or foul play. And like the autopsy conducted on Aaron—the baby brother Joyce would never meet—no clear cause of death. Because the autopsy revealed no clear cause of death, the infant's demise could not be considered a result of natural causes.

So after consulting with other experts, a Pennsylvania coroner changed the death certificate, which now listed asphyxia by smothering as the cause of death and homicide as the manner of death. With this, at least one murder charge in Pennsylvania seemed a foregone conclusion. Pennsylvania authorities issued murder warrants for the deaths of Joyce Anne Denochick and Autumn Dawn Spencer just days before Spencer's murder trial was scheduled to begin in Michigan.

Diane Spencer, it appeared, would have a thorough tour of the American court system.

Meanwhile, Spencer traveled to the Center for Forensic Psychiatry in Ypsilanti, Michigan, to undergo psychological evaluations. Before Spencer's preliminary hearing could occur, doctors needed to ascertain if she suffered from any mental illness that would leave her incompetent to stand trial for the murder of her son. During subsequent interviews with a psychiatrist, Diane Spencer denied knowing what, if any, role she had in her son's death, even though in her confession she admitted to the murder. Although she now seemed confused about Aaron's death, the psychiatrist's report declared her "in good contact with reality and free from symptoms of psychosis." Diane Spencer was "aware of the charges" pending against her.[12] She could and would face a jury in a murder trial.

During *The People v. Spencer*, the prosecution had no shortage of evidence: the smoking gun of the apnea monitor printouts and the defendant's confession, which the presiding judge declared legally obtained and admissible.

The defense countered the prosecution's rather loud evidence by depicting Diane Spencer as a pathetic figure who relapsed into cocaine use after the loss of yet another child. In her testimony, Spencer offered an explanation for her confession. Her confession, she suggested, resulted from her tremendous guilt. She felt responsible because she could not resuscitate Aaron after he stopped breathing.

During her testimony, she rehashed the version of Aaron's death she initially told investigators before confessing to murder. The morning Aaron died, she woke up at 4 a.m. to feed him, but he didn't eat well. To comfort the infant, who appeared to be congested, she walked around the room, cradling him in her arms. At some point, she fell asleep on the couch with Aaron. When she awoke, she discovered that Aaron had stopped breathing and that she had not reattached the sleep apnea monitor.

She attempted CPR, then in a panic called for help. She again tried to revive Aaron but failed—this was the source of the heavy weight on her shoulders that was removed with her confession.

The loss of Aaron, she explained, affected her deeply. At the hospital, even after Aaron was declared dead, she did not want to let him go and clung to the child's body. Her sense of guilt appears evident in her testimony when she explains the confession. "When Aaron died, I went through a lot of—what could I have done? What should I have done? What did I do wrong? When Chris Bertran had done CPR on my son, he lived. I did CPR on my son, he died. To a degree, at that point, I felt responsible . . . I did not—I know what I felt, and what I believed, and that is that I love Aaron very much, and that intentionally, or unintentionally, or at any other way, that I would not have taken my son's life. My son was my life. But, the more that it went on, and the more accusations that were made, and the more I was relapsing, and failing, and screwing everything up, I thought, well maybe. Maybe they are right. . . . I knew within me how I felt about Aaron, how I was with Aaron, how I took care of Aaron, and that throughout his life my efforts were always to protect Aaron, to take care of Aaron. Attempted to do CPR on Aaron, and failed."[13]

But what about the bizarre apnea monitor printout?

In her testimony, Diane described Aaron's death and offered an explanation for the "smoking gun"of the apnea monitor printout: "It was all quick, it wasn't slow, and it wasn't waiting around, and it wasn't, I'm going to sit here and wait until Aaron is dead, and I didn't turn that monitor to see if my son was dead, I turned it on to see if I could get a pulse, to see if he was alive."[14]

Her version of events that night explained why the monitor was not attached and the sequence of being turned off and on repeatedly, but it does not explain one fact gleaned from the monitor's memory chip: the time that elapsed from when the monitor showed Aaron had flatlined to the time Spencer called the police. Why did she wait an hour? The printout did not lie, which left one conclusion: Diane Spencer was lying. Again.

The prosecution's evidence was too convincing; the smoking gun of the apnea monitor printout and Diane Spencer's confession seemed to scream "guilty," and the jury listened. After a three-and-a-half-hour period of deliberation, the jury returned its verdict: guilty of first-degree murder. A year and a half after she smothered Aaron, Diane Spencer received her legal penance: life in prison without the possibility of parole.

Diane Spencer's mental state was not raised as a defense in her trial, but the information about the case suggests that she may have had the rare condition known as Munchausen by proxy syndrome. Chief Dan Miller is convinced; during his investigation, he found out that Diane used to inflict injuries on herself for attention—Munchausen syndrome without the "by proxy."[15]

Still, psychological tests proved that she was in touch with reality when she committed the murder, that she could understand the charges against her, and that she could help in her own defense; in other words, Diane Spencer was legally sane to stand trial for the murder of Aaron Spencer. The narrow legal definition of sanity in Michigan creates a wide corridor for people with many types of mental illnesses to pass through into the courts and, if convicted, into the prison system. Even if Diane Spencer does have this rare condition, this does not excuse or even explain the murder of three children, especially if she deliberately caused their deaths.

If those suffering from Munchausen by proxy syndrome use others as vehicles to obtain a type of attention, killing the vehicles would leave them stranded and without the desired attention. On the other hand, a death might occur by accident if the mother miscalculated while creating symptoms. Diane Spencer's confession gives no clue as to a motive; her statement that she had to kill them only suggests that she felt a certain degree of compulsion, not that she accidentally killed them while creating symptoms of fictitious illnesses.

Yet her conviction, like the first part of a two-part television show, represented just the first installment of the legal saga—a story "to be continued" in a Pennsylvania courtroom. Diane Spencer traveled from Michigan to Pennsylvania to face the two murder charges pending there. If convicted in Pennsylvania, she would face the ultimate penalty for her crimes: a possible sentence of death by lethal injection.

The linchpin of the Pennsylvania case—Diane Spencer's December 1990 confession to Michigan state police—was obtained in Michigan. Although the officers who obtained her confession violated no Michigan law, Pennsylvania law differs from Michigan law with regard to interrogation methods. In Pennsylvania, those questioning a suspect must inform that suspect about what questions they will ask *before* the interview, rather like a teacher providing the test questions before giving the test. Before they can question a suspect of another crime, they must again inform that suspect of his or her rights before proceeding. Unlike their counterparts in Pennsylvania, Michigan detectives need not advise a suspect a second time before questioning about other alleged crimes.

Before the 1990 interrogation in Lansing, Michigan, Diane Spencer waived her right to have legal counsel present. The officers questioning Spencer told her that they would ask her questions about Aaron's death but never informed her that they would ask about her daughters' deaths in Pennsylvania. Diane Spencer's confession, while legally obtained in Michigan and thus admissible in court, would have been considered illegally obtained in Pennsylvania and thus inadmissible in court. Without the confession, Pennsylvania authorities dropped the dual murder charges. The presiding judge ordered Diane Spencer to return to Michigan, where she began serving a life sentence for the murder of Aaron. She avoided a date with the executioner due to a legal technicality.

The dismissal of the Pennsylvania charges provided Spencer's defense with a compelling argument for an appeal of her conviction. Diane Spencer based her appeal on the timing of the warrants—warrants that no longer existed. The Pennsylvania murder warrants came just three days before Diane Spencer's trial began in Allegan County. The timing, the defense would argue, proved prejudicial to Diane Spencer. National media covered the alleged Pennsylvania murders, raising a question about the possibility of obtaining a nonbiased jury.

Emotions tend to run high during murder trials involving child victims, and jury members do not need prompting from a biased news media.

Her appeal failed; Diane Spencer will spend the rest of her life in prison for the murder of her son, Aaron. And what about her alleged victims in Pennsylvania, whom she admitted smothering? Their deaths lack the closure of a conviction and potential death penalty. Diane Spencer has just one life to give for her crimes, and that life will be committed to a Michigan prison.

For those who have met her, Diane Spencer does not appear to be a monster, even though she did something that many would consider monstrous. Yet, as retired Michigan state police detective Ron Neil (see "The Hand That Feeds") points out, she must be incarcerated. If she goes free, the cycle will occur again . . . and again . . . and again . . .[16]

At the time of writing, Diane Spencer resides in the Robert Scott Correctional Facility—a prison for female offenders in southeastern Michigan. It is a place that Gwendolyn Graham must also call home (see "M-U-R-D-E-R?"). Time in prison for perpetrators of crimes against children can be hard time indeed, and Spencer's stay in the prison system has not been without incident. While in an Allegan County jail awaiting trial in 1990, she became involved in a scuffle with another inmate, which led to an assault on a correctional officer who intervened. For this offense, she received a sentence of sixty days in jail.

This would be the first in a series of incidents that characterizes Spencer's first decade in the state prison system. Although the last few years have been without incident, her early years of incarceration were marked by a series of infractions for various types of misconduct including numerous fights. And shortly after she lost her appeal, Spencer tried to escape, but guards caught her attempting to go over the fence.

Another, more serious situation occurred in the Robert Scott Correctional Facility in 1995. A guard wandering by her cell during his usual rounds found Diane Spencer naked and tied spread-eagle to her bed with a towel jammed into her mouth. Someone had beaten her.

Perhaps the hardship of Diane Spencer's prison life is a reality best told by a few photographs. In her OTIS (Offender Tracking and Information System) photograph taken in 2003, over a decade after her conviction, she is smiling, although her time in prison has transformed her: the curly chocolate brown hair now formed into cornrows—a contrast to the image that accompanied a newspaper story about the investigation over a decade earlier.

Almost seventeen years later, Detective Neil shakes his head as he studies the photograph on the December 12, 1990, front-page story in the *Grand Rapids Press*.[17] For Neil, the photograph of a mother who appears to dote on her young child underlines the horrific nature of her crime: the unbelievable truth that Diane Spencer murdered her son.

The photograph also provides a visual summary of the case. In the photograph, taken the August just before Aaron's death, Diane Spencer holds her son up for the camera. She presents him to the photographer, their heads pressed against each other: the proud, loving mother and her child. She is smiling while Aaron has a more serious gaze. He is the object of her affection.

But in light of the suspicion that Diane Spencer suffered from Munchausen by proxy syndrome, the photograph takes on a secondary meaning; Aaron is not the subject of her affection but rather subject to her obsession. And this possibility gives the photograph a terrible subtext: Diane holds Aaron up as if presenting him to the photographer, but in another context, in another time, she is presenting Aaron to his pediatrician for an illness she imagined. And she smiles.

A month after the photograph was taken, she loses him . . . or sacrifices him . . . or saves him, depending on what version the reader chooses to believe. "You have no idea how much I loved him," she told Detective Ron Neil repeatedly during an interview. Indeed, she loved him to death.

## Notes

1. Daniel Miller, City of Wayland chief of police, personal interview with Tobin T. Buhk, May 2, 2007.

2. Information on Munchausen by proxy syndrome from Kerry Buhk, PhD, clinical psychologist, personal interview with Tobin T. Buhk, October 17, 2006.

3. Daniel Miller, police report from September 28, 1990.

4. Ron Neil, Michigan state police detective (retired), personal interview with Tobin T. Buhk, August 16, 2006.

5. Ibid.

6. Daniel Miller, personal interview with Tobin T. Buhk, May 2, 2007.

7. In the Wayland police station's evidence locker, the author, Tobin T. Buhk, had the opportunity to study the various journals Diane Spencer completed during stints in drug rehabilitation programs on May 2, 2007, and July 30, 2007. The journals tell the story of Diane Spencer's youth and her experiences with family and substance abuse. According to the notes Chief Dan Miller took during Spencer's discussion with John Palmatier, at one point during the interrogation, Diane Spencer became very angry and at that time discussed the abuse she suffered as a child. She also told a forensic psychologist about the abuse and verified her accusations during her trial (trial transcript, volume 3, p. 134).

8. John Hogan and Theresa D. McClellan, "Authorities Look Again at Deaths of Mother's Two Girls," *Grand Rapids Press*, December 13, 1990.

9. Daniel Miller, personal interview with Tobin T. Buhk, May 2, 2007.

10. Ron Neil, Michigan state police detective (retired), personal interview with Tobin T. Buhk, August 16, 2006.

11. Ibid.

12. Quoted in John Hogan, "Report OKs Trial of Mom Accused of Killing Son," *Grand Rapids Press*, July 17, 1991.

13. *People v. Spencer*, trial transcripts, vol. 3, pp. 136–37.

14. Ibid., p. 129.

15. Daniel Miller, personal interview with Tobin T. Buhk, May 2, 2007.

16. Ron Neil, personal interview with Tobin T. Buhk, August 16, 2006.

17. The photograph described accompanies the story by John Hogan, "'Tragic Coincidence' May Have Been Three Murders," *Grand Rapids Press*, December 12, 1990.

## Head Case

"Oh, don't forget, this is a real head, ladies and gentlemen," a voice from the tape declares.[1] The statement starts off a forty-five minute videotape and is just the beginning of a running commentary laced with profanity.

The audience listens in stunned silence to the home movie soundtrack. They have likely never heard anything like it, real or imagined. Not even in their nightmares. They cannot see the video picture; the television connected to the VCR playing the homemade video is facing away from them and covered.

The audience cannot see what the star of the home video is doing behind the cover, but they know. They know from the medical examiner's testimony. They might feel a sense of relief that they do not have to watch the film and perhaps carry from the courthouse images that would forever remain burned into their memories, like a computer file that one cannot delete: images of a teenager skinning and mutilating the decapitated head of his victim. A reality so horrific, so bizarre, so macabre, it first appears surreal, like a practical joke taken too far.

Yet it *is* real. It must be, or they wouldn't be here sitting in judgment of a seventeen-year-old boy instead of at the accounting firm, car dealership, or whatever jobs the jury members temporarily left when the trial began.

The voice of the teenager swears and laughs hysterically, accompanied by a soundtrack of heavy metal music. He carries on an imaginary conversation with the head, which he calls "Eddie."

The jury members cannot see the source of the voice in the video, but they can look across the courtroom and see the young man sitting next to his defense attorney. This is no ordinary audience and no ordinary screening. These twelve individuals face the dubious and difficult task of judging the movie star's sanity. Later that day, they will go to a room adjacent to the courtroom and ponder the question of sanity debated by experts who couldn't seem to agree about the defendant's mental health.

In Michigan, to be criminally or legally insane, the defendant must be considered mentally ill. Then it must be shown that he either did not know or recognize his actions as wrong, or he could not control himself even if he did realize the wrongfulness of his actions. For days, the jury listened to forensic psychiatrists ponder this legal definition and debate its application to the defendant.

One could argue that to do what the defendant did to his victim, he would have to be insane, but legal insanity and insanity don't always mean the same thing.

Kent County prosecutor William Forsyth decided to play the audio portion of the video as rebuttal evidence for the defendant's insanity defense, and the screening took place just before closing arguments on the last day of the trial. Audiovisuals can be very convincing . . . and potentially prejudicial. The visual images of the defendant skinning a human head could unfairly prejudice a jury, but playing the soundtrack, which Forsyth posited as evidence of Federico Cruz's legal sanity, might not. Cruz had apparently turned off the video recorder when his parents came home (a fact substantiated by earlier testimony), which indicated that he understood the need to hide the mutilations from them. When he resumed filming, he states, "Welcome to another . . . episode of the murder show." At one point in the video, he suggests that others should try it, "just make sure you don't get caught."[2] These statements seemed to indicate that Federico Cruz did not qualify as criminally insane.

Yet would the defendant's own words convince the jury that the seventeen-year-old perpetrator of the unspeakably horrific crime should go to prison for the remainder of his natural life? Or a mental institution for psychiatric treatment?

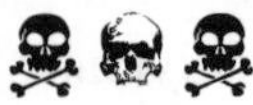

David Crawford had done it before; he had walked away from his group home in which he voluntarily lived. Perhaps he wanted to escape emotional doldrums . . . perhaps, stuck in the emotional horse latitudes, he wanted a change of wind to take him away . . . perhaps, like a swimmer caught in a rip tide, a wanderlust carried him away . . . perhaps this artist-to-be (he dreamed of drawing cartoons for Disney) found in nature the lifeblood for his creative engine and he needed an infusion . . . perhaps, like many youngsters, he just desired a change of scenery . . . whatever the motivation, young David Crawford left Wedgewood Acres—a home for mentally and emotionally challenged youths in a southern Grand Rapids suburb—to attend vocational classes but, unlike the other times, he would never return.

After buying food and cigarettes for him, a friend dropped seventeen-year-old David Crawford in Sparta Township, a rural area in northern Kent County, around noon on Thursday, April 25, 1996. Some residents of the township, which numbered about eight thousand in the spring of 1996, work the farms and the apple and peach orchards dotting the landscape, while others commute to jobs in the city of Grand Rapids a few miles south. It is a place where the country mixes with the city; where one can find a subdivision of homes alongside a road frequented by tractors moving along at twenty miles per hour, to the chagrin of busy commuters stuck behind them.

Crawford traveled south along railroad tracks—a sort of nature hike home. After about two and a half hours, he came across a boy who asked for a cigarette. The boy may have seemed like a kind spirit, but little did Crawford know, he had just met a monster . . .

David Crawford did not return to Wedgewood Acres Thursday night. Crawford's family, not the court, had placed him in the group home, so he enjoyed the privilege of attending an off-campus school that offered vocational classes. He had a history of absenteeism during his short time at the group home, so when he failed to return Thursday, no one considered him a potential victim of foul play.

Friday passed into Saturday, which passed into Sunday, which passed into Monday, and still Crawford didn't appear. On Tuesday, a missing person's report was filed with the police. Something must have gone wrong.

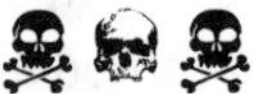

Meanwhile, across town in the rural community of Sparta, a macabre story unfolded over the weekend. Sixteen-year-old Federico Cruz told friends a story about murder, a story so horrific, it left them wondering if it was fiction or nonfiction. Was Cruz's murder tale merely a perverted bravado manifest as some dark fiction, or did the kid many considered the neighborhood bully actually commit murder?

Thursday evening, Cruz showed up at a friend's house with evidence of the deed. He carried with him a plastic grocery bag. He told the group of teens assembled in the basement—a band that had gathered to play—that he had made a video of himself mutilating his victim's head, cutting off various facial features before skinning it. He didn't bring the video, but rather more tangible evidence of the crime: the victim's skull.

Cruz removed the bloody severed head, which he called "Eddie," from the shopping bag and set it down. His friends stared at "Eddie" in disbelief; the head—without ears, nose, skin, or scalp, with eyes that stared at nothing—must have been a ghastly, almost unbelievable sight, something from a horror movie. Cruz placed "Eddie" back in the plastic bag, then picked up a guitar and began to play. According to one friend, Cruz worshipped the hip hop band Cypress Hill, whose emblem was a skull named Eddie.[3]

Cruz seemed proud of the murder; indeed, trial testimony of friends and acquaintances, who recounted their experiences for a jury over two years later, indicates that Cruz bragged about the murder. He even offered to give a friend one of the victim's ears.

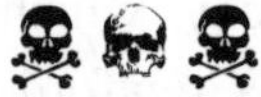

It didn't take long for the news of murder to travel. A parent of a friend to whom Cruz gave the video watched the ghastly images and turned it over to the police on Saturday. In the early morning hours of

Tuesday, search warrant in hand, police visited the Cruz home in Sparta Township, where the teenager lived with one of his three sisters and his parents. If they could find either the butcher knife used in the video or the clothes worn by the home movie star who did the mutilating, they would have concrete, conclusive evidence linking the teen with the video and possibly the murder.

*If* it was real at all. They prayed it wasn't.

The day investigators discovered that the "murder" was nonfiction began as a frigid, rainy morning. The sun had not yet risen, but when it did come up, it would cast light on a horrific skeleton in Federico Cruz's closet.

During the search, one of the investigators spotted a bag lying on the ground outside of Federico Cruz's bedroom window. He lifted the bag, judging its weight, before opening it. A balloon of hope that the head in the video was not a real human head had buoyed the officers, but the contents of the bag, like a jab with a sharp knife, burst that balloon. Cocooned inside several layers of paper and plastic bags was what remained of a human head—"Eddie" from the video.

Cruz did little to create a reasonable doubt about his involvement in the murder; in fact, when confronted by police, he did little to conceal the crime. Calm and not visibly agitated when interviewed, he told the investigators where he dumped his victim's headless corpse. When the sun rose, the investigators made the short trek. It was a frigid, overcast morning, and the light rain made it feel even colder than the 35-degree temperature. In a swamp behind the house, they found the body, still wearing tennis shoes, blue jeans, and a blue shirt. The damage to the corpse left little doubt that the investigators had just discovered a murder victim.

In a subsequent interview, Cruz told investigators a chilling tale about the murder of an unsuspecting kid who happened to wander past the railroad tracks behind his house.

*At about two-thirty in the afternoon, Cruz spots the teenager ambling down the railroad grade behind his house. He approaches the boy.*

*"Can I bum a cigarette?" he asks, noticing the pack of Marlboro cigarettes in the boy's front pocket.*

*The boy plucks the pack from his pocket, taps it against his wrist, and offers the cigarette. Cruz takes it and places it between his lips.*

*"Have a light?" he asks. Again, the boy obliges the request.*

*"Ever see weed before?"*

*The boy seems interested. He slowly shakes his head.*

*"Follow me." Cruz leads him into a forested area.*

*"These are all mine," Cruz notes, spreading his arms out to the sides.*

*The boy walks toward the little plants, accidentally stepping on one.*

*The attack comes as a complete surprise. Cruz buries his fist in the boy's stomach, and the boy doubles over in pain. Cruz continues to punch the boy in a frenzied barrage of blows, which drops him to the ground. Wild with fury, he kicks the boy until his victim is almost unconscious. His attack has left the boy writhing on the ground in slow, almost rhythmic movements.*

*Cruz steps on the boy's throat and presses all of his weight down, using his Nike high-top tennis shoe as a murder weapon. A slight, muffled gurgle comes from his victim, who cannot breathe. Desperate for air, the boy grabs Cruz's shoe. He becomes weaker, and his arms thrash about the ground, grasping for something, anything that will help him. After a few minutes, everything fades to darkness.*

Cruz told police that he pressed the sole of his Nike high-top gym shoe on the boy's neck for twenty minutes, which is what killed him. After the murder, he dumped the body in the swamp behind his house. He returned later that evening with a butcher's knife. He removed the head, taking it with him as a sort of trophy, and left the headless corpse. He told investigators that he wanted to obtain a genuine skull he could use as a decoration.

Yet from whom did he obtain his "trophy"? Who was the boy? Investigators began their search for an answer to this question as John Doe's body traveled to the Kent County Morgue for an autopsy.

Investigators needed forensic details to support Federico Cruz's version of the murder. The damage left in the wake of the killer's attack, illuminated by the fluorescent lights of the Kent County Morgue, would provide clues that could be used to reconstruct the crime.

All autopsies begin with a description of the victim and wounds, and the description of John Doe took a considerable time to detail; the autopsy report detailing the extensive injuries and describing the postmortem examination runs sixteen pages!

When it comes to death, a fantastic array of ways to leave the world exists. If variety is the spice of life, the medical examiner never suffers from a bland diet. If one spends enough time in a morgue, one will see some bizarre ways in which people have died and some creative ways in which murderers have dispatched their victims. Some killers do not stop at murder; they continue to degrade their victims by mutilating the bodies.

A medical examiner might spend his whole career without witnessing a murder as bizarre and ghastly as this one. John Doe's body arrived at the Kent County Morgue in two pieces; the torso came dressed in running shoes, bloodstained blue jeans, and a bloodstained blue button-down shirt, in the front pocket of which was a pack of Marlboro Light cigarettes. The jeans bore identifying marks: the letters "DC" on one front pocket and the name "David Crawford" in the lining of the other—perhaps John Doe's name?

The face looked less like a face than a prop from a Hollywood horror film: a crimson mass barely recognizable as a human head. The mutilations left little more than muscle over skull with some patches of skin still clinging to it around the eyelids and a strip running across the bridge of the nose. The nose itself was gone. The lips were missing. The ears had been removed, as had been the scalp. The head had been skinned, with almost all of the skin and subcutaneous tissue of the face and head removed. The eyes, however, remained.

At the scene, investigators managed to find a few pieces excised from the head, which accompanied John Doe's body: a portion of his left ear, approximately two inches long by an inch wide, and a large, ten-by-five-inch swath of his scalp. The clean edges of the ear and scalp indicated that someone had removed them with a sharp blade. All of these wounds were inflicted postmortem; John Doe did not feel them. They were carried out in a basement in front of a video camera—horrific mutilations preserved in a home movie.

The torso contained the forensic clues as to what caused John Doe's death as well as additional evidence that the killer mutilated his victim postmortem. The circumference of the neck contained a number of "hesitation marks" indicating that the person who severed the head from the torso paused at intervals, a movement consistent with sawing the head off with a butcher knife, as Federico Cruz said he did.

During autopsies of deaths that involve stab or gunshot wounds, each wound track is probed and detailed for the official record. No fewer than seventeen stab wounds marked the victim's torso. A murderer's graffiti, these wounds were inflicted postmortem when the killer repeatedly jabbed his knife into his victim's body.

Cruz admitted to investigators that he attempted to remove the victim's heart and spinal column—a claim substantiated by damage to the victim's torso. The killer created a massive, gaping wound about two inches wide and approximately six inches long running from the sternum to the upper midsection. The jagged edges of the wound indicated that the killer used at least five strokes with the knife to create it. The wound was such that it looked like the killer had attempted to remove something—the heart—in a hasty and amateur impromptu surgery. These mutilations made Federico Cruz seem like a reincarnated Jack the Ripper, who also mutilated his victims and removed various organs in impromptu surgeries.

An additional six stab wounds appeared on the right side of the victim's back between the right shoulder blade and the right buttock, bringing the total number of stab wounds to seventeen. Like he did on the front of the body, the killer cut a gaping wound in the middle lower back; this was perhaps the site of Cruz's aborted attempt to remove the spinal column.

All of these wounds and mutilations occurred after the victim had died, but what had caused his death? Marks on the victim's body provided clues. Several contusions on John Doe's upper chest exhibited a strange pattern of curved lines that looked as out of place on a human body as crop circle patterns in a cornfield. A pattern of contusions on the right front shoulder or deltoid consisted of a circle surrounded by faint lines around it. The pattern just above the right clavicle was also circular with several lines around it; other contusions on the left side of the neck and upper chest were in a sawtooth pattern. These marks were caused by the tread on a shoe when someone stomped his foot on the victim.

Like marks on a bullet from a gun's rifling, the patterns can be matched to a weapon, in this case a tennis shoe. Detectives brought a pair of Federico Cruz's shoes—Nike high-tops—to the morgue for comparison. The tread pattern fit the pattern tattooed onto the victim's body. Again, the forensic evidence supported Cruz's version of the murder: he told investigators that he stepped on the victim and pressed the sole of his shoe down on John Doe's neck, causing extensive bleeding or hemorrhaging in the neck tissues. John Doe died of asphyxia by blunt force trauma to the neck.

But whom did Federico Cruz murder? Who was John Doe? Cruz told investigators that he didn't know the victim. And the mutilations rendered the head unidentifiable. Police had been unable to find a match for the victim's fingerprints, and no missing persons report matched the victim's profile, because the victim wasn't reported missing until after police had found the body. Thus, when the video surfaced a few days before the discovery of the body, no one knew about the missing teenager from across town who had disappeared after not returning from his classes.

The name and the initials written into the victim's pants provided one clue. The victim's body provided a few more. The victim had a recently healed fracture in one of the bones of his leg, and he had undergone an operation to remove his appendix. It didn't take long to match the missing boy with the body found in the swamp. David Crawford broke his leg in an accident a year earlier when a car hit him and he had had his appendix removed. On Wednesday, forensic odontologist Dr. Roger Erbaugh provided the confirmation when he compared Crawford's antemortem dental records (x-rays) to the victim's teeth.

They matched.

The headless corpse belonged to David Crawford, which meant that "Eddie" was David.

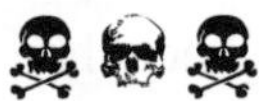

Where had the small town's version of Jack the Ripper come from, and what had motivated such a brutal crime?

A glance at Federico Cruz's family raises more questions about the murder of David Crawford than it answers; he came from a very good family who seemed to be living the American Dream.

Jose Cruz came to Michigan after serving in the Vietnam War. He met and fell in love with a woman while he worked in a migrant camp. Jose and Antonia Cruz had what seemed like an ideal family. Federico's older sisters had left the nest, attended college, and had begun their own lives. In 1996, two children had yet to leave the nest: Federico and his younger sister.

Federico earned excellent grades in school, but when he turned thirteen, he began a journey down a road away from domestic harmony. He began using drugs. He started with marijuana—the staple of his drug diet—which he used almost daily. His substance abuse would escalate to experimentation with the harder stuff: inhalants, LSD, and crack cocaine. His parents enrolled him in a substance abuse treatment program, but it didn't take: he left the program after only a week and a half.

The boy had also developed something of a violent streak. Since

Federico loved sports, his parents bought him a punching bag, but it did not seem to help. In his early teens, about the time when Cruz's criminal history began, he spent a short period of time in a psychiatric hospital, where he was diagnosed as bipolar, or manic-depressive. He was heard talking to himself.

By the age of sixteen, Federico Cruz already had a criminal record. Some lifelong criminals have careers that lead to book-length police records that read like crime novels. Others read like novellas. Cruz's brief criminal history reads like a short story.

While some described Cruz as gentle and friendly, others considered him something of a bully with a volatile, sometimes unpredictable temper. He once stole a neighbor's bicycle. And he once attacked, without provocation, a kid who attempted to date a girl Cruz liked.

Cruz formally entered the justice system at fifteen when charged in juvenile court with breaking and entering, assault, and malicious destruction of property. The charge began a pattern of violence that reached its apex with the murder and mutilation of David Crawford. At about the same time that these charges occurred, he was expelled from Sparta High School and began taking classes at an alternative-education high school.

Another assault charge followed, and another, in which Cruz allegedly elbowed a Michigan state trooper who had detained him as a suspect in a theft. The teenager seemed out of control, an admission his parents made in court; they told the court that they did not want their son to live with them at that time.[4]

For a brief period of time, Cruz washed dishes at an area restaurant, but the manager fired him after only a few months on the job. Four months later, a still-unidentified assailant murdered the restaurant manager, forty-five-year-old Robert Myers. After the Crawford murder, investigators studied the Myers murder for a possible link to Federico Cruz, but they found none.

The modus operandi of the two crimes didn't seem to match; whoever killed Myers sneaked into the house and shot him while his children slept in their bedrooms. No defilement of the body. The murder seemed to be the work of a professional assassin, perhaps an employee of Murder, Inc., not that of a deranged teenager who appeared to delight in mutilation. That the slain manager of the restaurant fired an employee who later would murder and mutilate a random victim appeared to be a thought-provoking coincidence only. The Myers murder still resides in a file marked "unsolved."

At some point, Cruz began listening to the band Cypress Hill, and perhaps his fascination with this group explains the most horrific element of this case: the severed, skinned head of his victim.

According to friends who testified at Cruz's preliminary hearing, the youth loved Cypress Hill and its mascot skull, Eddie. Eddie's ghostly visage appears on most of the band's CD covers and paraphernalia, and testimony suggests that a Cypress Hill poster and "Eddie" motivated the murder and subsequent decapitation. Perhaps Cruz wanted to obtain an "Eddie" in the flesh, or perhaps "Eddie" told him to do it . . .

With the autopsy concluded, Federico Cruz faced the dual charges of first-degree murder and the mutilation of a body. Charged as an adult, he faced life in prison without the possibility of parole. Or a lengthy stint in a psychiatric hospital, if Cruz's defense could prove that he was innocent by reason of insanity. His ultimate fate would rest with a jury that would base its decision on testimony about the defendant's mental health.

According to Federico Cruz, the voices in his head told him to do it. Although others could not hear these voices, they had heard Cruz responding to them.

People who knew Cruz periodically heard him talking to himself or to some imagined entity, the sentences in the conversations often punctuated with hysterical laughter. These conversations would continue during his incarceration and would add to the evolving debate about Cruz's sanity, particularly how it affected his ability to stand trial and his culpability in the murder of David Crawford.

A state forensic examiner visited Cruz in his Kent County jail cell and talked with him for several hours. He witnessed some strange behavior. Cruz periodically began laughing for no reason. He talked to himself or appeared to converse with someone not present. He whistled and made animal noises.

Cruz told his examiner that he heard voices. These voices, which sometimes emanated from the television or music, told him to harm or kill others—a command that he said he came closer and closer to following. He made a chilling admission: his parents were lucky to be alive. The voices told him to hurt them, too. Recently, he explained, he heard screaming in the night that he believed came from a demon or the devil and that disrupted his sleep.

The behavior appeared real and not faked, a fact supported by video from surveillance cameras that captured footage of Cruz talking to himself. And Cruz did not appear to be attempting to manipulate the circumstances. The forensic examiner declared Federico Cruz incompetent to stand trial and recommended to the court that it send Cruz to a psychiatric hospital. Legal competency to stand trial requires that the defendant not only understand the charges he faces but also that he is able to assist in his own defense. Cruz could possibly understand the charges, the examiner noted, but at the time he could not assist in his own defense. The court agreed: Cruz was incompetent to stand trial. Legal competency, however, can change over time.

Cruz traveled to a state psychiatric hospital where he would stay for a period of months for observation. Doctors took him off behavior-controlling drugs. He had fewer conversations with imaginary partners, and the instances of spontaneous laughter occurred less often, but the voices remained. And Cruz saw faces in the walls and objects floating through the air.

The aggressive behavior also remained. During his stay at the psychiatric hospital, Cruz was involved in no fewer than six fights. In one of the fights, by his own admission, Cruz intended to kill a man with a pool cue. He told a psychologist that he often felt an impulse to kill.[5] And on two occasions, he attempted suicide, once while in a seclusion cell, where he tried to hang himself with a T-shirt. He also suffered from a mysterious and sudden lapse of memory with no specific physical or mental cause to explain it; he didn't remember the murder of David Crawford, although he was aware of the murder charges he faced.

Despite his behavior, a second report, generated following a December 1996 interview, declared Federico Cruz competent to stand trial. He clearly understood the charges pending against him, and unlike a few months earlier, he now could assist in his defense. He was fit to stand trial. The debate about Federico Cruz's legal sanity, however, had just begun.

Even if he was he legally sane now, was he legally sane in April when he committed the murder? Did he understand right from wrong when he attacked David Crawford and pressed his high-top shoe on his victim's neck? And even if he did, did he lack self-control?

A judge ordered another evaluation to determine if Cruz understood right from wrong when he committed the murder. While everyone awaited the results of the test, Cruz, whose new temporary home was the Kent County jail, became involved in another incident that appeared to be a third suicide attempt. He fell or jumped off an elevated walkway and landed on the floor seventeen feet below. He was alone, which eliminated the possibility that someone pushed him. The incident forced a reevaluation of his competency to stand trial. Again, a forensic examiner declared him competent; during the interview, though, Cruz explained that ghosts inhabiting his cell pressured him into jumping.

With his competency to stand trial again established, the defense and prosecution began preparation for what would likely be a very contentious and heated trial. Trial preparation led to another heated legal debate: should the prosecution be allowed to show the tape of Cruz mutilating his victim's head? The gruesome nature of the home movie could make jurors sick, which could negatively affect the trial's outcome. Cruz's defense attorney argued that the gruesome contents of the tape would unfairly bias the jury and he moved that the judge should ban it.

Even if the trial judge allowed the prosecution to play the tape, Kent County prosecutor William Forsyth planned on using the tape only if necessary as a rebuttal for an insanity defense. The tape contained evidence that indicated Cruz's legal sanity, that he knew what he was doing and that it was wrong. Particularly damning was a statement Cruz made on camera in which he suggests others should not do what he is doing because they would get in serious trouble. On the tape, Cruz also indicates that he originally planned to attack a different person but decided to instead attack a complete stranger.

The defense maintained that Cruz was innocent by reason of insanity, and the tape, of which Forsyth warned jurors in his opening statement, seemed to prove it. One could argue that only someone with some serious mental issues could do what Federico Cruz did. Yet mental illness and legal insanity are two different concepts. To find Cruz legally insane, the jury would have to determine that he was mentally ill. But he could be considered mentally ill yet still legally sane, *if* he understood right from wrong and/or if he could control himself from committing acts he knew to be wrong when he murdered David Crawford.

The jury members had to consider the issue of sanity very carefully, because they could make one of four possible decisions: innocent, not guilty by reason of insanity, guilty, or guilty but mentally ill. If they found him not guilty by reason of insanity, Cruz would dodge a lifetime prison sentence and go to a psychiatric hospital and possibly one day regain his freedom. If they found him guilty but mentally ill, Cruz would go to prison to serve a sentence of life in prison without the possibility of parole, but he would receive the psychiatric treatment considered necessary.

The jury heard both sides from mental health professionals. The prosecution presented witnesses who testified about Cruz's legal sanity. One witness for the prosecution claimed that Cruz was sane when he murdered David Crawford. He apparently could control his impulses, since he requested a cigarette then led his victim into the woods. And he could apparently ignore the voices that told him to kill family members or acquaintances—by his own admission, he backed off on the "demons'" demands to kill his parents. *If* he heard voices.

A prosecution psychologist even testified that she believed Cruz exaggerated or even faked his symptoms.

During its case, the defense countered with an expert witness who claimed that Cruz was insane at the time of the murder. He heard voices, demons, Cruz called them, which drove him to kill David Crawford. He believed himself to be possessed by these demons, so at the time he did not realize the murder was wrong and felt compelled to commit it. Therefore, he was not legally sane and thus was not criminally responsible for the murder. These voices or demons persisted to speak to him while he was incarcerated. Their bloodlust apparently not satiated, they turned on Cruz and told him to harm himself, which he attempted three times while incarcerated. He tried to silence the voices by reading from the Bible or praying.

Ironically, the loudest voice in the trial came from the defendant himself. To counter the insanity defense, Forsyth turned to the tape Cruz made of himself mutilating his victim's head. Forsyth had decided to play only the audio portion of the tape for the jurors—a decision supported by the trial judge despite the objections of Cruz's defense that it would prejudice the jury.

In his cross-examination of the psychologist who testified for the defense, Forsyth suggested that Cruz realized the wrongfulness of the murder, evident in the fact that he led his victim into the woods, where no one would see them. Cruz's home movie would provide the clincher. It contained clues that indicated the defendant's legal sanity; at one time while filming the mutilations, he apparently turned off the tape when his parents came home—an action that suggested he knew wrong from right at the time.

Other statements supported this notion: "welcome to another . . . episode of the murder show"; "just make sure you don't get caught."

It would take less than two hours for the jury to return their verdict: guilty on both counts, first-degree murder and the mutilation of a body. The insanity defense failed.

David Crawford's mother, Juliet Crawford, stated in court that about a month before her son's murder, he "had kind of a vision": an angel visited him and told him that something bad would happen, "but God would take care of him."[6] A few days before his murder, perhaps motivated by his "vision," he wrote the following lines:

> God has changed my life to something good,
> His angels are by my side.
> He has made it so I understood.
> My soul is full of pride.
> I am starting to see
> That my life is turned around.
> And now that I'm a Christian
> I know I'm Heaven bound.[7]

This poem was read at his funeral and would make a fitting epitaph for the life tragically cut short. David Crawford's dreams of becoming a Disney artist ended when he was brutally murdered by a demon masquerading as a boy . . . or a boy masquerading as a demon.

Federico Cruz liked the band Cypress Hill. Some the band's songs make a provocative summation of Cruz's short biography of crime, which reached its climax with murder:

> "Ultra Violent Dreams" (from 1991's *Cypress Hill*)
> "Light Another" (from 1991's *Cypress Hill*)
> "Stoned Is the Way of the Walk" (from 1991's *Cypress Hill*)
> "How I Could Just Kill a Man" (from 1991's *Cypress Hill*)
> "Insane in the Brain" (from 1993's *Black Sunday*)

## Notes

1. Quoted in Peg West, "Prosecutors Play Tape to Counter Cruz Defense," *Grand Rapids Press*, December 18, 1997.

2. Ibid.

3. Ibid., "Cruz Bound over for Trial in Murder, Beheading Case," *Grand Rapids Press*, May 14, 1996.

4. Theresa D. McClellan, "'Nothing We Could Do with Him,'" *Grand Rapids Press*, May 14, 1996.

5. Doug Guthrie, "Teen Suspect in Beheading Case Fit for Trial, Report Says," *Grand Rapids Press*, January 18, 1997.

6. Quoted in West, "Slaying Victim's Mom Knows Son Is with God," *Grand Rapids Press*, December 31, 1997.

7. Quoted in Ken Kolker, "Friends Remember Murder Victim as Open, Giving," *Grand Rapids Press*, May 5, 1996.

# 6. burying the evidence

It is difficult if not impossible to prove a murder without a murder victim. No body, no victim. Savvy murderers understand this and sometimes go to strange, macabre lengths to bury their crimes by hiding the bodies and within them any evidence or proof a murder occurred.

They create makeshift cemeteries and hide their victims in caves, behind walls, in cisterns, under gardens, and just about any other place one can imagine . . .

They dump their victims' bodies in lakes and rivers, usually weighted down by something heavy like cinder blocks or dumbbells. Michigan, the "Great Lakes State," provides a murderer with numerous hiding places for his or her victim or victims; one such case led to the imposition of a death penalty on a man whose victim rose to the surface of a lake in a national forest. The cinder blocks he used to anchor her body could not hold her bloated corpse on the bottom.

If he dumped her body in the Pacific Ocean, he may have literally gotten away with murder. A bizarre case that occurred in 1935 in Australia provides a vivid illustration of the lengths to which a killer will go in attempting to conceal his crime and the difficulty of securing a conviction without a corpse. A fisherman snagged a tiger shark and took the fish to an aquarium, where a week later it threw up an arm with a length of rope knotted around its wrist. The rope raised the specter of murder, and investigators managed to trace a tattoo on the arm—two boxers—and identify the victim: an ex-boxer who had gone missing two weeks before.

When the victim disappeared, he was living in a rental house. Suspicions fell on his roommate, who had tangled with the law before and lived under the cloud of a pending fraud charge. Conspicuously absent from the rental's inventory: a tin trunk. Despite the fact that authorities never recovered the trunk or the rest of the body, a murder trial resulted. The accused managed to dodge some circumstantial evidence and won acquittal and possibly, through his concealment of the body, got away with murder.

A famous criminologist who studied the case concluded that the roommate dismembered the body on a mattress (also conspicuously missing) and placed the pieces in the tin trunk-turned-coffin. Except the arm did not fit, so he removed the arm, tied it to the trunk, and dumped it into the Pacific. A short time later, a marauding and hungry tiger shark swallowed the arm.

Other killers obliterate their victims' bodies so that, in case of discovery, authorities would not be able to identify the victim. They slice off fingertips and batter faces to destroy their victims' identities (see the sections in "Identity Crisis"). Or they employ other measures. The British serial killer John George Haigh sealed his victims into barrels of acid to destroy their bodies and evidence of his murders. Not all attempts to destroy evidence are as extensive as Haigh's. A common stratagem employed by murderers to obliterate evidence is the house fire.

Killers will often engineer house fires to obliterate crime scenes and victims and to disguise a murder as an accident, but often the fires do not completely destroy the evidence of murder. They will also stage accidents to dress a murder scene in the clothes of an accident. One killer staged a car accident to conceal the fact that he murdered his business partner. The head injuries were more consistent with a blow to the head than the blunt force injuries one would expect to see in the head of a car accident victim, and a bone fragment discovered at the office confirmed that the deathblow occurred there.

Another wily killer attempted to conceal the murder of his wife as a suicide. He could not, however, conceal the fact that she was shot twice in the head—a forensic impossibility and the key piece of evidence that led to his first-degree murder conviction.

Sometimes their ploys work, but as these examples illustrate, sometimes they don't. When these stratagems fail, the victims' bodies travel to the morgue, where the medical examiner determines the cause of death, establishes the manner of death as homicide, helps identify the victims, and discovers forensic links that often bind the victim to his killer. And the ME's closet becomes more crowded . . .

## Sex, Lies, and Cement (and Counterfeiting): Caveat Emptor

Prisoner number 180741 passes time in a cell in the Carson City Correctional Facility. A diminutive man of five feet seven and one hundred twenty-five pounds with narrow shoulders and sandy-colored hair that has receded to midscalp, he does not look like the Hollywood vision of a coldhearted killer.

And according to Prisoner 180741, he isn't a killer. Like many other convicts, he maintains his innocence of the crime that led to his murder conviction and sentence of life without the possibility of parole. He believes that he stands inside a frame built by law enforcement officers, prosecutors, and the testimony of a frightened seventeen-year-old witness, who, desperate to avoid a lengthy prison sentence, sacrificed his life for hers.

An innocent man doomed to life in a cage, cuckolded by the testimony of his friend and ex-girlfriend? Or a devious, manipulative criminal who used several aliases including "Angel" and who engineered a murder to cover up a counterfeiting scheme?

If you place your left hand on the table, you have created a rough map of Michigan's lower peninsula. About in the center of your palm's backside, approximately in the center of Michigan's lower peninsula, sits Carson City, a small town with just a thousand residents. An aerial view of the area would look like a quilt with deep green squares interspersed with rust and earthen-colored squares: deciduous and evergreen forests mixed with farmland. Carson City is the type of place a person goes to forget the hustle and bustle of big-city life, to slow the hands of time, to be bored. It is a place where time passes slowly. For the inmates behind two rows of razor wire in the Carson City Correctional Facility, this place is all about time, and it passes slowly.

For Harry Bout, time must pass very slowly indeed.

Yet this story does not begin here.

The story begins over twenty years earlier in the basement of a small house on the west side of Grand Rapids, about three blocks from the water artery bisecting the city. The chocolate brown waters of the Grand River enticed settlers, and the village of Grand Rapids was born in the 1830s. Skilled carpenters, many of whom lived in small houses on the west side, flocked to the furniture factories that sprang up on the river's shores. The village has evolved into a sprawling metropolitan area of a million residents and is Michigan's second city (Detroit is the most populous).

If it could talk, the house on Broadway would tell of European immigrants who walked a few blocks to the west side furniture factories and toiled from sunup to sundown for meager wages. It would also narrate a story of murder and international intrigue.

This murder mystery is a *CSI* episode waiting to be written. It has all the ingredients of a thriller: a spectacularly horrible and violent murder as the centerpiece around which loiters a cast of enigmatic, unsavory characters and a plot involving sex, counterfeiting, and international intrigue. And four hundred pounds of cement. The perpetrator's claim to innocence, some believe, may contain some element of truth, and his arrest and conviction involve allegations of police corruption, prosecutorial misconduct, and international treaty violations.

Following a tip provided by a man who knew the secret kept in the house's cellar, investigators arrived at the Broadway residence at about one in the morning of April 5, 1985. They came with a search warrant, pickaxes, chisels, sledgehammers, and the belief that Onunwa Alphonsus Iwuagwu, missing for just under a month, lay buried in concrete in the basement.

Iwuagwu's wife, Charlotte, reported his disappearance when the forty-year-old Nigerian immigrant failed to return after a night out with friends on March 7. He simply vanished without a trace until investigators discovered his car—a brown 1978 Chevrolet Chevette—parked near an Indianapolis, Indiana, airport about four weeks later.

From their informant, investigators learned that Iwuagwu hadn't taken a trip to Indiana or even left the city, but he had made a trip to the basement of the Broadway house. Mobsters in old movies threaten someone with cement shoes. Whoever killed Iwuagwu, investigators had reason to believe, gave him a cement coffin: the killer or killers disposed of the body by placing it in a sump pump hole and encasing it in concrete.

The house was owned by Mary Ann Schut, who lived there along with an elderly renter named Evelyn Schneider. The two women seemed the least likely people to occupy a house that concealed a murder victim. If the Nigerian lay buried in the basement, as the police informant claimed, how did he come to reside in the house occupied by the two seemingly innocuous ladies? Police had reason to believe that Harry Bout, Schut's twenty-six-year-old son, and Bout's live-in seventeen-year-old girlfriend, Dawn Bean, had something to do with Iwuagwu's disappearance.

The tiny, cramped basement—approximately four feet by five feet and with a ceiling of under six feet in height—made the excavation difficult, as the team of investigators chipped at the concrete slab throughout the night. After just a few strikes with a sledgehammer, a body appeared, but only after six hours of laboring did the team manage to remove the corpse from its impromptu crypt made from four hundred pounds of cement. The naked body was curled into a fetal position and was in a state of advanced decomposition, its head wrapped in a plastic bag likely to prevent the spillage of blood from the three gunshot wounds to his head. Almost a month after his disappearance, Onunwa Iwuagwu, known to friends as "Al," had surfaced.

The autopsy revealed that he had sustained three bullet wounds to his head. The fatal wound passed through the top left of his skull, struck the bottom right side and ricocheted, deflecting back into the brain. When some bullets strike a hard surface like bone, they flatten on impact and take the shape of a mushroom. A "mushroomed," nonjacketed bullet from a small-caliber gun (.32) was recovered in his brain. The path of the bullet—from above downward and from left to right—suggested that someone fired the shot while standing above the victim or by holding the gun over the victim's head and firing downward.

Two other bullet entrance wounds in the scalp indicated that Iwuagwu was shot a total of three times in the head. Unlike the fatal bullet, which remained encased in the victim's brain, these two bullets deflected off the skull and exited through the entrance wounds; they did not penetrate the victim's brain and were not recovered during the autopsy. One bullet struck from the front left side of Iwuagwu's forehead, an inch and a half above his left eyebrow. This bullet left small lead fragments around the wound. Another struck him in the back of his head (the occipital scalp) and also bounced out of the entry wound. Soot covering this wound suggests that the perpetrator fired the gun from very close, perhaps a few inches away from Iwuagwu's skull.

Another strange wound, which was inconsistent with a gunshot homicide, appeared on Iwuagwu's body: a three-and-a-half-inch incised wound on the back of the victim's knee. The lack of bleeding in and around the wound indicated that this injury occurred after death (postmortem). The perpetrator or perpetrators, the wound suggested, attempted to dismember the body, perhaps as a means of disposing of it.

With the autopsy completed, Onunwa Iwuagwu traveled from the morgue to a local funeral home. Despite the ghastly appearance and horrific stench from the advanced state of decomposition, the body went on display because Nigerian tribal customs required a viewing of the body. Yet his postmortem journey had not yet reached its terminus: he would make one last trip to his native Umunomo Ihitteafoukwu, Nigeria, for burial.

The forensic evidence uncovered at the autopsy appeared consistent with the narrative that had led the police to the Broadway house and the location of Onunwa Iwuagwu's body. The trail that eventually led police to the house and its ugly secret began a few hours earlier in an interview room, in which a man told a macabre story of sex, lies, and cement.

Police questioned Elvin Shaver—a longtime friend of Bout's—about Iwuagwu's disappearance. During a subsequent interview, he told them that he knew the whereabouts of the missing Nigerian businessman. By Shaver's own admission, he helped conceal the murder by assisting in the burial of Iwuagwu; he did not, he maintained, participate in the murder.[1]

They placed a deal on the interview table. Shaver agreed to provide investigators with the location of Iwuagwu's body, his killer, and a recounting of events that he witnessed the night Iwuagwu disappeared. In exchange for his cooperation and testimony at the subsequent trial, he received an assurance that whatever sentence he received for his role in concealing the body—a charge of accessory after the fact and a potential five-year prison term—would be served in a federal prison concurrent with whatever penalty he received for parole violation. He had done time in a federal prison for passing counterfeit banknotes.

The plea bargain was a good deal for Shaver, because as part of the agreement, the prosecutor would not pursue him as an alleged habitual offender—a tag that could have thrown him in a prison cell for the rest of his life.

It was an easy bargain for authorities to make—they would receive everything—a body, a murderer, a motive—in exchange for little in return.

Caveat emptor?

According to Shaver's version of the events that occurred on

March 7, Harry Bout called him to the Broadway home where, in one of the upstairs bedrooms, Onunwa Iwuagwu lay facedown, a pan placed under his head to contain the blood from the gunshot wounds.[2] Shaver and Bout had known each other for eighteen years and both spent time in prison on counterfeiting convictions. Now, according to Shaver, Bout desperately needed help from his friend—help in covering up a murder he had just committed.

As Shaver related to the police—a story he repeated during the preliminary hearing and during the subsequent murder trial—Bout explained the dynamics of the murder to him upon his arrival at the Broadway house: Dawn Bean, Bout supposedly told Shaver, stood at the top of the stairs and enticed Iwuagwu to the upstairs bedroom with the promise of sex. Iwuagwu was quickly hooked. He took off his clothes and followed Bean upstairs. Bean had allegedly reeled him into the bedroom and signaled Bout, who shot the unsuspecting man three times in the head.

According to Shaver, he agreed to help Bout dispose of the body. They carried it to a downstairs bathroom where Bout attempted to dismember the body with a rusty knife, but after the initial incision (the cut at the back of Iwuagwu's knee), they decided that a better plan would be to place the body in the sump depression in the basement of the Broadway house and conceal it with cement.

Then, according to Shaver's version of events, Bean drove Iwuagwu's Chevette to an Indianapolis airport with Shaver and Bout following in Bout's car. Upon their return, they bought four bags of concrete mix and covered the body.

As for Bout's motive, Shaver supplied details for this aspect of the crime as well. Shaver testified that in a late-night meeting at a cemetery prior to the killing, Bout told him that he was planning the murder because Iwuagwu had obtained counterfeiting plates from Bout and either he or someone back in Nigeria was planning to use the plates to print fake US currency. Shaver explained that Bout feared authorities would discover the counterfeiting plot and connect the plates to him. Iwuagwu, Bout told Shaver, exploited that fear and was blackmailing him.

In fact, Harry Bout did have a history of counterfeiting.[3] The US Secret Service conducted a yearlong investigation, after which, in January 1983, Harry Bout faced eleven counts on a federal indictment for printing $78,000 in counterfeit $20 bills. Bout's funny money had even found its way to Dallas, Texas. During his tenure as a counterfeiter, Bout used at least six aliases, including "Angel," Jim Broadmore, Andrew Fishman, Jonathan Fishman, and Alex Sterling.

History, at least for Harry Bout, had repeated itself. In 1983, another informant, as part of a plea bargain, exposed Bout in counterfeiting charges when authorities arrested that informant for passing counterfeit twenties. Now, Elvin Shaver's narrative exposed Bout to criminal charges for the murder of Iwuagwu. There is no honor among thieves.

In 1983, Bout had an out. He made a deal of his own. He confessed to two of the counts on the indictment; in exchange, the US attorney's office in Grand Rapids dropped the other nine counts and assured him that he would spend no longer than a year in prison. In addition, the US attorney's office in Detroit agreed to not investigate Bout's alleged activities in their jurisdiction. Bout made a good deal—each of the charges to which he confessed in US District Court carried a maximum prison sentence of fifteen years. Bout traded a possible thirty for one.

The axiom *caveat emptor*, or buyer beware, applied. In 1983, the US attorney purchased a confession, but *if* Shaver's story about the Iwuagwu murder proved accurate, once Bout was free, he again set up shop as a counterfeiter. This time, however, his web may have included Onunwa Iwuagwu. The chief suspect in the disappearance and murder of Iwuagwu began to look more like a con man and possible kingpin in a counterfeiting scheme who turned to murder to protect his illegal money machine.

Bout and Iwuagwu had in fact known each other from legitimate business dealings. Iwuagwu had accumulated twenty rental properties, and Harry Bout did maintenance work on some of the properties. According to the story Shaver told police in early April 1985, when Shaver arrived at the Broadway address, Bout admitted to murdering

Iwuagwu because he had obtained counterfeiting plates from him. Iwuagwu's widow, Charlotte, steadfastly denied her husband's involvement in a counterfeiting scheme, but the Secret Service investigated a scenario in which he planned on taking profits gleaned from counterfeit US bills back to Nigeria.

This time, however, no deals would be made, at least not with Harry Bout.

Shaver's story and the discovery of Iwuagwu's body placed Harry Bout and his seventeen-year-old girlfriend, Dawn Bean, in handcuffs. They faced a trio of charges: first-degree murder, conspiracy to commit murder, and using a firearm during a felony. In short, if convicted this time, Bout would spend the rest of his life in prison.

The Broadway home provided more evidence to support elements of Shaver's story. In the upstairs bedroom into which Dawn Bean allegedly lured Iwuagwu, the carpet backing contained bloodstains that indicated the murder occurred there. A bloodstained kitchen knife provided corroboration to the fact that Bout attempted to dismember the body; a metal trashcan and a wooden dowel, both found with cement residue, supported Shaver's story of the four bags of cement, the sump hole, and the disposal of Iwuagwu's body. In the house that Bout shared with Bean (they lived together at the Broadway house but relocated shortly after Iwuagwu's murder), investigators found two .32-caliber shells.

Investigators also located an employee at a local lumber store. According to the employee (who also testified at the trial), Bout asked him how much cement he needed to fill a hole two feet square and four feet deep. When told he would need five bags, he asked for four bags. "I've got filler," he said.[4] The filler was Onunwa Iwuagwu.

So far, all of the evidence supported Elvin Shaver's story. The prosecution, it appeared, had made a good deal by obtaining Shaver's testimony.

It didn't look good for Harry Bout.

All of the evidence seemed to point to Bout as a coldhearted killer, except for one piece of evidence that, if Bout was guilty, was difficult to explain and difficult to dismiss.

The Broadway house itself provided the one piece of evidence that appeared strangely incongruous to the murder case against Harry Bout—a key witness whose testimony seemed to cast a shadow of reasonable doubt over Bout's role in the murder. Evelyn Schneider, the fifty-seven-year-old woman who rented the upstairs bedroom—the room next to the one in which Iwuagwu died—testified that while lying in bed that night, she heard a gunshot from the stairwell and saw Harry Bout run up the stairs, with a shotgun, not a .32-caliber pistol, in hand. He passed her open bedroom door and walked toward the adjacent bedroom—the room in which the murder occurred—and then she heard two more shots. She testified that she heard Bout say, "Dawn, are you alright."[5]

If true, her story placed Bout somewhere else in the house during the murder, which placed two people in the room: Onunwa Iwuagwu and Dawn Bean. Indeed, at the trial, Harry Bout alleged that Dawn Bean had murdered the Nigerian businessman and that his only role in the whole affair was helping to dispose of Iwuagwu's remains.[6]

But could Schneider have seen someone coming up the stairs from her bed? Did the structure of the house support her statement? This vital question would resurface during the subsequent trial.

The trial, however, was delayed for two months. During preparations for the trial, Bout fired his lawyer, and the trial date was canceled and rescheduled. Originally, Bout claimed that he murdered Iwuagwu in self-defense. When the new trial date arrived, Bout's new lawyer pitched a new version of events that occurred in the upstairs bedroom of the Broadway house.

*The People v. Harry Bout* took place in front of a packed courtroom gallery of spectators and reporters, who listened as the various witnesses slung accusations at each other like poisoned darts.

The prosecution's two star witnesses: Elvin Shaver and Dawn Bean, who like Shaver, had agreed to a plea bargain with authorities. Once a suspect in the murder, Bean would now face a jury as a prosecution witness.

Shaver repeated the story he told investigators. Bout murdered

Iwuagwu to cover up a counterfeiting scheme. As if the counterfeiting wasn't a strong enough motive, Bout, Shaver told the jury, believed the murder would result in his acquisition of the Nigerian's real estate holdings.

To win a first-degree murder conviction, the prosecution had to prove that the crime was premeditated. The friend-turned-witness for the prosecution provided details about this aspect of the case as well. Bout, Shaver explained, spoke about the murder months in advance. He discussed murder plots and methods of disposing of Iwuagwu's body. Bout showed him a .32-caliber pistol about six weeks before the crime occurred and said he bought it for the purpose of murdering Iwuagwu.

And when Shaver arrived at the Broadway house, Shaver told the jury, Bout admitted to the murder.

Dawn Bean had told investigators a different version than the one that Bout had allegedly told Shaver the night of March 7—a version she repeated at Bout's murder trial. If, as Bout allegedly told Shaver, Dawn Bean played the role of the teenage vixen and lured Iwuagwu to the bedroom with the promise of sex—a willing accomplice to murder—she would belong next to Bout facing a premeditated murder charge and possible sentence of life in prison without the possibility of parole.

Yet, she claimed, she knew nothing of Bout's plan to murder Iwuagwu.[7] She testified that she thought the three of them went to the bedroom for a ménage à trois—a threesome—and when they entered the bedroom, Bout shot Iwuagwu. She admitted to helping Bout dispose of evidence, including Iwuagwu's car because, she testified, she feared Bout.

Bout, she testified, had even attempted to orchestrate their defense from jail: he wrote her letters directing her to claim that Iwuagwu attempted to rape her and that Bout shot him in self-defense when Iwuagwu lunged at him with a knife. Ironically, Bout himself had provided evidence that seemed to support Bean's testimony. During the preliminary hearing, Bout attempted to pass a note to a family member of Dawn Bean in the courtroom gallery, but a police officer intercepted it. The note contained instructions to Dawn Bean. She was to claim that Iwuagwu had sexually assaulted her; Bout would then claim that he shot Iwuagwu as an act of self-defense.[8] Bout, the note suggested, was attempting to fabricate evidence to support his claim of innocence.

In reality, Bean noted in her testimony, Bout had asked her as early as February to help him dispose of his alleged blackmailer, but she refused. Her version placed the onus of murder on Bout and Bout alone.

For a third time, one of Bout's associates, this time his girlfriend, had betrayed him with authorities, who offered her a deal that only a fool would reject: they charged her with accessory after the fact—a charge that carried a maximum five-year sentence—in exchange for her testimony against Harry Bout.

Caveat emptor? Did the prosecution make a good deal? Harry Bout would provide his answer to this question when he testified in his own defense.

In his testimony, Bout offered yet another version of events that led to Iwuagwu's death.[9] According to Bout, Dawn Bean agreed to sex with Iwuagwu, who in turn offered to arrange for Bout to have sex with a female acquaintance of Iwuagwu's. When he heard shots from the upstairs bedroom, Bout grabbed his mother's shotgun, loading it as he raced up the stairs. (It is at this point that Evelyn Schneider testified she witnessed him at the top of the stairs.) Inside the room, he claimed to have seen Dawn Bean with the gun in her hands and Onunwa Iwuagwu dead on the floor. In Bout's version, Bean allegedly shot Iwuagwu because at some point she changed her mind about the sex, but he forced the issue. Bout's only wrongdoing in the affair, he maintained, was in helping Bean conceal the corpse.

Thus, the real killer, Bout alleged during his testimony, was one of the prosecution's two star witnesses. Bout's story placed the .32 that killed Iwuagwu in Dawn Bean's hand; the deal with the prosecution, according to this version of Iwuagwu's murder, released her from murder charges. Subsequently, Harry Bout found the .32 thrust into his hand and found himself facing life in prison.

Yet Bout's story had experienced an evolution of sorts, a fact that leeched away some of his credibility and threw suspicion on the version he now told the jury. During an early phase of the case, Bout claimed that he, not Dawn Bean, shot the Nigerian in self-defense. In his testimony, Bout offered an explanation for this change in stories.

This story, he now told jurors, had been fabricated at the advice of the attorney who represented him during the arraignment. No one would believe that sweet, innocent teenager Dawn Bean murdered anyone in cold blood, so, Bout alleged in his testimony, his former attorney helped him to fabricate the self-defense story. They even allegedly created a murder weapon—a knife—to sell the story. According to Bout, a photograph of the knife was sent to Bean so she could later identify it, and at the attorney's alleged direction, Bout wrote letters to Bean about the self-defense scenario.

As an interesting twist of the usual courtroom dynamic, the attorney would answer the allegations as a prosecution rebuttal witness. The trial judge ruled that the attorney-client privilege vaporized with Bout's allegations, so his former lawyer could testify about what they discussed. The attorney denied any involvement in a fabrication. Bout, he testified, told him that he killed Iwuagwu in self-defense but at one point characterized the prosecution's case as accurate, an admission that the lawyer interpreted to be an admission of guilt.

Bout originally pointed his finger at Elvin Shaver, the lawyer testified, then changed his story to self-defense. Only after he learned that Bean would testify against him, the lawyer noted, did he finger Bean for the murder.

Things didn't look good for Harry Bout.

Yet Schneider's testimony corroborated Bout's version, *if* she had been able to see someone coming up the stairs from her bed. The prosecution called two witnesses—Grand Rapids police officers—who testified that she could not have seen someone coming up the stairs and passing in front of the door to her bedroom if her head was near the bed's headboard (she testified that she was trying to go to sleep when she heard the shots).

The defense presented witnesses who indicated a person in the spot Schneider claimed to be *could* see someone coming up the stairs. While the jury did see photographs and diagrams of the floor plan, the presiding judge denied a defense motion to visit the house and crime scene, a decision that, according to Michigan law, is at the judge's discretion. The jury would have to decide the issue from the photographs and the testimony.

Schneider's testimony did raise a few questions that were probed by the prosecution. After she saw Bout with the shotgun, why didn't she get out of bed to investigate? Surely, she had reason for concern. No, she replied, she thought the young tenants were having a party.

Why didn't she tell investigators about what she saw when she gave her statement the day they found Iwuagwu's remains? She responded that she was upset and didn't remember.

The crime scene and forensic evidence also created an intriguing inconsistency with Schneider's testimony. Schneider claimed that the first shot came from the stairwell, where she saw Harry Bout with a shotgun. Yet crime scene technicians found no evidence anywhere in the house that a shotgun was fired, and the autopsy revealed that Iwuagwu sustained three wounds from a .32 at close range. So if Schneider did see Bout on the stairwell with the shotgun *after* hearing the first shot, it seems impossible that he pulled the trigger of the gun that murdered Iwuagwu, unless Schneider erred in remembering what she saw that night. Despite the inconsistencies, Schneider's testimony lent some credibility to Bout's story.

The jury deliberated for seven and a half hours, during which time they contemplated the testimony of Dawn Bean, who admitted to being in the house (and in the room) during the murder and to helping conceal the body; Elvin Shaver, a witness with a checkered legal past who admitted to helping conceal the body; and Evelyn Schneider, the tenant who claimed to have seen Bout run up the stairs after she heard the first shot.

Schneider's testimony was like a penny on the railroad track: it seemed to derail the train carrying Harry Bout straight to state prison.

Jurors asked to see the floor plans and photographs of the Broadway house during their deliberations. Still, the jury could not eliminate the question marks surrounding Schneider's testimony. Nevertheless, Schneider's testimony, while it raised some doubt, apparently didn't raise enough doubt.

The jury didn't buy Bout's claim of innocence and found him guilty of all counts. Sentencing followed: Bout would spend the rest of his days in a Michigan cell. Elvin Shaver received two-and-a-half to five years. Dawn Bean received a sentence of one year and a stern warning from the judge who sentenced her: "If you stub your toe or get into further trouble I'll deal with you severely," Judge Stuart Hoffius warned.[10]

Case closed. The denouement to this murder mystery occurred when the jury read its verdict in August 1985.

Or so it appeared.

A revelation of sorts occurred. In December 1987, Elvin Shaver recanted his testimony and made shocking allegations. Police officers, he claimed in an affidavit, threatened him with a life sentence as a habitual criminal if he did not cooperate with testimony that depicted Bout as a coldhearted murderer and architect of Iwuagwu's demise.[11]

Shaver's allegations offered yet another twist in this already serpentine case.

According to Shaver's affidavit: his explanation of the motive that Bout murdered Iwuagwu to avoid blackmail and potential exposure as a counterfeiter?

Forced.

His story about Bout's admission of the murder on March 7, 1985?

Coerced.

The fact that Bout discussed the murder before March 7, 1985?

Not a fact.

The officers, he alleged, even resorted to strong-arm tactics and pushed him around in a back hall. In short, the prosecution's key witness now admitted to lying under oath.

Michigan courts, though, have typically viewed recanted testimony with a healthy dose of suspicion. For good reason—caveat emptor. What may appear genuine may in fact be a sham. Counterfeit. One coconspirator, for example, "rolls over" on another coconspirator in return for a reduced sentence, a plea bargain, or immunity. After a conviction, the coconspirator with a deal recants his testimony, creating reasonable doubt and a basis for at least a new trial and at most an acquittal or a vacated sentence. Did Elvin Shaver have a crisis of conscience and attempt to give his friend an "out"? Honor among thieves, perhaps? Or was he telling the truth this time?

Other statements Shaver made suggested that his new "truth" about police corruption lacked merit. In a letter he allegedly wrote to Bout, he admitted that he conjured the story that detectives bullied him in a hallway and made several other peculiar statements that called his allegations as well as his trial testimony into question: "They did not fabricate about (you) being blackmailed over the counterfeiting because that is what I told them." "You know Harry, they wanted you so bad and so I told them what they wanted to know to help myself. So I lied to get a deal. I am very sorry, Harry." "Well, Harry, I believed in my mind that you did do the killing that I actually made myself believe that you talked about it before and after. But since I had the chance to think about it you really never said anything about killing."[12] Elvin Shaver, it now appeared, didn't even know what Elvin Shaver knew. Lies and truth became so entangled, they were inseparable.

For Harry Bout, Shaver's recantation and admission that he lied represented new evidence and justified a new trial, so he appealed his conviction. The State of Michigan Court of Appeals heard his case and in 1987 returned his case to district court.

Bout would receive another day in court in May 1987. In an unforeseen twist, the prosecution's star witness in the 1985 murder trial would now testify for the defense. Elvin Shaver, though, had one more surprise; when Bout's defense attorney asked questions about his recantation, he repeatedly invoked the Fifth Amendment. Why this change of heart, again? Perhaps he feared that if his statements deviated from those he made in the 1985 trial, he would face additional charges for perjury. His refusal to testify drew the ire of the court and resulted in a contempt charge that added an additional sixth months to his sentence of two and a half to five years he was serving for his role in the burial and subsequent cover-up in the Iwuagwu murder.

Judge Hoffius denied Bout a new trial based in part on the mountain of evidence (including testimony from Bean and Shaver) presented at the 1985 trial that pointed to Bout as the murderer: "I have seldom heard such overwhelming evidence as to the guilt of the defendant," he stated.[13]

Yet ironically, Shaver's refusal to testify and the fluid nature of his "fact" cast some doubt on the story he told investigators in 1985. Once a lie is exposed to air, any truths around it corrode and appear suspect.

Bout returned to his cell and the case file returned to the file cabinet, but it refused to stay there.

Nearly twenty years after the discovery of Iwuagwu's body, Bout obtained a new lawyer and in 2004 another day in court in yet another attempt to finagle a new trial. This time, Bout alleged that his defense attorney in the 1985 trial convinced him to write notes that indicated guilt despite his innocence, which warranted a new trial.[14]

And since his 1985 conviction, Bout's defense claimed, Elvin Shaver was not the only one talking. A former neighbor alleged that Dawn Bean, the prosecution's other key witness in the 1985 trial that led to Bout's conviction, bragged about killing Iwuagwu.[15] Cecil McKinney met Dawn Bean when he lived a few doors down from her on Broadway, and over the years, attempted to stay in touch. In 2003, he swore in an affidavit that Bean not only confessed to the murder but she bragged about it in a conversation they'd had. He also claimed that in 1983 or 1984, he had given her a .32-caliber handgun that she carried in her purse.

Her supposed conversational partner, though, had a long criminal record, which cast doubt on the veracity of the allegation. Circuit Judge Donald Johnston commented on the evidentiary value of statements made to a career criminal: "If you found 12 of the dumbest people in Kent County, they might believe his testimony."[16]

And unlike Shaver, Dawn Bean, the prosecution's other star witness in the 1985 murder trial, did not recant her testimony about the events that occurred in the house at 1572 Broadway when Onunwa Iwuagwu was murdered. Because she did not change her story, it became more credible. Yet not changing her story also fit into Bout's allegations. Changing her story could place the .32 that killed Iwuagwu in her hand, and murder has no statute of limitations. A conviction would take her from freedom straight to jail without passing Go: powerful motivation to stick to her story. The forensic evidence, however, appears to support her version of events.

Result: no new trial.

Meanwhile, Bout's protests of innocence, publicized on various Web sites, had garnered some international support and caught the eye of the Dutch consulate. Representatives of the Dutch consulate and press gathered to watch the 2004 hearing. Bout, born in the Netherlands and brought to the United States as a child, was technically a Dutch citizen and therefore protected under an international law ratified in 1969 by the US government: the Vienna Convention on Consular Relations. Article 36 concerns the rights of foreign nationals detained for crimes and guarantees the accused the right to contact their consulate to procure help in their defense; the country detaining the prisoner must also inform him of this right.

The Dutch consulate became concerned that the Grand Rapids police had violated Article 36 by not allowing Harry Bout to contact the Dutch consulate. Penalties for first-degree murder are much harsher in America than in the Netherlands. Bout will spend the rest of his life in prison without the possibility of parole. Yet if he had committed first-degree murder in the Netherlands, by 2004 he would have completed his sentence. To paraphrase a common saying, do the crime in a country, do the time in *that* country, and the time in America is longer than the time in the Netherlands.

The Bout case was not the first time an entity of the US government became entangled in Article 36 of the Vienna Convention on Consular Relations. In January 1982, two German citizens faced charges of murder and attempted murder following a bank robbery in Marana, Arizona. For their crimes, Karl and Walter LeGrand received a trial, a conviction, and a visit to the executioner. Authorities in Arizona, though, failed to inform them of their right to seek assistance from the German consulate; subsequently, this violation of Article 36 did not emerge during their appeals, which ultimately reached the US Supreme Court but failed to release them from death row.

Just over a decade later, in 1992, the LeGrands learned of the rights guaranteed by the Vienna Convention on Consular Relations. They notified the German consulate and raised appeals on the basis that the Arizona authorities, in failing to notify them of their rights, violated international law. They lost their appeals, and the Arizona Supreme Court set their execution dates for February 24 and March 3, 1999. Despite efforts by the German government, Karl LeGrand's execution went according to schedule. After the first execution, the German government made application to the International Court of Justice (ICJ) to hear a case in which US authorities violated the Consular Convention—international law. The application included a request to stay the execution of the second LeGrand brother. The ICJ granted Germany's request at the eleventh hour—March 3, 1999—the date scheduled for Walter LeGrand's execution.

The ICJ, however, could not break Walter LeGrand's date with the executioner. Both the governor of Arizona and the US Supreme Court denied a stay of execution, which proceeded according to schedule. The LeGrand brothers paid the Arizona penalty for capital crimes. Despite the deaths of the principal actors in this drama, the ICJ heard the case during which Germany asked for guarantees that the United States would not again deprive German nationals of the rights provided by Article 36. In this proceeding, the United States agreed it had violated Article 36 in the LeGrand case. This admission didn't help the LeGrands or others who made similar claims.

Article 36 would reemerge in later cases like a stomachache that would not subside. The Commonwealth of Virginia executed Angel Breard—a citizen of Paraguay and Argentina—despite allegations of

Article 36 violations. And in 2004 yet another judge denied Harry Bout's petition for a new trial. Unlike the LeGrand brothers and Breard, though, Harry Bout does not sit on death row; Michigan does not use judicial execution.

The forensic evidence uncovered during the autopsy proves that someone, using a medium-caliber weapon such as a .32, shot Onunwa Iwuagwu three times in the head. But who? The answer to that question hinges on which story, or rather which storyteller, to believe. The prosecution's case relied on a parole violator who exchanged a tale of murder and intrigue for a promise that whatever sentence he received be served in a federal prison concurrent with the penalty for the parole violation, and a seventeen-year-old girl who made a deal, turned state's evidence, and testified for the prosecution. The defense relied on the story of a convicted counterfeiter and a woman who did see or could not see, depending on whose chain of witnesses one believes, Bout running up the stairs after the initial shot was fired.

The jury chose the former, and Bout received a life sentence for first-degree murder without the possibility of parole. He will never again pass Go.

The tangle of lies, like vines covering a brick wall, is virtually impossible to see through; the truth, like the wall, is there, somewhere, behind the vines, but one cannot see it. A few lingering questions, therefore, remain.

What exactly did the elderly resident of Bout's mother's home see from her bed on the night of March 7, 1985? Evelyn Schneider's testimony is the linchpin in Bout's claim of innocence. She was the only one in the house without a questionable reputation; Bout is a convicted counterfeiter and murderer, and Bean and Shaver both admitted to assisting Bout in concealing the crime and both made deals with the prosecution. Yet, at the 1985 trial, police officers testified that Schneider could not have seen someone coming up the steps from her bed. Did she make a mistake? Or did they? Some even believe that *mistake* is not the right word. Allegations of police misconduct hover in the atmosphere of this case like foul breath.

Yet if Harry Bout did not murder his Nigerian acquaintance, who did? According to Harry Bout, the next logical suspect would be Dawn Bean. According to Shaver's testimony at the preliminary hearing in 1985, she was the only other person in the house at the time of the murder and she testified to being in the bedroom when the murder occurred. Bout claimed during the 1985 trial that she committed the murder; Bout's allegations imply that the prosecutor's deal gave her the ideal chance to bury her crime in false allegations, to mix a different sort of cement into which she pushed her one-time boyfriend. Did these alleged lies bury Harry Bout in a verbal quagmire?

The authorities continue to believe that the answer to this question is a resounding *no*. Bean has never recanted her testimony, and the 1985 jury found her a credible witness.

In addition, the forensic evidence suggests a premeditated crime rather than a crime of passion or an accident, and thus tends to undermine Bout's allegations and his claim of innocence. During his testimony at the 1985 trial, Bout claimed that Bean had agreed to sex with Iwuagwu and was upstairs with Iwuagwu alone. Bout raced upstairs after he heard shots fired. The shooting, according to Bout, occurred as a result of a sexual assault.

In such a scenario, if the woman changes her mind about sexual intercourse and the man presses the point, she might use a handgun to protect herself. Or she might produce the handgun as a deterrent and a shooting might occur if the man attempts to grab the pistol or a struggle ensues. Such a scenario would fit one or two bullet wounds to the chest or abdomen but not three gunshots to the head. The positioning of the gunshot wounds are consistent with someone shooting the victim from behind, like someone lying in wait for the Nigerian to enter the room.

The cries of innocence for Harry Bout, however, continue to be shouted, although it appears likely that no one in the courts is listening. The loudest come from several Web sites, one of which offers several pages of evidence supposedly proving Bout's innocence.[17]

At his trial, Bout admitted to helping conceal Iwuagwu's body, but to this day he maintains that he had nothing to do with the murder. Much of Bout's claim to innocence hinges on the structure of the Broadway house and what one elderly woman could or could not have seen. What did Evelyn Schneider see from her bedroom the night Onunwa Iwuagwu was murdered?[18]

For some, this and other questions about that fateful night in 1985 remain to be answered, and for some, these questions lead to the most important question of the all: is Harry Bout's claim of innocence real or counterfeit?

## Notes

1. John Barnes, "Suspect's Note May Bolster Evidence in Slaying," *Grand Rapids Press*, April 17, 1985.

2. Elvin Shaver gave this version of events surrounding the murder during the preliminary hearing. Details of Shaver's testimony from ibid.

3. Harry Bout's criminal history from John Barnes, Arn Shackelford, Elizabeth Slowik, and Tom Rademacher, "Police Hint Slaying, Phony Bills Linked," *Grand Rapids Press*, April 6, 1985.

4. Quoted in Barton Deiters and John Agar, "Convicted Killer's Story Sways Dutch, but Judge Is Unmoved," *Grand Rapids Press*, June 22, 2004.

5. Quoted in Barnes, "Bout Jury Hears Witnesses Tell Conflicting Stories about Killing," *Grand Rapids Press*, August 7, 1985. The Web site "The Harry Bout Story," available at http://www.injusticeline.com, provides an in-depth discussion of the photographic evidence, including a short video and several still shots of the house interior.

6. Barnes, "'I'm Not a Murderer,'" *Grand Rapids Press*, May 24, 1987.

7. Ibid., John Barnes, "Girlfriend of Murderer Bout Gets Year in Jail, Judge's Warning," *Grand Rapids Press*, October 1, 1985.

8. Ibid., "Suspect's Note May Bolster Evidence in Slaying," *Grand Rapids Press*, April 17, 1985.

9. Ibid., "Murder Suspect Bout Blames Murder on Girlfriend," *Grand Rapids Press*, August 6, 1985.

10. Quoted in ibid., Barnes, "Girlfriend of Murderer Bout Gets Year in Jail, Judge's Warning."

11. Ibid., Barnes, "'I'm Not a Murderer.'" Interested readers can find Shaver's 1986 affidavit and other relevant information about the case on the Web site "Free Harry Bout," available at http://www.geocities.com/freeharrybout.

12. Quoted in ibid. During a lengthy interview, Harry Bout showed *Grand Rapids Press* reporters the letter Shaver allegedly wrote to Bout.

13. Quoted in ibid., "Bout Is Denied New Trial as Top Witness Clams Up," *Grand Rapids Press*, May 30, 1987.

14. Deiters and Agar, "Convicted Killer's Story Sways Dutch, but Judge Is Unmoved."

15. Cecil McKinney's affidavit can be found in its entirety on the aforementioned Web site, "Free Harry Bout."

16. Judge Johnston is quoted in Deiters and Agar, "Convicted Killer's Story Sways Dutch, but Judge Is Unmoved."

17. The aforementioned Web site, "Free Harry Bout," contains an evidence section. Here interested readers can find several apparent affidavits concerning the case.

18. Interested readers can find on the aforementioned Web site pictures and video clips depicting the inside of the Broadway house and the view from Evelyn Schneider's room. Clips can also be found at the Web site "The Harry Bout Story," *Injustice Line*, http://www.injusticeline.com (accessed January 8, 2006).

## The Hand That Feeds

Mary Moynahan's hand displayed an enigmatic injury: abrasions covered her left hand, which had been fractured in several places. The injury left investigators bewildered. Detective Ron Neil recalls the moment when he learned the grisly truth about the injury.

> I went up to Dr. Cohle's office and asked him what might have caused the injury to her hand. Dr. Cohle walked over to a file cabinet and placed his hand in the drawer.
>
> "What do you think about this?" Dr. Cohle asked as he closed the drawer on his hand. His solution made sense.[1]

Her killer, it appeared from the injuries, forced Mary Moynahan's hand into a drawer and repeatedly slammed the door shut, which would have caused intense, agonizing pain to the seventy-eight-year-old. Why would the killer torture her in this manner?

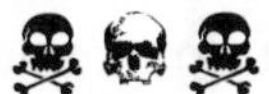

Hastings, Michigan, is a small, rural town that is equidistant from the metropolitan areas of Grand Rapids to the north, Battle Creek to the south, and Kalamazoo to the southwest. It is a town at the crossroads, literally, and as such it has become a popular bedroom community for busy commuters. Although cornfields have disappeared under subdivisions, the area maintains the feel of a small farming community. Winding roads snake through hills covered with deciduous forests as thick as ivy on a wall. Every few miles, a silo, like a defiant finger, sticks out above the treetops as if to say, "I'm still here." And faded red barns that once held farm machinery still stand like elderly residents and seem to invite passersby to sit under their roofs and listen to stories of times past.

Indeed, if buildings could talk, they would tell anecdotes about the personalities that peopled this landscape, mostly farmers. One particular house in Hastings would tell a horrific tale that rocked the small community when a big-city crime shocked residents.

Hastings is also the place retired Michigan state police detective Ron Neil calls home. A twenty-six-year veteran with the state police, Neil retired in 1997 after a distinguished career in which he progressed through the ranks from trooper to investigator to detective sergeant. In Lansing, the state capital, he became a member of the organized crime unit. In his six-year tenure, he investigated major conspiratorial-type crimes, spending much of his time undercover investigating crimes such as a money-laundering scheme in the pornography industry. Next, he worked as an investigator for the attorney general's office, progressing to the rank of first lieutenant and then to Michigan state police post commander.

In his retirement and from a home he helped to build on seventy-six wooded acres, Neil runs Lair Investigations, a private detective firm that specializes in investigating cases of insurance fraud. He named his business for his lifelong fascination with the wolf. The name is appropriate; Neil spends his time watching, observing, and catching those who attempt to defraud insurance companies by feigning injuries. He works about a hundred cases a year.

One such case involved a man who allegedly fell while building a garage—an accident that supposedly shattered his ankle when a truss failed. As a result of the fall and his shattered ankle, he consulted an orthopedic surgeon, who fixed the ankle. Like the truss that led to the accident, the surgeon failed. Or so the man claimed. He sued both the truss company for producing a faulty truss and the surgeon for malpractice. If successful, the claimant would enjoy a multimillion-dollar payday.

The two insurance companies offered to settle for $250,000, but the claimant did not take the offer. Not when he could make much more money with a win in court.

At this point, the attorney representing the doctor hired Neil to do surveillance on the claimant. An investigation typically begins with a background study followed by observations. In this case, Neil parked his van in an inconspicuous spot to watch and film the malingerer in his own habitat. The claimant's property was a veritable junkyard of stuff, such as snowmobiles and old cars. From his van, Neil observed the claimant putting up what seemed like thousands of Christmas tree lights. He also did several other things that seemed like labors of Hercules for a man with a bad ankle: he climbed onto the roof and wrote "Noel" on it, and he placed an extension ladder on an electrical pole and climbed it with a decorative star in one hand and a cordless drill in the other.

Neil watched the scene unfold, amazed at the injured man's limberness. The man couldn't quite get high enough on the pole, so he placed all of the weight on his left ankle (his "bad" ankle) and reached to attach the star; this was all caught on videotape for the court to consider later.

Later that evening, Neil, under the guise of a bystander looking for directions, approached the claimant. On tape from a camera in his van, he caught the claimant admitting that he, by himself, placed over sixty thousand Christmas tree lights on his property.

At trial, the same claimant assumed a different posture; he entered the court with a cane, limping, hobbled by his shattered ankle from the collapsed truss. The claimant and his attorney were given the videotape to review during a court recess, after which the attorney returned and informed the court that the claimant had decided to drop his lawsuits. Ron Neil watched in fascination as the claimant threw away his cane on the courthouse steps, his limp suddenly disappearing. As Neil points out, sheer greed—the lure of a much larger cash settlement in court—kept him from pocketing a quarter of a million dollars. This is *not* an abnormal case, but the wolf prevents such fraud from paying off. Such stories could make a fascinating book, as could the many cases that Neil helped crack in his tenure as a state police detective.

Indeed, Neil's fascination with the wolf is an apt metaphor for his life's work; for twenty-six years, Detective Neil protected his community by investigating and bringing to justice criminals and human predators who perpetrated the most horrific crimes; the wolf thus protected the lair by tracking and capturing those whose actions jeopardized its safety. One such case involved two elderly sisters who vanished without a trace in March 1987, in Neil's community of Hastings.

Five years earlier, Mary Moynahan had moved to the rural commuter community to be close to one of her sisters, Eloise Smelker. She lived in a ranch-style house about four miles from Hastings. Her younger sister, Dorothy Perkins, who lived in a senior citizens apartment complex in the Lansing suburb of Haslett, periodically made the short trek west to visit her sister. The two sisters enjoyed each other's company immensely and often played cribbage together. Tragedy struck during Perkins's last visit, however, which came in February 1987.

Perkins had been with Moynahan for two weeks and planned to return home on Saturday, February 28. When she failed to appear by Sunday, her children, worried, informed police Sunday evening and asked that they check the house for Perkins, who had perhaps stayed an extra day with her sister and didn't notify anyone—the best possible scenario. An officer traveled to Moynahan's house at about nine o'clock in the evening. The porch light was on; Perkins's car sat in the driveway, but Moynahan's Lincoln Town Car was gone. And so were the two sisters, who appeared to have traveled somewhere together.

Yet subtle clues inside the house suggested that although the two sisters were not present, they had not willingly gone anywhere, either. Perkins's son and daughter, who lived in the Lansing area, traveled to Hastings on Monday morning and visited their aunt's home. Inside the house, they did not find the disarray of broken dishes and overturned furniture that would suggest a struggle. Nothing appeared to be missing, making robbery unlikely. In fact, everything seemed in order: dishes done, beds made, and Dorothy Perkins's suitcase packed and ready for the return trip to Haslett. Yet they found something odd: the women's winter jackets. If the sisters had gone somewhere in March in Michigan, certainly they would have taken their coats with them.

They had just vanished. It was as if a hole opened in the earth and swallowed the two sisters.

An official missing persons report followed on Monday morning, and the Hastings police began an investigation for the two women who, to outsiders, must have seemed like opposites; Moynahan, eight years older than her sister, kept to herself and seemed comfortable melting into a crowd, while Perkins, the gregarious one of the pair, liked to chat. Through interviews, investigators managed to piece together a time line leading to the women's disappearance.

Friday morning, between eleven and noon, the pair visited a local salon, which Moynahan frequented, to have their hair done. Later that day, they visited a hardware store, and between two and three, a jewelry store, where an employee said they looked at glassware. A neighbor told police she spoke with the sisters at around four. The last time anyone spoke to the women was at seven that night. Between eleven and eleven-thirty, a neighbor noticed lights on inside the house. The same friend and neighbor who spoke with the sisters at four on

Friday tried again to contact them between five and seven on Saturday without success. Therefore, sometime between eleven on Friday night, February 27, and five o'clock Saturday afternoon, February 28, the earth opened up . . .

Residents of the small community began to grow increasingly concerned, as no evidence of the sisters' whereabouts had surfaced. An ominous storm cloud seemed to have settled over their idyllic community, as many feared that the two women had met some tragic fate.

Police searched the woods around the Moynahan residence but found nothing, no clues as to where the sisters went or what may have happened to them. They expanded their search to a ten-mile radius of the surrounding area using helicopters to scour the landscape for Moynahan's missing Lincoln.

Perhaps the sisters traveled to a restaurant in a neighboring community and had an accident en route. Perhaps the driver had a heart attack and they struck a tree, or perhaps a deer darted out in front of the car . . . but the Lincoln, like the sisters, seemed to have been swallowed whole. Besides, friends and family characterized the two elderly women as the types to eat at local restaurants and take direct routes. A "Sunday" drive was uncharacteristic, and if the two sisters were alive and well, why had they not attempted to contact anyone? But then hope tends to weave illusions that cover and obscure more likelier, more sinister possibilities . . .

. . . like murder. Mary Moynahan was selling her ranch and had advertised the home in local newspapers. The advertisements gave her address and telephone number, which greatly raised the number of people, and thus suspects, who may have visited the home.

Police checked Moynahan's banking activity in Hastings for large withdrawals for some clue as to the sisters' whereabouts. Still, they found nothing. Not a trace.

Then on Wednesday, following a query by investigators, airport security found Moynahan's Lincoln Town Car parked at the Kent County International Airport in Grand Rapids, thirty miles north of Hastings. The car was impounded and searched for evidence, but its presence at the airport raised a bizarre question: had the sisters, perhaps weary of the winter weather, decided to take an unannounced vacation to a warmer clime? Perkins's packed suitcase and the winter coats left at Moynahan's residence seem strangely incongruous with this scenario, as did the sisters' penchant for familiarity and routine. A spontaneous, spur-of-the-moment jaunt just didn't fit their profile.

And the discovery of the Lincoln at the airport seemed to solidify suspicions of foul play. The abandonment of a victim's car at a public place—where it could sit for days, weeks, even months before discovery and buy the killer time to conceal the crime or to flee—is a common stratagem employed by killers. As was seen in "Sex, Lies, and Cement," Onunwa Iwuagwu's car was dumped at an Indiana airport. In "The Sea Shall Give Up Her Dead," Judith Matisse's killer (if indeed she was murdered) left her car outside of Comerica Park, where the Detroit Tigers play, only to be accidentally discovered several months later.

Back at Mary Moynahan's home, family members of the missing sisters continued their investigation and had discovered something that might include a clue to the sisters' whereabouts: Moynahan kept meticulous records of her business dealings. Moynahan's late husband owned a Ford dealership and invested in real estate. When he died, he left his wife with a significant estate and some of his entrepreneurial spirit. Like her late husband, she dabbled in real estate, which led her into an association with a Hastings-based builder named Keith Prong, who had constructed her home. At about the time she purchased the home from Prong, in 1982, Mary Moynahan decided to become a silent investor in his business, Keith Prong Builders, Inc. Moynahan's records included papers that detailed the sums she loaned the developer to build houses.

Prong, a general contractor, had a flawless reputation as a builder. He specialized in the construction of homes in the mid- to upper-price range. He appeared to have a burgeoning business in construction, but appearances can be deceiving; few knew the depth of the hole of debt he had dug for himself. He borrowed from a variety of sources, including the elderly resident of Hastings.

In 1987, Barry County, which includes the city of Hastings, did not maintain a detective to investigate a missing persons report. So Michigan state police detective Robert Golm—whom Ron Neil calls "the most thorough investigator I've been around" and someone who "had the mind to place himself in a suspect's shoes"—was called by the sheriff's department to assist them.[2] It has been said that the best investigators must have the ability to think like criminals. Detective Robert Golm possessed that ability. Now the wily veteran, nearing his April retirement date, applied his experience and skills to the vexing case of the missing sisters.

Detective Golm led a team of investigators who probed the missing sisters' finances. They searched through Moynahan's financial records and discovered a chronicle of Moynahan's business relationship with Keith Prong. The papers gave Prong a strong motive: he owed a significant sum to Moynahan, which led detectives to interview the builder. During questioning, Prong confirmed that the two conducted frequent business. The relationship brought suspicion onto Prong like a searchlight onto a fleeing convict. Keith Prong left the interviews on Monday a prime suspect in the disappearance of the sisters.

And Golm discovered another very suspicious piece of evidence connecting the builder to Moynahan: a check written to Prong dated Friday, February 27: the same day she disappeared and the last time anyone saw the sisters alive. Moynahan's check contained a curious anomaly: while Mary Moynahan had very neat handwriting, the writing on the check appeared shaky, as if she penned it while under some duress. Had she written the check while someone, perhaps Keith Prong, held a gun to her head? Or persuaded her in some other way?

He certainly needed the money.

An investigation into Prong's finances revealed a chronicle of financial woes. The thirty-four-year-old developer and father of four had failed as a businessman. Moynahan represented just one of many creditors Prong owed money; by January 1987, he found himself buried under a mountain of debt. He filed for chapter 7 bankruptcy, claiming a debt of $86,834 with net assets totaling just over $11,000.

His credit card debt alone totaled $22,911. His bankruptcy application listed twenty-eight creditors; it did not, however, list as a creditor his silent partner—Mary Moynahan.

A sinister scenario emerged: a desperate, financially insolvent builder has a meeting set with his silent financial backer, who is expecting payment and is about to suspend her business relationship with him. He decides that the solution to his problem is to murder his chief creditor, except a complication arises—the presence of Dorothy Perkins. She knows about her sister's meeting with the builder and could finger him after her sister disappears. Her knowledge has sealed her fate. She has to go. So he goes to Moynahan's residence, perhaps to squeeze her for more money, then to eliminate one of his financial problems and also the only other woman who knew of the meeting. He murders both of them.

With his prime suspect in mind, Detective Robert Golm made a shrewd deduction. If Prong killed the women, where would he have secreted the bodies and thus the evidence of his crime? Perhaps on one of his properties. Golm focused his attention on a site for which Prong had received a building permit on February 19: a home Prong was building in Middleville—a town a few miles northwest of Hastings. The hunch paid dividends: Golm interviewed someone who reported hearing a tractor or some type of heavy machinery running at the site during an odd hour. The noise in fact came from a backhoe—a piece of equipment used for the digging and filling of holes.

According to Neil, the bodies would still be hidden today had it not been for the sharp instincts and investigative talent of Detective Robert Golm. "If not for Golm," Neil is convinced, "those bodies would not have been found."[3]

Golm traveled to the site, which contained the foundation of a home under construction by Prong. Something seemed amiss; the fact that the wall had already been backfilled didn't make sense. Typically, Detective Golm knew, walls were not backfilled until the weight of the house sat on the foundation, and this house had not yet been built. The site contained *only* the foundation.

An extensive search of the site followed. The search of the property could be characterized by the adage "there is always one place you have not looked." Investigators dug around the entire perimeter of the house to find the clandestine graves of the elderly sisters; the site looked more like a moonscape pocked by craters than a residential plot. In the last place they looked—at the corner on the inside of the foundation under ten feet of dirt—they found what they were seeking. The missing sisters were no longer missing.

On Tuesday evening, March 10—almost two weeks after they vanished—the earth opened up and disgorged the bodies of Mary Moynahan and her younger sister, Dorothy Perkins. Forensic odontologist Dr. Roger Erbaugh (see "The Sea Shall Give Up Her Dead") confirmed the identification of both victims through a comparison of antemortem and postmortem dental charts. Investigators had found the two sisters from Hastings twelve days after they went missing.

The appearance of their bodies left little doubt that they were murdered: both women wore makeshift burial shrouds made of plastic bags taped over their heads with gray electrical tape. Both women's hands were bound behind their backs with electrical tape. And their killer or killers took pains to cover up the crime by dousing the bodies with kerosene—an attempted red herring to throw tracking dogs off of the scent.

One could detect a faint scent of kerosene on the victim's clothes as they lay on the stainless steel tables to be photographed and awaited the last medical examination they would receive in the mortal world.

The white plastic bag covering Dorothy Perkins's head, which appeared to be a trash bag, was speckled with blood. A strip of black electrical tape around the neck fastened the two layers of plastic to Perkins's head, and strips of gray duct tape over the white plastic covered her eyes and mouth, although suffocation was not the cause of death. When the bag was removed at the Kent County Morgue, a grotesque image emerged: bright crimson blood covered her face and saturated her hair. Only after her head was rinsed and her scalp shaved did the extent of her fatal injuries become clear: a dozen gashes in her scalp indicated that her killer or killers struck her head with a blunt object. Twelve times. Enough force to crack her skull, creating a linear fracture on the left side of her skull.

In addition to her massive head injuries, Dorothy Perkins sustained injuries to her left hand before she died: two fractured fingers, abrasions, and soft tissue damage. The damage to her hand was consistent with a scenario in which she threw up her hand in a defensive posture, as if in a vain attempt to protect herself from the blows that ended her life. The damage is also consistent with a scenario in which her killer or killers tortured her by slamming her hands between two hard surfaces. She also sustained three fractured ribs, but the absence of hemorrhaging around the ribs suggests that these fractures occurred after she died, perhaps as a result of the transportation and burial of the body.

Mary Moynahan entered the Kent County Morgue with her head wrapped tightly in a brown plastic bag on top of two layers of blood-speckled white plastic secured by gray duct tape and black electrical tape. Her hands were bound behind her back with black electrical tape.

Three scalp lacerations indicated that, like her sister, Moynahan also sustained blows to her head. The blows did not cause a skull fracture or bleeding inside of her skull, however, so Mary Moynahan did not die as a result of the head injuries. Perhaps her killer strangled her.

If her killer throttled her to death, the delicate horseshoe-shaped bone in the neck, the hyoid bone, would likely be fractured, although the absence of fractures does not exclude the possibility of a manual strangulation. If a murderer uses a ligature (such as a belt or an extension cord) to strangle his victim or covers the neck with a towel or blanket before manually strangling his victim, the damage might not appear. No damage appeared in Moynahan's hyoid bone or cornua (posterior projections) of the thyroid cartilage. No hemorrhaging appeared on her neck or in the neck structures. No pinpoint hemorrhages (petechial hemorrhages) appeared on her neck or in her face or eyes. In short, no evidence existed that her killer throttled her to death.

But her killer had wrapped a plastic bag tightly over her face. Had this been done before death? A complete autopsy revealed no other cause of death. No bullet or stab wounds, no poison or narcotics in her system. With the absence of any other cause of death, the fact that the plastic bags were secured tightly on her head with the electrical tape indicated that Moynahan's murderer asphyxiated her by forcing a bag over her head.

The autopsy did uncover another injury. Like Perkins, Moynahan's hands were damaged: two fingers on her left hand and both the radius and ulna bones in the right wrist were fractured. These injuries indicated that before death, she sustained some type of blunt force injury. For some reason, her killer or killers struck several blows with a blunt object on her left hand and her right wrist.

The day after the discovery of the bodies—Wednesday, March 11—detectives led Keith Prong, handcuffed, into custody. Because Detective Golm was due to retire at the end of April 1987, Detective Neil inherited the case.

The financial links binding him to Moynahan and the discovery of the bodies on his property left Keith Prong facing three counts: one count of premeditated murder and two counts of felony murder. To prove the charge of premeditated murder, prosecutors needed to prove that the builder *planned* to murder Moynahan and Perkins. According to Michigan law at the time of the crime, felony murder consisted of murder committed during the commission of another felony, which in this case appeared to be extortion, as investigators believed that Prong went to Moynahan's home that night to obtain money. The evidence they had collected left little doubt, but the degree of premeditation would become clear only after Prong gave his chilling confession to investigators as part of a plea bargain.

Facing overwhelming evidence, Keith Prong's attorneys wanted to make a deal. He would plead to two counts of second-degree murder in exchange for a full confession to the crime. A full confession . . . no detail omitted.

Yet one detail bewildered Detective Neil: the damage done to the sisters' hands, in particular Mary Moynahan's left hand. Neil traveled to the Kent County medical examiner's office to review and discuss the autopsy photographs. Perhaps the excavating equipment caused the damage to her hand, Neil wondered. The wounds, however, were not consistent with this scenario. The hemorrhaging on her hand suggested the damage occurred antemortem, while her heart still pumped the blood that would cause the bruising at the injury site.

But the wounds could have occurred when someone slammed her hand into something like a door jamb or a desk drawer. This raised an intriguing but not provable scenario: Moynahan wrote out the check with her right hand while someone repeatedly slammed her left hand in a drawer. She was right-handed, and the check dated the day she disappeared was in writing that looked shaken. One can imagine the scene: the elderly woman on her knees, tears running down her cheeks, as her assailant slams her fingers repeatedly in a drawer. In her right hand she clutches a pen and, despite the pain, does her best to write a legible check.

With his plea bargain accepted, Prong tells what Detective Ron Neil characterizes as a "remarkable" story of what occurred that cold Friday night.[4]

He parks his pickup truck at a storage facility where he kept construction supplies. In the back of the truck is his ten-speed bicycle. He has prepared a weapon: a pipe with duct tape on it for a handle. Prong slides the pipe up his sleeve, where he carries it during the five- to six-mile bike ride to Moynahan's residence.

Unlike an earlier story he'd told investigators—that he went to the house to force Moynahan to write a check—he now tells them that he planned on killing her. The murder is premeditated.

The degree of premeditation in Prong's confession is chilling. He plans everything from the murder weapon to disposal of the bodies.

> *He parks his truck, which has the sign "Keith Prong Builders, Inc." on its side door, by a garage he rents. He ties around his waist rope that he will use to tie up his victim and brings plastic sheets that he folds up and tucks into his coat. He rides the bicycle to the residence.*

*According to his scheme, he is going to place the victims in the trunk of Moynahan's car and drive the bodies to a site where, in a few months, a new house will be built ten feet on top of the graves. Had Detective Golm not discovered the location, the home would have effectively covered the graves, its owners perhaps haunted by poltergeists, and the Perkins family would never have found out what happened to their relatives.*

*He strikes Dorothy Perkins several times on the head with the pipe mace he has created and forces a plastic bag over Mary Moynahan's head. He suffocates her, but apparently not before he extorts more money from her: he forces her to write a check in the amount of $10,000. The check is dated the same day that the women disappeared and leads investigators past the scent of the red herrings Keith Prong dragged over his trail.*

*Prong places the bike he rode to her house in the backseat of Moynahan's Lincoln. He wraps the bodies in the plastic shrouds he brought and places them in the trunk. With check in hand and bodies in trunk, he drives Moynahan's car to his truck, where he transfers the bodies from one vehicle to the other. He takes the bodies out of the Lincoln, puts them in the back of the pickup, cocooned in plastic, and covers them with a few pieces of plywood.*

*Leaving Moynahan's car at the transfer point, Prong drives his truck home carrying the bicycle and the dead bodies of his two victims in the bed. He parks the truck on the street in front of his house. Leaving the bodies in his truck parked on the street (!), he rides the bicycle back to the storage area where he left Moynahan's car. He drives her Lincoln to the airport to create the appearance that the sisters took a flight out of the area, and takes a taxi back to Hastings.*

*At home, with his pickup containing the sisters' bodies still parked on the street, Prong has dinner with his wife and kids and goes to bed. At some point, he realizes that he has left the truck on the street. He knows the Hastings ordinance against leaving a vehicle on the street over night. If police tow or even ticket his vehicle, they might discover the bodies, so he gets out of bed and pulls the truck into his driveway. He returns to bed and goes to sleep.*

Neil recalls the interview with Prong as if it occurred yesterday.

> "Keith," I asked him, "how did you sleep?"
> "Ron, I slept like a baby," he responded.

Prong's response speaks volumes about his state of mind after committing two vicious murders.[5]

> *The next morning, Prong drives his truck to the Middleville house site and places the bodies alongside the outside foundation wall. Using a backhoe, he covers the bodies (the sound heard at an odd hour and reported to investigators). After he buries the bodies, he goes to the bank and cashes the $10,000 check, leaving the one telltale footprint on his trail that he failed to cover.*

The check also led Detective Neil to ultimately question Prong about the damage to Mary Moynahan's hand.

Ron Neil believes that torture was not part of Prong's plan. When Prong arrived at the Moynahan residence to extort more money from the elderly matron, Neil speculates, Mary was not cooperative. "I'm convinced that he slammed her hand in the drawer to force her to write the check," Neil says. The handwriting on the check was "shaken"—not her usual, neat handwriting.

What really happened? Only one man knows for sure, but would he talk?

When Neil interviewed Prong, he brought along a picture of the bruises on Moynahan's hand. At the end of the interview, he showed the photo to Prong and asked him to tell him about the bruises.

"When I showed him the photo, he said 'I don't want to talk any more,'" Neil recalls.[6] Prong refused to explain the damage to his victim's hand, despite the fact that his plea bargain depended on an accurate, detailed chronicle of the murders.

When Detective Neil prompted Prong with the likely scenario that the damage could have been caused by slamming the hand in a door, Prong repeated his statement that he would not discuss the hand, leading to a fascinating question. If he confessed to a premeditated crime in all its chilling detail, why, at the risk of losing his plea bargain sentence, would he refuse to discuss the damage to Mary Moynahan's hand? If he did slam her hand into a drawer, why would he omit this seemingly trivial detail?

Detective Neil offers this explanation: "Because you don't torture old women."[7]

The coldhearted killer with ice water running in his veins—a man responsible for bludgeoning one elderly woman to death with a metal pipe and asphyxiating her sister with a plastic bag—refused to own up to using physical violence in forcing Moynahan to write a check.

The forensics evidence uncovered at the autopsy, however, suggests that he forced her hand . . . literally.

The plea agreement (two second-degree murder sentences with the possibility of parole) sent Keith Prong to prison for sixty to ninety years. Prong could conceivably leave prison a parolee. The victims' family members, when asked about what they envisioned as apt punishment, said that Keith Prong should remain in prison at least until he reaches the age of Mary Moynahan when she died. The trial judge accommodated this request and sentenced Prong to a term that made him ineligible for parole until he reaches the age of seventy-three—the age of Moynahan when he murdered her.

This story has a fascinating footnote, an interesting subplot. According to Neil, Keith Prong did not begin his crime résumé with the murder of the two sisters. The pickup he drove that night to transport the bodies to his building site—that he parked on the street and moved into his driveway to avoid discovery—was stolen. So were the previous three pickup trucks he drove. Keith Prong: builder by day and car thief by night. He became such an adept car thief, in fact, that he evaded prosecution for some time; he would steal a car, drive it to Detroit, and leave the car. He would go to metro-area Detroit car dealers, find pickups, test-drive them, and never return. He would have already obtained a license plate for the type of vehicle he planned to steal, so he knew the car type he was looking for; he would simply drive off with the vehicle and switch plates. Amazingly, no one ever caught him. In fact, some of his construction equipment was stolen as well.

At the time of this writing, Prong is fifty-six years old and has spent nearly two decades in prison. He resides in the Carson City Correctional Facility. Now the former builder's neighborhood includes characters like Harry Bout (see "Sex, Lies, and Cement").

"His wife didn't know anything about any of this," Neil explains, referring to the car-swiping scheme. "His life was a life of deceit."[8]

A life of deceit that culminated in a horrific crime when, like a rabid dog, Keith Prong bit the hand that fed him . . . and then perpetrated a double murder.

**Notes**

1. Ron Neil, Michigan state police detective (retired), personal interview with Tobin T. Buhk, August 16, 2006.
2. Ibid.
3. Ibid.
4. Ibid.
5. Ibid.
6. Ibid.
7. Ibid.
8. Ibid.

## "I Shot the Drug Dealers, but I Swear It Was in Self-Defense"

Local police found the deserted car, a rental, parked on the side of a remote dirt road in Bingham Township, Michigan, on May 12, 2004. When they looked inside, they discovered bloodstains and evidence of a violent struggle, including gunshot holes, skull fragments embedded in the passenger side door, and a tooth. Upon further investigation, police traced the car through the rental agency in Chicago to a name: Raul Ramirez, a resident of Texas.

Investigators traced the movements of Raul Ramirez before his disappearance. They learned that Ramirez and Manuel Longoria landed at Chicago's O'Hare Airport nearly two weeks earlier, on April 30, rented the car, and drove it to Traverse City. Later that day, Ramirez checked into a Traverse City hotel. Apparently dissatisfied, he and his travel companion checked out . . . and disappeared.

Michigan's lower peninsula looks like a left-hand mitten. The pinkie finger represents the Leelanau Peninsula. The gap between the pinkie and ring finger represents Grand Traverse Bay, at the base of which is Traverse City. The entire area represents a paradise for the naturalist (there is in fact a town named Paradise), with the majesty of its deciduous and evergreen forests, yellow-sand beaches, giant sand dunes, and innumerable lakes. For the urban dweller, the area provides a much-needed retreat from the traffic and hurried existence of the city.

Within a hundred-mile radius of Traverse City—a resort haven and the crown jewel of the area—one can access the quaint lakeside villages of the Leelanau Peninsula; the massive perched sand dunes (unique in the world) of Sleeping Bear Dunes National Park; North and South Manitou Islands, uninhabited islands that form part an archipelago of islands along Lake Michigan's western coast and part of the national park; or the more sophisticated, metropolitan atmosphere of Traverse City and its network of coffeehouses, specialty shops, art galleries, and boutiques. If feeling lucky, one can visit one of the area's Indian reservation gambling casinos.

During the winter months, skiers shush through snow-covered evergreen forests and bask in the pleasures offered by one of the area's resorts.

During the summer months, divers explore the many wrecks of the Manitou Underwater Preserve, kayakers make the short trek from South to North Manitou or along the Manitou Strait past the perched dunes of the Sleeping Bear Dunes National Forest, swimmers soak in the area's inland lakes, and hikers and campers disappear into the forests. During the first week in July, just about all of them converge on Traverse City to partake in the Cherry Festival and indulge in everything cherry, from the expected (cherry pie), to the different (cherry-flavored tea and beer), to the bizarre (cherry-flavored BBQ sauce).

And then they return to the resorts and the cottages lining the lakes to celebrate the Fourth of July. A bird's-eye view of the area reveals hundreds of glittering blue dots—inland lakes, like tiny blue sapphires, that are ringed by forest. Cottages and residences line the shores of these lakes like so many sunbathers at the beach. It is to one of these residences, on Bass Lake, that Raul Ramirez and Manuel Longoria traveled in their rental car on May 1, 2004. They would never return—alive.

Somewhere in this paradise of lakes, rivers, forests, and resorts, they simply vanished. Despite efforts by law enforcement to locate them, they remained underground—figuratively and literally.

Six days after the discovery of their abandoned rental car, on May 18, 2004, Raul Ramirez and Manuel Longoria surfaced from shallow graves near a property owned by the O'Non family, their bodies bearing mute testimony to their violent deaths. The blanket of cold earth that had covered them for the two weeks prior to their discovery preserved their remains and made a determination of time of death difficult.

Just how many injuries they sustained would become clear when their bodies traveled south to Grand Rapids and an autopsy was performed at the Kent County Morgue. Bullet holes riddled both bodies, and the killer or killers had also stabbed and beat Ramirez, causing extensive damage to his face, including a gash from a knife blade.

In cases involving gunshot wounds, each bullet hole is examined in detail: its location on the body meticulously described, as well as the wound characteristics, including the presence or absence of gunpowder and soot around the wound, and the size and shape of the circumferential sum of skin that is scraped where the bullet entered the body.

The medical examiner must determine the path of each bullet, what internal injuries it caused, and if it caused a fatal injury. Autopsies of victims shot numerous times can be very time consuming and painstaking because the nature of the injuries can illustrate what the victim experienced in his or her final moments of life and what object or objects the killer used.

For example, a depressed skull fracture, which looks like a spider's web, would indicate that the victim sustained a blow to the head with an object like a hammer, whereas a long, thin skull fracture would suggest that the killer used a blunt object such as the side of a two-by-four. In this manner, the medical examiner can reconstruct the crime from the inside out. The descriptions of the injuries can also indicate the degree of savagery in the crime and provide prosecutors with valuable evidence when making their case, as they did in the double homicide of Ramirez and Longoria.

One gunshot tore through Ramirez's arm and severed his spine. Had he survived, the bullet would have turned him into a paraplegic and relegated him to a life in a wheelchair. Another shot struck him in the chest. He also sustained a stab wound to his face, and his face and torso had been battered by a blunt object with such force that whoever struck him must have wound up like a baseball batter before swinging (a key fact that would provide vital evidence at the subsequent trial). Despite the grisly damage caused by the two gunshot wounds, which may have been fatal, the bullets didn't kill Raul Ramirez; he lived for one to two minutes before his killer ended his life by striking him in the head and then in the liver with a blunt object, likely a baseball bat.

Longoria sustained four gunshot wounds, two of them fatal. One shot went through his body, tearing through his right arm before continuing its path through his liver, lungs, and heart. The other fatal shot entered through the back of his head, behind his left ear, and traveled through his mouth, blowing out several teeth before exiting through his nose. In the rental car, investigators found shards of skull embedded in the passenger side door and a tooth. Although a DNA test was not conducted on the material (a bone of contention at the subsequent trial), only Longoria's wounds could have caused the embedded skull fragments. And only Manuel Longoria lost a tooth.

The wounds examined during the autopsy revealed a grisly sequence of events. The killer shot Ramirez twice and Longoria four times. The shot to the back of Longoria's head suggested that the killer either removed him from the car, or, while he was still in the car, stood over him and administered an execution-style coup de grâce.

Ramirez was still alive, bleeding from the bullet wounds that would have eventually killed him, when he was pulled from the car. His killer sliced his face with a knife and took several full swings with some type of blunt instrument. The amount of force needed to create the damage found on Ramirez's head and liver suggested that the killer needed a full range of motion to administer the blows. If he struck while Ramirez still sat in the car, he could not have generated the sufficient force needed to lacerate the liver.

Who committed the brutal double murder? And why? The search for answers led investigators on a trail that would bring them to a drug ring and a trial that would shock the small resort community.

Suspicion fell on twenty-one-year-old Matthew O'Non, an acquaintance of the two Texas men. During interviews, O'Non's name came up repeatedly, but authorities could not establish what role, if any, he played in the murders because they could not find him; he had also vanished.

O'Non was not new to the justice system; four years earlier, he pled guilty to breaking and entering, and a parole violation involving an assault landed him in a state prison. Now, investigators believed, O'Non and his girlfriend, Kristin Drow, had fled Michigan, and an FBI-led manhunt followed.

Two months later, on July 27, the FBI Phoenix Task Force tracked down and arrested O'Non in Glendale, Arizona. Drow had returned to Michigan and was questioned by the police, who did not consider her a suspect at the time. Meanwhile, Matthew O'Non was living in Arizona under an assumed name. When they arrested him, agents found among his possessions two books on identity altering.

The bodies of Ramirez and Longoria were found near O'Non's family's cottage, O'Non knew the victims, and he had fled the jurisdiction and lived under an alias. If he had no involvement with the slayings, why did he flee Michigan and assume a new identity?

He would answer these questions in court. During their investigation, the authorities had accumulated enough evidence for prosecutors to build a powerful case against O'Non for first-degree murder, and from their investigation emerged a sordid story about an alleged Texas-to-Michigan drug ring involving the trafficking, sale, and distribution of both marijuana and cocaine. O'Non had supposedly obtained from Ramirez and Longoria, his alleged suppliers, over fifty pounds of marijuana worth an estimated $30,000, on credit. The debt, according to Matthew O'Non, led the two Texas men to the Bass Lake cottage, where the killings occurred. O'Non admitted to shooting the men, but just how the deaths occurred would become a matter of contention between the defense and the prosecution. Yet one fact remained: Raul Ramirez and Manuel Longoria died horrifically violent deaths at the cottage.

The defense and the prosecution presented very different scenarios about what occurred at the Bass Lake cottage on May 1, 2004.

O'Non's defense, orchestrated by attorney Craig Elhart, in its opening argument conceded that O'Non peddled drugs and that he killed both Ramirez and Longoria at the cottage, but that O'Non acted out of self-defense. O'Non's attorneys painted the picture of a twenty-one-year-old petty drug dealer in league with heavy hitters from Texas. The young drug impresario simply got in too deep. He began to fear for his life and the lives of his family after his failure to pay for the more than fifty pounds of marijuana he obtained on credit from Ramirez and Longoria, who hounded him about payment with harassing phone calls that turned threatening. He supposedly attempted to sting the alleged drug dealers by setting up their arrest, but when his plot failed, he feared that they would respond with force.

For protection, Matthew O'Non purchased an AK-47 from a friend (as a convicted felon, he could not legally purchase a firearm). His version of the story that unfolded on May 1, 2004, depicts Ramirez and Longoria as two angry drug dealers sent to Michigan to kill him. O'Non testified that Longoria called him on the morning of May 1 and threatened him. Later that day, he claimed, the two men arrived unexpectedly at the Bass Lake cottage intent on killing him. Longoria exited the rental car and fired shots at O'Non, who retreated to the cottage, returning fire with his AK-47. He shot and killed the alleged drug dealers, but it was in self-defense:

> *Matthew O'Non, surprised by the arrival of Ramirez and Longoria, in fear for his life, goes outside in his boxer shorts, carrying the AK-47 for his own protection. Longoria notices the weapon, springs from the passenger seat, firing his handgun and then ducking for cover from O'Non, who returns fire with the assault rifle. O'Non doesn't miss, and he kills both Longoria and Ramirez. Fearing prosecution, he removes the bodies from the rental car, and wraps the corpses in the tarps and ropes that he bought at an area supermarket (initially purchased at the request of his parents, who wanted him to remove a pile of woodchips). Fearing retaliation by the Longoria family, he flees to Arizona.*

The defense also offered explanations for O'Non's actions after the killings—actions that seem to call into question the notion that he acted in self-defense. He covered up the killings because he feared that Longoria's family would retaliate and the police would not believe his story. That is why Matthew O'Non wrapped the victims in tarps, buried them, disposed of their firearms, and fled to Arizona.

The prosecution, led by Leelanau County prosecutor Joseph Hubbell, outlined a different scenario, one supported by the forensic evidence and a surprise witness.

> *Matthew O'Non, clad in dark clothes, directs the two Texas men to the Bass Lake cottage on May 1, 2004, perhaps luring them to the residence with a promise to pay his debt for the marijuana. When they arrive, he ambushes them, spraying bullets at Longoria, who is sitting in the driver's seat. The attack occurs rapidly, but when he realizes what is happening, Manuel Longoria raises his arm as if to shield the barrage of bullets, one of which enters under his armpit and tears*

> *through his body. O'Non takes a step or two to the side and fires at Ramirez, who sustains two lethal gunshot wounds, one of which severs his spinal cord, paralyzing him. O'Non fires another round into the back of Longoria's head, killing him and sending shards of bone into the passenger's side door. He then pulls Ramirez from the car, and in a frenzy, slices him with a knife, causing a one-inch long cut in his face, and strikes him with an object like a baseball bat or a board in both the torso, lacerating his liver, and in the head—causing the blow that kills Raul Ramirez. The entire attack takes less than two minutes. He buries the bodies and flees to Arizona.*

To prove first-degree murder, which in Michigan carries a sentence of life without the possibility of parole, the prosecution must prove that the defendant acted in a "premeditated" and "deliberate" way in killing the victims. The prosecution sought to prove the murder charge through the prior relationship that existed between O'Non and Ramirez and Longoria; how O'Non acted before the killing; the circumstances of the killing; and how O'Non acted after the killing. If the prosecution failed to prove that O'Non acted in a "premeditated" and "deliberate" way in the killings, he could receive a second-degree murder conviction and a drastically shorter sentence. Another possibility loomed: if the jury believed the self-defense story, O'Non could win an acquittal and walk out of the court a free man.

In addition to an entirely different version of the murders, the prosecution portrayed a different Matthew O'Non than did the defense—he was depicted as a cold, calculating, and seasoned drug dealer who had purchased drugs from his Texas connection in the past. Unable or unwilling to pay for the fifty-plus pounds of marijuana, he orchestrated an ambush. He lured them to the Bass Lake cottage, and when they arrived he pounced, sending a rain of six bullets into the rental car, murdering them. Greed and not self-defense motivated his actions.

Common sense also undercut O'Non's self-defense claim, which depicted the two victims as assassins. If Ramirez and Longoria traveled from Texas to kill the young drug dealer, as O'Non suggested in his testimony, why would Ramirez rent a car in his own name? And would they just drive up to the Bass Lake cottage? No, they more than likely would have used stealth to approach the cottage. They would have sneaked onto the property under the cover of darkness, armed with pistols muted by silencers. But the prosecution came to the trial armed with more than common sense: they had powerful forensic evidence.

A key part of O'Non's self-defense story hinged on one central question: was Manuel Longoria in the car when he was shot? If Longoria was not in the car, perhaps he did fire the first shot, and O'Non was the defense not the offense.

Crime scene investigators used ballistic rods to follow the trajectory of the bullets fired, and the prosecution presented this evidence to the jury. The ballistic rods indicated that the bullets fired at the car came from two positions just a step or two apart. The bullet trajectories indicated that O'Non first fired the AK-47 at the driver, took a few steps to the side, and fired a second salvo at the passenger. If O'Non had been retreating from gunfire when he fired the shots, the pattern would have appeared differently, most likely more scattered. The ballistic rods seemed to support the likelihood of Matthew O'Non springing on his unsuspecting guests, showering bullets at the rental car, incapacitating one, sidestepping for a better angle, and shooting at the other. The ballistic rods suggested that both men had been in the rental car when they received their wounds.

The forensic evidence uncovered in the autopsy also supported the prosecution's versions of events; the medical evidence suggested that O'Non and not the Texas men perpetrated the attack. Graphic autopsy photographs shown to the jury provided a chronicle of the injuries and how they were inflicted. This chronicle contradicted elements in Matthew O'Non's self-defense scenario, such as Longoria's position during the shootings.

In his opening statement, defense attorney Craig Elhart suggested that Manuel Longoria left the passenger side of the rental car and fired at Matthew O'Non, but the forensic evidence suggested that Longoria received his injuries while still in the car and sitting on the driver's side.

Only Manuel Longoria lost teeth, and investigators found a tooth in the car. And, although investigators did not conduct a DNA test on the shards of bone (a curious omission noted at the trial by O'Non's defense attorney), only the shot to the back of Longoria's head could account for the skull fragments embedded in the passenger-side door. None of Ramirez's wounds would have left this evidence. If Longoria had been out of the car when shot, the bone fragments inside the car door become difficult to explain.

Furthermore, the bullet wound under Ramirez's armpit suggested a defensive posture; someone firing a weapon would not likely throw up his arm as if to shield himself from some harm, nor would someone who leaped from the car, gun blazing, as the defense suggested.

While the bullet wounds on Ramirez's body indicated that he was also shot while still in the car, the force needed to cause the internal damage to his liver most likely would have required the killer to have enough room to wind up and take a full swing. In other words, the forensic evidence suggests that O'Non most likely pulled Ramirez from the car to inflict such a blow. And he did it within a minute of the gunshots.

The numerous skull fractures also indicate that the killer must have battered Ramirez with some type of blunt object. These vicious injuries supported the prosecution's version of events: they made it easier for the jury to envision O'Non as a cruel, calculating murderer rather than a terrified would-be victim who fired his weapon to protect himself after the Texas duo opened fire.

*If* a gun battle occurred with Matthew O'Non retreating from the barrage of shots fired by the Texas men, Ramirez and Longoria must have discharged weapons, but no handguns were found, raising the question of whether or not Ramirez and Longoria even possessed weapons. In the cinematic version of Agatha Christie's *Death on the Nile*, Hercule Poirot intimidates the killers into confessing by threatening to conduct a hot wax, or moulage, test. When a person discharges a firearm, tiny particles of primer residue become lodged on the skin. The hands can be swabbed with cotton-tipped applicators, which can be chemically tested for gunshot residue.

The defense attacked the failure of investigators to conduct such gunshot residue tests on the hands of the victims, which could have indicated that the men fired weapons and supported the self-defense story. Yet primer residue may also be found on the skin of people near the weapon that is fired. And the residue can be easily wiped or washed off. Because of the unreliability and nonspecificity of the primer residue tests on the hands, many crime labs, including the FBI and Michigan state police labs, don't conduct them.

And if either Longoria or Ramirez did fire guns, why did O'Non dispose of them, as their presence would make or break his self-defense story?

Also curiously absent was any evidence of gunfire at the scene. And certainly such a pitched gun battle would leave damage such as stray bullet holes or spent cartridges, unless O'Non did a very thorough job in sanitizing the site . . . or the two Texas men never fired their weapons, *if* they even had weapons.

The prosecution also presented a few curious bits of evidence that suggested premeditation, such as video surveillance cameras at an area supermarket that captured the image of Matthew O'Non purchasing the tarps and ropes in which he would later cocoon the bodies of his victims.

Matthew O'Non, though, had an answer for everything when he took the stand to testify. The ropes and the tarps, which indicated premeditation? His parents asked him to purchase the tarps and ropes to help dispose of a woodchip pile, not to dispose of murder victims. The bushes near the bodies were planted earlier as a memorial to his relationship with Kristin Drow, not after the murders to disguise the makeshift burial.

Yet one thing was difficult to explain: the lack of evidence suggesting Ramirez or Longoria even carried, let alone fired weapons. A pitched gun battle would have left some evidence, such as pockmarks from wayward bullets striking trees or the house, or gun casings around the scene. The discovery of just one bullet casing would lend some credibility to the self-defense scenario.

And, it appeared, that one bullet casing *was* found on the property.

Faye Robyn O'Non, Matthew's mother, who, since 1998, worked as a corrections officer for the Grand Traverse County Sheriff's Office, testified that she had found a bullet casing on the Bass Lake cottage property but discarded it—unfortunate, because the bullet would have provided physical evidence, even if just a shard, to support her son's defense. *If* the bullet existed. She neglected to mention the existence of this alleged bullet when the FBI questioned her.

Even Matthew O'Non contradicted his own self-defense scenario. In his testimony, he explained that he pulled the bodies from the car, which contradicted his version of events in which Longoria sprang from the car, shooting at him. And he did not offer an explanation for the knife gash to Ramirez's face—another injury that becomes difficult to believe in a scenario in which O'Non protected himself from would-be hit men. The forensic evidence and the defendant's own testimony belied the fact that the deaths resulted from an act of self-defense.

His voice wouldn't be the last one the jury would hear.

Later on the day that Matthew O'Non took the stand, the prosecution's surprise witness also would take the stand and counter O'Non's tale of self-defense. The witness was Kristin Drow—O'Non's girlfriend and codefendant at the preliminary hearing. Drow initially pled the Fifth Amendment when questioned by the prosecution during the trial, but after she made a deal with the prosecution—her truthful testimony in exchange for not facing charges in the killings (she would face charges as an accessory after the fact for her role in disposing of the bodies)—she agreed to tell the jury what happened.

Drow's latest rendition of the events that night was a different version than she initially told authorities; she admitted under oath that on previous occasions she had lied to the police and the FBI about what occurred at the Bass Lake cottage on May 1. Her admission about her earlier subterfuge represents a certain degree of honesty, but in admitting to lying, her credibility became suspect, especially when considering the prize offered by the prosecution in exchange for her testimony. The paradox of a witness who deceives authorities and then testifies for them can be summarized this way: "I lied before, but I'm not lying now . . . honest."

Credibility aside, the jury would hear Kristin Drow's testimony. Five days after she refused to testify by invoking her Fifth Amendment rights, and later on the day the jury heard O'Non deny that he killed the drug dealers to avoid making payment for more than fifty pounds of marijuana, Drow took the stand and told a story not of self-defense but of an ambush. Matthew O'Non, she testified, gave Ramirez and Longoria directions to the Bass Lake cottage on May 1. According to Drow, O'Non planned the ambush and prepared the ropes and tarps because he did not want to pay for the marijuana he allegedly obtained from his Texas connection.

When the two arrived, O'Non left the cottage. Drow testified that she heard a male voice say, "No, don't," followed by gunfire.[1]

After two hours of deliberation, the jury returned a verdict. Matthew O'Non, now twenty-two years old, stood to hear his fate; guilty of premeditated first-degree murder. He would receive a life sentence without the possibility of parole. Kristin Drow would receive a minimum of twenty-four months as an accessory after the fact.

The O'Non case created a tsunami that swept up and carried away others, including Matthew O'Non's mother, Faye Robyn, and father, Nicholas. Faye Robyn testified that she threw away a bullet casing she found on their cottage grounds. The bullet, ironically, may have supported her son's self-defense story. Or it was a fabrication intended to give credence to her son's version of events. In either case, one certainty remains: she never told investigators about the cartridge. Her suspension and dismissal soon followed, as did more serious allegations.

In January 2005, Leelanau County prosecutors brought formal charges against Matthew O'Non's mother, Faye Robyn, and father, Nicholas, for a litany of alleged felonies. Faye Robyn faced six counts, and Nicholas five counts, including perjury, obstruction of justice, and accessory after the fact to a felony. Their alleged involvement included the failure to report the discovery of the bullet casing and failure to report that at a family meeting Matthew O'Non told them about the killings and the subsequent burials on the Bass Lake cottage property.

Other damning allegations were made against the O'Nons in the felony complaint. According to the complaint, Matthew O'Non told Kristin Drow that following the murders, his father disposed of the AK-47 murder weapon and buried the marijuana north of the cottage's property line (investigators found Matthew O'Non's fingerprints on the tarps used to bury Ramirez and Longoria, but not on the packaging of the marijuana), then advised Matthew to move the bodies. In addition, the felony complaint alleged that Nicholas O'Non delivered letters written by Matthew O'Non to Kristin Drow, instructing her to give false testimony supporting the self-defense scenario (she testified that the victims did not possess weapons).

After Matthew O'Non's conviction, evidence continued to emerge of a drug trafficking network. In October 2005, four residents of Leelanau County, including Matthew O'Non and his brother Christopher, were indicted by a federal grand jury in an alleged drug trafficking ring based in scenic Sutton's Bay on the pinkie finger that is the Leelanau Peninsula. The probe named Matthew O'Non as a drug kingpin for a ring that peddled large amounts of marijuana in the area.

Just over two years after the murders, the O'Nons made the case a family affair. In May 2006, Nicholas O'Non cut a deal with the prosecution. He swapped all of the other charges for a guilty plea and admitted to tampering with evidence. Just after Matthew O'Non's arrest, Nicholas and his wife traveled to Arizona and met Justin Judd, with whom Matthew O'Non stayed while evading capture in Phoenix, Arizona. There he asked Judd not to tell investigators that Matthew's brother Christopher had helped Matthew flee the jurisdiction and the state. As for Faye Robyn's involvement, Nicholas stated under oath that she walked away from the conversation at this point.

He also admitted to carrying letters from Matthew O'Non to Kristin Drow. The letters, which Matthew O'Non wrote while incarcerated in Arizona, were falsely addressed to O'Non's attorney (so their contents were covered under attorney-client privilege). Later, Nicholas O'Non admitted, he helped Drow to burn the letters, which he believed carried instructions about her testimony (Drow testified that the letters directed her to say that the two Texas men shot first). He received six months in prison for his role in the cover-up.

In early September 2006, Christopher O'Non received eight years in a federal court for his role in the drug operation: two counts of maintaining drug houses, one within a thousand feet of an elementary school. Five days after her son received his sentence, Faye Robyn O'Non would stand and face the jury at the end of her trial for three counts: perjury in a capital crime, witness intimidation, and conspiracy to witness tampering. The verdict: guilty on two counts, perjury and witness intimidation, but not guilty on the third count of conspiracy.

Despite O'Non's claim that she did not lie, the prosecution managed to convince a jury that Faye Robyn O'Non fabricated the story of finding the spent bullet shell from a handgun on her property. The reason? Her motive? Simple: to create substance for her son's claim that the Texas men shot at him first and that their deaths resulted from self-defense.

When a person testifies in a trial, his or her words become etched into the stone of the court record, which at any time, like an echo that can be heard years later, is preserved for further reference. Discrepancies that might appear like tiny cracks in the original trial over time can widen into giant fissures that destroy the integrity of a witness's story. Faye Robyn O'Non told the jury of her son's murder trial that when she found the spent handgun bullet shell, she had visited the family cabin to water the flowers. This tiny detail—that she traveled to the cabin to water the flowers—might appear insignificant, but in her trial, it became a fissure in her story.

The prosecution obtained weather reports indicating that it rained heavily the day she said she found the spent shell. Odd to water the flowers after an inch of rain blanketed the area. Did she not notice this torrential rainstorm? Were the flowers still thirsty? Or did she lie?

This seemingly insignificant discrepancy stretched Faye Robyn's credibility. Her story about the handgun bullet, however, was a much more dangerous prevarication: if it had created a reasonable doubt for the jurors in Matthew O'Non's case, a guilty man may have gotten away with murder.

The jurors also believed that she attempted to change the testimony of Justin Judd. When he made a deal with the authorities, Nicholas O'Non reported under oath that during their trip to Arizona, his wife exited the conversation when he asked Judd to "forget" to tell investigators about Christopher O'Non's role in helping Matt flee the jurisdiction.

Yet Judd testified that Faye Robyn O'Non did take an active part in attempting to alter his testimony. According to Judd, Faye Robyn told him several times that he knew nothing, which was her attempt at prefabricating his statement to investigators. Instead of telling investigators that Matthew O'Non confessed the murders to him while in Arizona, he was to tell them that he knew nothing. Judd's story created a discrepancy between what he said under oath during the trial and what Nicholas O'Non reported under oath as part of his plea agreement regarding how much of a role Faye Robyn O'Non played in the attempted cover-up. The jurors believed Judd's story.

The fifty-one-year-old received a sentence of between thirty-six and one hundred and eighty months—between three and fifteen years—for perjury and an additional fourteen to forty-eight months for witness tampering.

In his signature tune, Bob Marley sang, "I shot the sheriff, but I swear it was in self-defense." Self-defense is a common stratagem employed to mask premeditated murders. Despite forensic evidence contradicting his claim, Matthew O'Non tried this defense . . . and failed.

## Note

1. Quoted in Ian Storey's "Former Girlfriend Testifies to Plans," *Traverse City Record-Eagle*, March 16, 2005, http://www.record-eagle.com/2005/mar/16onon.htm (accessed November 12, 2006).

## Who Murdered the Ice Woman?

On January 15, forty-eight-year-old Kathy Vroman left the Country Car Company in Milford, Indiana, where she worked as a receptionist . . . and vanished.

She went to work in the morning but never returned home. Concerned, her husband, William Vroman, filed a missing persons report. Vroman told police that he last saw his wife when he dropped her off at work at nine that morning, and the owner of the dealership told police that she had left the dealership in a Chevrolet Astro van at 12:30 p.m. William Vroman also worked for the dealership, but he later testified that on the morning of the fifteenth, business was slow so he left to look for work in Elkhart.

The afternoon that Kathy Vroman disappeared, the dealership appeared to be clean and tidy. Conspicuously clean. Almost sterilized. Even a car salesman who visited the dealership at about 1 p.m. on January 15 noted how oddly clean and orderly the dealership appeared. He noticed that the ubiquitous piles of paperwork that typically litter a used car dealership did not appear in the Country Car Company. And the place smelled of disinfectant. The stench was so strong it burned the nostrils. At the subsequent murder trial, this car salesman would recount that when he visited the dealership, Jason Fisher, who ran the Country Car Company, was sweating "like a whore in church."[1]

Someone had recently cleaned the dealership, but something had been missed. William Vroman and a Country Car Company employee, George Aldrich, had seen what looked like spots of blood on a doorway at the dealership and called the police. Investigators visited the used car dealership and with the owner's permission looked around; they found suspicious spots that looked like blood. A search of the premise later revealed more evidence of blood spots and an empty bottle of hydrogen peroxide.

The apparent blood spots at the Country Car Company left investigators with the uneasy feeling that something sinister had happened to their missing person; they had found something that suggested she may have been involved with foul play.

But they didn't find her. Police scoured the vicinity but found nothing.

Kathy Vroman, it appeared, had disappeared into the night.

One day turned into another, and over a week had passed, but Kathy Vroman did not surface.

Then came the break they needed: a startling long-distance phone call from Florida. Kathy Vroman had been murdered, the voice on the other end of the telephone line told the Kosciusko County dispatcher. The caller knew, because her husband, Lawrence Grant, helped to conceal the body. Grant, who after Vroman's disappearance traveled to Florida, provided a rough map to the location of Vroman's body, which was passed to the Michigan state police.

In Florida, Lawrence Grant broke down and told authorities a macabre tale of murder most foul. Kathy Vroman had been murdered at the Country Car Company and her body had been dumped just across the border in Michigan. Grant also supplied a possible motive: Vroman's death may have occurred due to a disagreement over stolen cars.

Thus, the phone call from Florida opened a murder investigation, which in turn led to a robbery investigation, but did the robbery plotline at some point converge with the murder plotline? As investigators probed the background of their suspects during the parallel robbery investigation, they discovered the existence of an intriguing subplot connecting this motley cast of characters. And this subplot suggested a powerful motive for murder.

The month before Kathy Vroman disappeared, on December 2, 2000, the Rice Ford car dealership in Warsaw, Indiana, had $100,000's worth of 2001 model vehicles stolen; three vehicles gone. The chief suspects in the theft: Jason Fisher, William Vroman, Lawrence Grant, and George Aldrich. Jason Fisher owned the Country Car Company and employed Grant and Aldrich. William Vroman worked as a part-time salesman and mechanic for Jason Fisher and as a part-time truck driver for Jason's father, Ralph Fisher. And authorities were aware that other such thefts occurred in northern Indiana. The lines connecting these suspects appeared to form a ring—an alleged car theft ring with the Country Car Company at its center.

Did the alleged ring also include Kathy Vroman? Or did it swallow her? Was knowledge of the thefts motivation for the forty-eight-year-old receptionist's murder?

Investigators initially followed a line that Kathy and Jason Fisher argued over a sum of money that Kathy's husband owed the Fishers, and Jason shot her. The discovery of an alleged car theft ring suggested another possibility, and more questions: did she or her husband threaten to tell police about the car theft ring? Did Kathy Vroman's murder relate in some way to her participation in or knowledge of the car thefts? Was she silenced before she could tell the tale of the car theft ring? It would be a powerful motive for murder.

Investigators now possessed what appeared to be the outer frame of the puzzle. Inside the frame, a picture had begun to emerge: a man, whose face remained concealed behind a shadow of allegations and hearsay statements, stands behind the receptionist's body holding a small-caliber handgun. She was silenced because she knew too much. Now, detectives needed to find the pieces of the puzzle and fit them together, but they were missing the biggest piece: Kathy Vroman. And Grant would now give investigators that piece.

On the telephone from Wildwood, Florida, Grant told Michigan police that he and Jason Fisher traveled north into Michigan and dumped Kathy Vroman's body alongside a road in a wooded area. According to Michigan state police trooper Michael Thyng, Grant's recollection of the scene was reliable, but since he was unfamiliar with the area and the body was deposited in the middle of the night, he could not give precise directions to the spot.[2] What he did remember: they traveled north on 131 into Michigan through a small town (which Michigan state police assumed was Constantine), passed a Meijer's supermarket, and turned north. Michigan state police used the grocery store as a landmark and an intense search followed. The search, which involved units in the air as well as on the ground, took over twenty-four hours.

While Michigan state police searched for the body, local and Indiana state police investigators searched for the various pieces to complete the puzzle: evidence of how, where, and why the alleged murder occurred. The discovery of the missing van, which resulted from information Lawrence Grant provided, lent corroboration and thus credibility to Grant's story. Indiana police located the 1996 Chevrolet Astro van with dealer license plates parked at a truck stop near the neighboring community of Angola. Jason Fisher told investigators that Kathy Vroman left the car dealership for home in the van at approximately 12:30 p.m. on January 15. According to Grant, she did leave the dealership in the vehicle, but feet-first: the van was used to transport Vroman's body. The van provided more evidence that supported Grant's allegations. Inside, police found spots of "red stain" that appeared to be blood on the van's left and right floor mats, step, and right front door armrest. They also recovered a light-colored hair from the step.

Now that the missing person case had become a murder investigation, investigators didn't need a lengthy search for a chief suspect; they focused their attention on Jason Fisher. Lawrence Grant told authorities Jason Fisher admitted to him that he murdered Kathy Vroman. According to court documents, Ralph Fisher allegedly told the police about a similar admission; in a sworn affidavit, which would later become a source of controversy, the lead investigator in the Vroman murder stated: "During further investigation, Ralph Fredrick Fisher, generally known as Fred Fisher, reported that his son, Jason Fisher, had told him that he (Jason) had shot Kathy Vroman." The father also allegedly told police that he helped his son conceal the crime. In the affidavit, the lead investigator states, "Fred Fisher said that he helped Jason with the destruction of the evidence of the shooting."[3]

In addition to the damning allegations from Grant and Jason Fisher's own father, the younger Fisher was seen in possession of a .25-caliber handgun consistent with the type of weapon police would come to believe Kathy Vroman's killer used. The face in the puzzle picture, investigators now believed, was Jason Fisher's.

Police executed search warrants for the residences of Jason Fisher and William Vroman, but their searches produced no evidence of the murder. The Country Car Company was a more fertile ground; searches yielded more evidence that the used car dealership may have been the site of foul play. Investigators found evidence of blood on a doorframe, on the carpet of an office, and on the carpet of the lobby. They also found evidence that someone had removed carpets and applied Kilz stain-covering paint to some of the office floor space at the dealership. These clues pointed to the conclusion that Kathy Vroman had met a sinister end, but without a body, police would never know her fate. The police also didn't have a murder weapon. A lengthy search failed to locate the .25-caliber pistol that police believed killed Kathy Vroman.

They would find one key piece of evidence in the Michigan woods that left no doubt about the nature of the secretary's death.

In the early morning hours of Friday, January 26, Michigan state police officers led by Trooper Thyng converged on a wooded area in St. Joseph County, just across the Michigan/Indiana border, near the city of Three Rivers. Using Grant's vague directions, they searched among the deciduous trees and evergreens, eventually finding their target lying in a ditch about five feet from the road: the body of Kathy Vroman partially buried in a snowbank and covered with pine branches. Her body had been transported and deposited about twenty minutes north of Milford. The discovery of the body closed one file—the missing persons case—and opened another—a murder investigation.

Her body had been concealed under a snowbank covered by pine boughs, but over the eleven days from her disappearance to discovery, the snow covering her compacted and froze. So did her body, which police had to chip from the ground. Kathy Vroman arrived at the Kent County Morgue frozen solid. Stiff.

Before the autopsy could proceed, Kathy Vroman needed to thaw. Her body lay for three days at room temperature, surrounded by lamps to provide a little extra warmth, before she thawed enough for the autopsy to proceed. Heat lamps and fans could have sped up the process of thawing, but a rapid defreeze would also speed up the process of decomposition. So, pathology personnel waited.

The freezing also made it more difficult to establish time of death. When a body lies outside in temperate weather, a procession of insects, beginning with maggots or fly larvae, invades. The presence of these insects can help forensic scientists establish a time of death. Extremely cold weather can impede or even prevent this process, so in such cases time of death is determined not so much from scientific extrapolation and interpretation but from deductive and inductive reasoning based on shrewd detective work. Timing, they say, is everything.

An examination of her body revealed two gunshot wounds to her head—to her face and the back of her head—both inflicted while she was alive. The bullet that struck Kathy Vroman in the right cheek passed through the left common carotid artery before coming to a stop in her chin. This wound proved fatal; she bled to death. Another bullet hit her in the back left side of her head, tearing downward into her chest cavity. This bullet likely would not have killed her. No forensic evidence existed to prove which shot struck her first, but the placement of the bullets suggested a scenario: the killer faced Vroman and fired the first bullet into her cheek. As she lay bleeding to death on the floor, the killer administered a coup de grâce with the second bullet fired into the back of her head. The reverse could also have occurred: the killer shot Vroman in the back of the head, and while she lay on the floor, fired the second bullet into her face, from which she bled to death. Whatever the scenario, Kathy Vroman didn't commit suicide; someone murdered her.

Both bullets were recovered from the wound tracks and indicated that whoever murdered Kathy Vroman used a small-caliber handgun consistent with a .25-caliber handgun—the same type of weapon known to be in the possession of her husband, William Vroman, and Jason Fisher—the owner of Country Car Company and her boss.

Formal charges followed a day after Michigan state police discovered Vroman's body: Jason Fisher, twenty-two, faced a murder charge and a forty-five to sixty-five-year prison sentence or the death penalty.

His father, Ralph "Fred" Fisher, forty-six, faced charges of assisting a criminal and unlawful movement of a body.

Jason Fisher's alleged confederates in car theft also faced a variety of charges. Aldrich, twenty-eight, and William Vroman, thirty-two, faced dual charges of burglary and car theft for their involvement in the December robbery of the Rice Ford dealership. If convicted, they would serve sentences of two to eight years for burglary and six months to three years for car theft. Lawrence Grant, another employee of Jason Fisher and a suspect in the theft, was transported from Florida to Indiana to face charges in the car thefts.

The Vromans's closet, investigators would discover, harbored another skeleton. Their legal troubles did not stop at the Indiana border. The Vromans left upstate New York under a cloud of embezzlement. William worked as chief of the Herrings volunteer fire department, and Kathy worked as a secretary. After it became clear that the department was $60,000 in debt, authorities began an investigation, which ultimately turned into larceny charges (for at least $2,200) filed in New York while William Vroman faced prosecution in Indiana.

They relocated to northern Indiana in August 2000, but they couldn't run away from trouble. It didn't take long for trouble to find them in their new place of residence; less than six months after the move, Kathy Vroman lay on one of the stainless steel autopsy tables in the Kent County Morgue, and William Vroman faced criminal charges in addition to a comparatively minor charge for check fraud.

Jason Fisher waited in jail without bond while one by one criminal charges turned into convictions and prison sentences for his acquaintances. Lawrence Grant, who left for Florida shortly after Kathy Vroman's murder, pled guilty to assisting a criminal, unlawful movement of a body, and car theft. Five and a half years.

William Vroman made a deal with the prosecution. He pled guilty to burglary for his role in the Rice Ford robbery; the prosecution dropped charges of auto theft. He received a sentence of four years: two years incarceration and two years on probation. He (and the others convicted in the robbery) would find out that crime does not pay; the sentence included restitution to the Rice Ford dealership in the amount of $109,342.73, in addition to court costs.

Although he played no role in Kathy Vroman's murder, George Aldrich received the stiffest penalty in the Rice Ford robbery: eight years (the court would later reduce his sentence) for driving the conspirators to the Rice Ford dealership.

As for the elder Fisher, the prosecution dropped the charges of assisting a criminal and unlawful movement of a body. Ralph Fisher now faced a single count of conspiracy to obstruct justice. Jason Fisher, and Jason Fisher alone, it appeared, would face a jury for the murder of Kathy Vroman.

Jason Fisher awaited his December 2001 trial date in prison and began to prepare for his defense. The cumulative weight of the murder charge topped by additional charges of burglary and theft for his alleged involvement in the Rice Ford plot apparently began to have an effect. The investigation had revealed possible lines of criminal activity allegedly connecting the car thieves to Jason Fisher, and a picture emerged of the younger Fisher as the alleged ringleader. If found guilty of Kathy Vroman's murder, he would spend the rest of his life in prison.

Ten months in jail can be a long time indeed, but it is just a fragment of the life sentence that comes with a murder conviction. A life sentence can be a very long time for a twenty-something convict—about sixty years in fact—particularly if it is served for a crime he didn't commit.

In this case, investigators found and arranged puzzle pieces to form the image of a man—the leader of a car theft ring—standing over a victim he silenced to prevent exposure to authorities. But had they misplaced a piece? Did they have the wrong man holding the murder weapon? Jason Fisher would provide a shocking answer to this question.

In early December 2001, Jason Fisher gave investigators a shock: he was innocent of the charges and he had hired a reputable polygraph examiner and submitted to polygraph tests to prove the veracity of his story. According to a statement Jason Fisher gave to investigators, he saw his father, Ralph, shiny gun in hand, standing over Kathy

Vroman's body in the Country Car Company's office. This allegation suggested that father, not the son, murdered Kathy Vroman. He gave a book-length statement of 280 pages in support of his claim.

Yet, the case against Jason Fisher and the subsequent murder charges resulted in large part from statements made by Ralph Fisher and Lawrence Grant about Jason Fisher. Now prosecutors faced a situation: the accused in turn accused the accuser. How could they determine who was lying and who was telling the truth? Jason Fisher, his story perhaps buoyed by the polygraph results, convinced the prosecution that he didn't commit the murder.

According to Jason Fisher's statement, on the day Kathy Vroman died, his father came to the Country Car Company dealership to discuss business with William Vroman, who owed him a sum of money—repayment for an advance Vroman received for a truck delivery. William Vroman wasn't there, and an argument broke out between Ralph Fisher and Vroman's wife, Kathy. Jason explained that he became uncomfortable when the argument erupted.[4]

He left the room, he told police, only to return twenty or thirty minutes later to find Kathy Vroman lying on the floor with a pool of blood around her head. Ralph Fisher, Jason claimed, stood by Vroman's body, holding a gun. He did not, however, tell police that he had seen his father *shoot* Kathy Vroman. According to Jason Fisher, Ralph placed the pistol on a file cabinet and instructed Jason to call him on his cell phone in five minutes.

This story changed everything. The December trial was postponed and rescheduled. The prosecution would have a new court date and a new defendant.

The long arm of the law snagged Ralph Fisher, whose legal troubles were now compounded by a murder charge. The prosecution's case against Ralph Fisher had evolved through several phases: the initial charges of assisting a criminal and unlawful movement of a body were dropped and replaced with a single charge of conspiracy to obstruct justice. The murder charge then trumped the conspiracy charge, which was subsequently dropped.

The fickle nature of the prosecution's case led to some legal squabbles as Ralph Fisher prepared for his defense. Ralph Fisher's defense attorney noted that the prosecution's case was characterized by a vicious cycle of charges, arrests, dismissals, and more charges; according to Fisher's attorney, this negatively impacted his client's due process rights and represented a degree of "vindictiveness."[5]

The prosecution's changing theory also created some fascinating legal twists that would make an interesting *Law & Order* episode. While the state's first evolution of the murder case depended on statements by Grant and Ralph Fisher about Jason Fisher, the second evolution depended on statements by Jason Fisher about Ralph Fisher. Essentially the same evidence applied. Thus, the state's case against Ralph Fisher would result in the defense presenting a mirror image of the state's original case against Jason Fisher. A letter written by Ralph Fisher's defense attorney to the prosecutor provides a succinct overview of the situation: in it the defense attorney notes that much of the same evidence the prosecution intended to use against Jason Fisher would now, in a stunning twist, be used by the defense to prove Ralph Fisher's innocence.[6]

While potential witnesses prepared to sling accusations at each other in court, the defense made its own allegations about the manner in which the prosecution handled the case, much of them based on the probable cause affidavit from the chief investigator in the case. The affidavit, the defense argued, contained misstatements, specifically the statement "Fred Fisher said that he helped Jason with . . . the transportation of the body of the victim."[7] Not only was this statement false, the defense noted, the criminal charge related to this allegation—unlawful movement of a body—had been dismissed. The inclusion of this statement in the official court record amounted to no less than misconduct, the defense alleged.

The affidavit, which contains a lengthy statement from Jason Fisher pointing the finger at his father for the murder, also mentions the polygraph test: the investigator states that he had "also learned that Jason Fisher has passed a polygraph examination concerning these matters."[8] This statement, the defense alleged, was hearsay; the investigator "learned" that Jason Fisher passed the polygraph, implying that he didn't know about it firsthand, and the affidavit did not contain "reliable information establishing the credibility of the source."[9] Besides, polygraph tests are inadmissible in court.

And according to Ralph Fisher's defense attorney, the statement also suggested that "*all* of Jason Fisher's statements were verified by polygraph."[10] Since the affidavit became part of the official court record—in other words, open to public scrutiny—the media reported its contents, which, the defense claimed, prejudiced any members of the community against Ralph Fisher. The charges, the defense argued, should be dismissed.

They weren't.

Despite these objections, in March 2002, Ralph and not Jason Fisher would face a jury for the murder of Kathy Vroman.

The details about the murder remained clouded by various versions of the truth presented during Ralph Fisher's murder trial. Like roses, these "truths" concealed the thorns underneath that could cut and shred the prosecution's case. Testimony of the various conspirators and alleged conspirators turned the trial into a legal form of Truth or Consequences, with the jury as the audience, attempting to ferret out the truth from the various versions they heard. They couldn't all be telling the truth—someone had to be lying.

Jason Fisher took the stand on March 20, 2002, and repeated the story he told investigators. The prosecution could not present evidence from the polygraph or even mention it during the trial, so their star witness's story would have to be the linchpin of their case. The line of questioning included a bit of legal theatrics: Jason Fisher pointed to his father and identified him as the man he saw standing over Vroman's body holding a gun. Ralph Fisher closed his eyes as if to hide from his son's testimony against him.

According to Jason Fisher, in an office at the Country Car Company, Ralph Fisher and Kathy Vroman allegedly began arguing about a debt William Vroman owed to him. Jason Fisher, who testified he didn't feel comfortable around such arguments, left the scene. When he returned twenty to thirty minutes later, Kathy Vroman lay dead on the floor with a halo of blood on the floor around her head.

He left the office, ran to the bathroom, and threw up, and then called his father's cell phone. According to Jason Fisher, Ralph said he needed to move the body and "clean up the mess."[11]

Jason Fisher testified that he could not move the body any farther than the dealership's break room. He and Lawrence Grant (who by the time of the murder trial had already been sentenced for assisting a criminal and unlawful movement of a body) wrapped Kathy Vroman's body in a tarp and secured her legs by tying an extension cord around them. They carried her to a van and transported her to, of all places, a church parking lot where they met Ralph Fisher.

Ralph, according to his son, allegedly told them that they needed to "take care of Bill now," which, Jason testified, he believed meant that they were to kill Kathy's husband. Ralph hugged his son, Jason recalled, and allegedly told him to "get going."[12]

Jason Fisher testified that he could not carry out William Vroman's alleged death sentence. He called his father's cell phone, and new instructions allegedly followed: drive the van containing the body to the Wal-Mart Supercenter in Goshen, Indiana. In Jason Fisher's version, the van and Kathy Vroman's body would sit in the parking lot for several days before being moved once again, this time to Michigan.

Ralph Fisher, Jason alleged in his testimony, directed his son and Lawrence Grant to take the body to Ohio, douse it with acid, and set the automobile on fire, but instead, the two men turned north and deposited the body in a wooded section near the city of Three Rivers. They parked the dealership van that Kathy Vroman drove in a neighboring community—perhaps to create a red herring in the missing persons case—where investigators later found it. They tossed Kathy Vroman's coat and purse in a Dumpster. Jason Fisher also testified that he had dumped the murder weapon—the .25-caliber handgun—in a trash bin.

This is the sequence of events that occurred the day Kathy Vroman disappeared . . . according to Jason Fisher.

Under cross-examination, Jason Fisher appeared to have lapses of memory and responded with "I don't knows" and "I don't recalls." He also admitted that in exchange for his testimony, the murder testimony pending against him would be dropped.

If Jason Fisher's story was the truth, then Kathy Vroman may have died over a $900 debt that her husband owed Ralph Fisher. Or did she? William Vroman, who worked for both Fishers (he worked as a mechanic and salesman at Jason Fisher's dealership, and he worked as a truck driver for one of Ralph Fisher's businesses), testified for the prosecution. He admitted that he owed Ralph Fisher money, but he did not feel that the debt endangered his life.

In fact, he testified that later the day his wife disappeared, he and Ralph Fisher discussed the debt and came to an amicable agreement. Vroman's testimony made it seem highly unlikely that the debt led to murder. Perhaps the alleged argument was about another subject . . . the Rice Ford auto theft? Had Kathy Vroman or her husband planned or threatened to tell authorities about the heist? William Vroman testified that he planned on turning himself in to authorities for his role in the auto thefts, and authorities believed that the murder was tied to the auto theft.

The two prosecution witnesses would also disagree about other "facts" of the case. One thing on which they did agree: both men stipulated that a gun box, which held a .25-caliber handgun and which police found stashed in a Dumpster in Elkhart County, looked like the one used to house a pistol allegedly in Jason Fisher's possession at the time of Kathy Vroman's death—a gun consistent with the weapon used to shoot her. The gun box contained the serial number of the gun it held, which enabled investigators to trace the box to the gun dealer who sold the pistol to William Vroman. But who owned the weapon at the time of Kathy Vroman's murder?

Their agreement about the gun began and ended with the gun box. William Vroman, who admitted to initially purchasing the weapon for his wife—a chrome .25-caliber Phoenix Arms handgun—claimed that the gun belonged to Jason Fisher. He and Kathy lived for a while in a trailer on the Country Car Company lot, and he testified that he had traded the gun to Fisher for propane gas for the trailer.

Fisher, though, claimed that he only kept Vroman's gun for safekeeping when Vroman left town. According to the lead investigator, Jason Fisher told him that he had given the gun back to Kathy Vroman before she disappeared. Jason Fisher also told investigators that he discarded the gun in the same Dumpster in which they found the gun box, but despite an exhaustive search, which included sweeping several streams, police never found it. They could see the "smoke" from its barrel, but they never found the "smoking gun."

Vroman also testified that he last spoke with Kathy around 11:45 a.m., and when he drove by the Country Car Company around noon, he saw the Chevrolet Astro on the lot, but he did not see Ralph Fisher's blue Ford Expedition. This was around the time that Jason Fisher testified he saw his father, holding a handgun, standing over Kathy Vroman's body. In fact, Vroman noted during cross-examination, he first saw Ralph Fisher at the dealership at 5 p.m.

Despite these discrepancies, Jason Fisher's testimony seemed damning to Ralph Fisher's claim of innocence in the murder.

The son's testimony also made the father look like the mastermind behind the auto theft ring—a puppet master who allegedly manipulated and directed Jason Fisher, Lawrence Grant, George Aldrich, and others. Ralph Fisher, according to Jason, directed the thieves as to what vehicles to steal during the Rice Ford heist. For procuring a 2001 Ford Expedition, Jason Fisher claimed, Ralph Fisher allegedly paid him $5,000 and a vehicle worth $12,000. The elder Fisher, his son alleged, taught him how to conceal a stolen car with false identification, specifically, replacing VINs with those from older, salvaged models. Authorities had been investigating other car thefts in northern Indiana. Perhaps the Rice Ford heist was the last in a sequence of robberies.

Jason Fisher told a compelling story. His testimony started a fire that the defense would have to extinguish.

Ralph Fisher's defense posited a much different scenario: Jason Fisher, not his father, was the alleged criminal impresario, bent on controlling his miniature criminal empire at any cost. In the defense scenario, Jason Fisher allegedly hatched a plot to murder both Kathy and William Vroman because they planned to tell police about the Rice Ford theft. Jason Fisher, the defense alleged, decided that he could pin the murder onto his father's lapel, and his father would wear the label of "murderer" without complaint. It's the least a father could do for his son. And the defense posited that bad blood between father and son, which began with a divorce when Jason was seven years old, also factored into Jason Fisher's alleged choice of a scapegoat for his crime.

Jason Fisher, the defense attempted to show through several witnesses, was obsessed with the HBO series *The Sopranos*. He watched the show at the Country Car Company. Acquaintances testified that he patterned himself after Tony Soprano: he dressed like the show's main character and he slicked his hair back. In raising Jason Fisher's love of the show, the defense subtly suggested that he also emulated his television hero by allegedly eliminating informants; during questioning, one witness even testified that Jason Fisher admired the way snitches were dealt with on the show. If the defense allegations were true, Jason Fisher had a powerful motive for murdering Kathy Vroman: she knew about the Rice Ford theft.

The defense called a series of witnesses who one by one threw bucket after bucket of reasonable doubt over the fire created by Jason Fisher's damning allegations against his father.

Lawrence Grant admitted that he participated in the transportation and disposal of Kathy Vroman's body. When he arrived at the Country Car Company at Jason Fisher's beckoning, Kathy Vroman had already been killed and her body prepared for transportation. According to Grant, Fisher took him to a garage, where he witnessed a macabre sight: Vroman's body, cocooned in a tarp, her legs tied with an electrical cord. Someone had already placed half of her body into a makeshift coffin for transportation—a trash can. Grant, it appeared, would play a part in the crime by helping to take out the trash. This testimony contradicted Jason Fisher's story that Grant helped him move the body to the garage and prepare it for transport.

Grant's statements in part led to Jason Fisher's arrest and a murder charge in the first place; he told authorities that Jason Fisher admitted to him that he had murdered Kathy Vroman. Grant repeated his allegations in testimony: "He told me that he did it, that he shot Kathy."[13] Grant also testified that Jason Fisher told him that he shot Kathy twice, and that the experience was different than it appears on television.

Further, Grant testified that he first saw Ralph Fisher at the Country Car Company on the *evening* of January 15—hours after Kathy Vroman's murder. Grant also alleged that Jason Fisher threatened to kill him and his family if he refused to help him with the body, and that he also directed Grant to skip town. These statements presented a sharp inconsistency to Jason Fisher's testimony.

During his testimony, Jason Fisher had offered an explanation for Grant's allegations and the difference in their stories: Ralph Fisher, he alleged, paid Grant to make this claim. Grant did receive $500 in a wire transfer while en route to Florida after Kathy Vroman's murder—a fact confirmed by his ex-common-law wife, Judy Holmes, who also testified for the defense.

Judy Holmes, whose initial call sent Michigan state police officers into the forest to search for the "ice woman," testified that she and Grant left for Florida at Jason Fisher's request, but first stopped at Ralph Fisher's business to pick up money. She testified that they also received from Ralph Fisher a wire transfer of $500 while en route to Florida. This money did not represent a payoff, according to the defense; Ralph Fisher, the defense pointed out, was a generous man inclined to give economic help to his friends and family. He often helped out his son with cash loans.

In her testimony, Holmes also alleged that Jason Fisher had spoken of the murder ahead of time and initially wanted to shoot Kathy and William Vroman in their home as they slept because he feared that William Vroman, who felt guilty about the auto thefts, might go to the authorities. In addition, she noted that a short time after Kathy Vroman's murder, Jason Fisher asked her if she knew what happened to his receptionist. She did, she told him, and he allegedly responded: one less person to worry about. These statements went a long way toward establishing a reasonable doubt that Ralph Fisher murdered Kathy Vroman. Jason Fisher's allegedly loose lips, it appeared, might sink his father's murder charge.

George Aldrich testified that Grant removed the seats in the van used to transport Kathy Vroman's body before the murder—a fact that seemed to suggest premeditation. He also told the jury that Jason Fisher called him on the fifteenth and asked him to return to the Country Car Company to answer telephones. Kathy Vroman had left. Phone records indicate that the call occurred at 12:11 p.m.

And the defense presented the most convincing piece of reasonable doubt of all: an alibi. Ralph Fisher wasn't even at the Country Car Company when Kathy Vroman died. He could prove it; the defense could produce eyewitnesses who together formed a time line of Fisher's movements on January 15, 2001. This time line appeared to establish the fact that Ralph Fisher could not have been present at the Country Car Company when Kathy Vroman was shot.[14]

When did the murder occur? Timing is everything, especially for an alibi defense.

During trial preparation, Ralph Fisher's defense filed a notice of alibi that delineates Fisher's movements on January 15, 2001; it also requested that the prosecution provide a statement with three items of information: the alleged date, place, and time of the murder. The prosecution's response contains two of the three: the date (January 15), and the place (the Country Car Company).[15] Testimony, though, would provide this third element.

William Vroman last spoke to his wife at 11:45 a.m., which established one end of the time interval during which the murder most likely occurred. In his statement to police and subsequent testimony, Jason Fisher alleged that Ralph Fisher appeared at the dealership between 11:30 and 12:30 and that he saw Kathy Vroman's body twenty to thirty minutes later. Phone records indicated that William did speak with Kathy at 11:45 a.m. According to the story of the state's star witness, the murder would have occurred sometime in the next thirty minutes, making the other end of the time interval 12:15 p.m. Additional testimony and phone records supported this time frame; Jason Fisher allegedly called George Aldrich at 12:11 p.m., requesting him to come to the Country Car Company to answer phones.

The murder, this testimony suggested, occurred sometime between 11:45 a.m. and 12:11 p.m. According to the notice of alibi filed by Ralph Fisher's defense, Ralph Fisher was nowhere near the Country Car Company during this time frame.

Anthony Byers, who worked for Ralph Fisher and lived in his home, testified that he removed snow at Fisher's home in Elkhart County from around 7 a.m. to 8 a.m. Fisher was at home at the time, and together the two men left the residence and traveled to Fisher's business in Goshen—RAF Enterprises, Inc. Employees verified Fisher's presence at RAF that morning.

Fisher, according to Byers's testimony, left the business for around a half hour to forty-five minutes; Byers saw Fisher drive away, pulling a trailer carrying an auger. About thirty minutes later, Fisher returned with an empty trailer. The two men then loaded a skid loader onto the trailer and left for Burkholder Repair to return the equipment. On the way, they stopped to fill the loader with diesel. Fisher's wife, Ramona, produced a receipt showing the date—January 15, 2001—but not the time of purchase. They arrived at Burkholder, Byers estimated, at approximately 12:15 p.m. The owner of Burkholder—Levi Burkholder—testified that Fisher did return the equipment on January 15, a fact reinforced by an invoice dated January 15; the invoice also contained a notation that Byers requested to keep the skid loader a half a day longer than he initially planned. Burkholder did not, however, recall the exact time they returned the equipment.

Byers and Fisher returned to the Fisher residence at approximately 1 p.m.—well after the time established for Kathy Vroman's death. Byers also testified that upon their return, Ralph Fisher received a cell phone call from the Country Car Company; Byers recognized the number.

Telephone records indicated that Jason Fisher did call his father's cell phone. Yet if they were both present, as Jason Fisher testified, why did he call his father's cell phone? Jason Fisher claimed that after he discovered his father standing over Kathy Vroman's body, the elder Fisher instructed him to call his cell phone in five minutes, but Byers's testimony cast doubt on that statement.

In fact, the defense suggested, the phone records exonerated Ralph Fisher. The phone records indicated that from his home in Goshen, Ralph Fisher called his son at 11:30 a.m. and spoke for almost ten minutes (the earliest he could have left home was 11:39 a.m.). Kathy Vroman's murder, investigators believed, occurred sometime between 11:45 a.m.—the last time that William Vroman spoke to her—and 12:15 p.m. The call to Aldrich at 12:11 p.m., the defense posited, represented the end of the murder time frame. Ralph Fisher could not have driven from Goshen to the Country Car Company in Milford in six minutes!

The defense hired a private investigator to retrace the route Ralph Fisher claimed he took to the Country Car Company on the day Kathy Vroman disappeared—January 15, 2001. The same route took the investigator almost forty-four minutes. And unlike the investigator over a year later, Ralph Fisher would have made the trip in the slush and snow that is common in January in the Midwest.

In short, Ralph Fisher had an alibi.

The jury deliberated for just ninety minutes before they returned their verdict: not guilty. Ralph Fisher walked out of the courthouse a free man.

So would Jason Fisher. His testimony came with a price: he traded his testimony against his father for the promise that he would not face murder charges. After comparing Fisher's testimony against the statement he made prior to the trial and finding no discrepancies, the prosecutor agreed to drop the murder charge against him with prejudice—a legal term that means the prosecutor cannot refile a murder charge against Jason Fisher for the murder of Kathy Vroman.

This did not mean that Jason Fisher would escape the long arm of Kosciusko County's law. After his father's acquittal, he admitted his role in the Rice Ford theft and pled guilty to burglary and theft. He received a sentence of four years for burglary and a year and a half for theft, his term diminished by the time he had already spent behind bars. The court ordered him to pay $109,342.73 in restitution to the Rice Ford dealership.

Together, the car theft conspirators—Aldrich, Grant, Jason Fisher, and Vroman—received a total of twenty-two years in prison for their roles in the Rice Ford heist. Both Fishers avoided court convictions for Kathy Vroman's murder; the murder charge against Ralph ended in acquittal, and Jason Fisher's charge was dropped in exchange for his testimony at his father's trial.

To date, no one has served any time for the crime, leaving Kathy Vroman's murder without legal vengeance.

Ralph Fisher left the courthouse a free man in March 2002, but did he also leave as a wronged man, caught in a vortex of false allegations and a false arrest? In 2004, he filed a civil suit against Milford County and its sheriff based on a number of claims, including false arrest. It appeared that the investigation into Ralph Fisher's alleged guilt had holes, and not pin-sized holes but gaping tears.

The lead investigator, who had not worked a homicide investigation prior to the Vroman murder, admitted during testimony that he did not try to verify Ralph Fisher's alibi after it was filed because he didn't believe it; he did not study receipts and he did not interview Ralph Fisher's employees. The defense filed the alibi on March 1—seventeen days before the trial began, which the prosecutor characterized as a short time frame in which to investigate an alibi.

Another curious omission in the investigation: while Indiana state police kept the gun box in storage, no one involved in the investigation requested fingerprint tests done on the box. Rookie mistakes perhaps, but negligence that resulted in false arrest? Not according to the courts. All charges were dismissed in both federal and state courts.

Unsettling questions remain for many, and speculation occurs like the muted dialogue of partygoers who engage in discussion when their subject's back is turned.

Did Jason Fisher know that his father could produce a parade of witnesses who would state that he'd been nowhere near the Country

Car Company during the murder? Did the son know that the father would "beat the murder rap" and engineer his own release by exchanging information for dropped charges?

The prosecution believed that the answer to these questions was no. Although the specific details of Jason Fisher's polygraph tests are protected by the attorney-client privilege and thus not a part of the clerk's court file, the results apparently convinced the prosecution that the younger Fisher's story was true. Two different polygraph experts analyzed Jason Fisher's tests, and prosecutors compared the test responses with Fisher's testimony. The testimony matched, and the experts confirmed that he passed the test. Jason Fisher told the truth; he didn't murder Kathy Vroman.

Neither did Ralph Fisher. According to the jury and alibi witnesses, Ralph Fisher wasn't even at the Country Car Company that frigid day in January when Kathy Vroman died, and so he couldn't have killed her either.

Yet Kathy Vroman didn't shoot herself in the head twice; someone murdered her.

But who?

The case is frozen.

## Notes

1. Quoted in Rod Rowe's "Jury Verdict Expected Today," *Goshen News*, March 22, 2002, http://www2.goshennews.com/news/files/2002/3/3-22-2002/news2.html (accessed August 1, 2007).

2. Michael Thyng, Michigan state trooper and crime scene investigator for the major crime task force, telephone interview with Tobin T. Buhk, August 25, 2007.

3. On Thursday, August 23, 2007, the author examined the clerk's files for the state's cases against both Fishers: *State of Indiana, Kosciusko County, v. Ralph "Fred" Fisher*, Cause No.: 43C01-0201-MR-1; Court Documents, *State of Indiana, Kosciusko County, v. Jason M. Fisher*, Cause No.: 43C01-0101-CF-0090. The quoted statements are from the probable cause affadavit in the state's case against Ralph Fisher. Prior to Ralph Fisher's murder trial,

the defense objected to a portion of the following statement in the lead investigator's affidavit: "Fred Fisher said that he helped Jason with the destruction of the evidence of the shooting and with the transportation of the body of the victim." In both his motion for discharge and his motion to dismiss, Ralph Fisher's defense attorney cites the portion of the statement "helped Jason . . . with the transportation of the body of the victim" as a misstatement of fact and falsehood. He does not, however, specifically mention the other portions of the statement as misstatements.

4. The probable cause affidavit in the case against Ralph Fisher contains this statement Jason Fisher gave on December 6, 2001:

> A little [later] Kathy [Vroman] said my dad was on the phone then we talked but he wanted to talk to Bill [Vroman] and Bill wasn't here so he said he was going to come down to talk with Bill or Kathy. Then while we were talking Bill called on another line and talked to Kathy so when I hung up then a little while later maybe between 11:30—12:30 dad came and he started talking about Bill and wanting Kathy to call him when he called and said he wanted to talk with him when she was done, and Bill even asked if anyone was there and she said no, so when she hung up dad started arguing with her about Bill and wanted to talk with him, so I decided to go outside and get away from the arguing, by going out an work on the air bag in the expedition out behind the shop and tryed getting the bag out but I couldn't, so after awhile I gave up and went back inside through the garage and in through the breakroom into the lobby were I saw Kathy laying on the floor with her face down and sort of turned away and blood around her head on the floor and dad was just standing there in the front of the door way to my office with a gun in his hand and then he looked up at me and set the gun on the black file cabinet next to Kathys desk and said I got to go call me on my cell in 5 minutes, and lock the front door behind me. Then he walk out and got in the expedition [Blue] and drove off.

5. Defense attorney Thomas Leatherman's memorandum in support of motion to dismiss, filed January 28, 2002.

6. Defense attorney Thomas Leatherman's letter to prosecution, dated January 28, 2002.

7. Information for probable cause affidavit, filed January 2, 2002.

8. Ibid.

9. Defense attorney Thomas Leatherman's motion to discharge, filed January 28, 2002.

10. Ibid.

11. Quoted in Ruth Anne Lipka, "Jason Fisher Testifies against His Father," *Times Union*, March 20, 2002, http://www.timeswrsw.com/N0320020.HTM (accessed October 31, 2006).

12. Ibid.

13. Quoted in Ruth Anne Lipka, "Defense Rests in Ralph Fisher Murder Trial," *Times Union*, March 22, 2002.

14. Defense attorney Thomas Leatherman's motion of alibi, filed March 1, 2002. This document delineates Ralph Fisher's alibi. The following is quoted from the motion of alibi:

| | |
|---|---|
| 7:00 | home |
| 7:15–7:45 | plowing snow at home |
| 7:45–8:00 | travels to R.A.F. |
| 8:00 | arrives at R.A.F., greets employees & gets ready for work day |
| 8:15–9:51 | in his office at R.A.F. making & receiving phone calls & engaging in the general operation of the business of R.A.F. |
| 9:51–10:24 | travels to drop off rental |
| 10:31–11:07 | travels back to R.A.F. |
| 11:07–11:45 | in his office at R.A.F. making phone calls & engaging in the general operation of the business of R.A.F. |
| 11:45–1:00 | fills up rental skid loader with gas, redelivers rented skid loader, pays bill & travels to his home on CR-40 |

15. State's reply to defendant's alibi notice, filed March 8, 2002.

# 7. accidents

The flickering light of cherry red flares and the electric blue and red flashes of the police and emergency vehicles cut through the darkness of the moonless night and bounce off the wet highway pavement, making the entire area come alive. The flickering crimson of the flares, like invisible hands, holds back the eastbound traffic headed toward downtown. On the other side of the median, traffic has slowed to an almost imperceptible crawl for no reason other than the morbid desire of the motorists to witness, like voyeurs, the tragedy that occurred on the other side. The barrier, literally and figuratively, separates them from the accident scene.

In Michigan, these types of accidents occur often, but they usually involve deer attempting to cross highways. From spring through early fall, one can scarcely travel a length of highway without seeing a whole or partial deer carcass on the shoulder.

But this wasn't a deer.

Minutes earlier, a seventeen-year-old girl had run across the highway to make a meeting she'd arranged with her friends at a Steak 'n Shake on the other side. She would never make the meeting. The impact from the first car that struck her tossed her into the air. The driver of the second car likely didn't see her until she smashed into the passenger side of his windshield, leaving a bloody spiderweb fracture. This impact tossed her body like a rag doll, now unraveling at the seams, backward. A third and fourth vehicle—an SUV and a pickup truck—ran over her body, scattering body parts onto the shoulder.

The death scene investigator arrives at the scene to photograph and collect the body parts, which travel to the morgue where the medical examiner can piece together the accident, if not the body. The autopsy establishes cause of death and subsequently determines how long the victim suffered and if she felt any pain, which will determine the amount of general damages awarded in the potential civil suit that follows virtually every fatal accident. A toxicology screen will also reveal if the victim took any substances that may have contributed to the accident. The presence of heroin or a blood-alcohol level of .15, for example, could explain why she ran across a highway in the darkness. It would also lessen the culpability of those who hit her.

The autopsy revealed that she died instantly of massive blunt force injury to the head that left her skull in fragments. She died when the first car struck her, which removes the other drivers from any possible role in her death as well as any potential lawsuit. The toxicology screen also revealed the presence of alcohol and cannabinoids; this cocktail likely left her senses dulled and loosened the legal noose around the first driver's neck.

Sometimes accident victims come to the morgue with interesting forensic surprises. A police officer, dispatched to intercept a drunk driver speeding the wrong way down a highway, died when the vehicles of the two men smashed together in a head-on collision. The drunk driver died instantly of a head injury. The officer did not. The steering column of his car crushed his legs, trapping him while the car burst into flames. His charred body did not conceal the small hole in his temple caused by a .40-caliber bullet. Facing a painful death, he shot himself with his own service revolver.

By sheer number, a majority of the skeletons in the medical examiner's closet come from accidents that range from the mundane to the surreal to the bizarre. Most come from car accidents. Some come from interaction with animals. Others from work site accidents. One victim was almost severed in half at the waist when a large, two-story-tall door fell on him. Another, a civil engineer, died when a truck backed over him on a construction site.

Sometimes medical mishaps and accidents bring victims to the morgue. One such victim died from complications of a liposuction surgery.

Indeed, if the ME's closet is standing room only—overcrowded with skeletons—it is in large part because of accidents . . .

## Big Cats

The John Ball Zoo, named after one of the city's founding fathers, sits on a wooded hillside on the near west side. As far as zoos go, in proportion to the size of the Grand Rapids metropolitan area, it is undersized, like a toddler wearing an adult's clothes. Despite its diminutive size, the zoo has an interesting setting—it is perched on a hill and situated inside a forest. It is also the scene of a horrific death that occurred in December 1985 . . .

Zookeeper Donna Reed,* in the thirty-third week of her pregnancy, ambles through the winter holding cages of the South American exhibit, making her rounds and checking each of the animals. In early December, the cold, icy hand of winter has gripped the area, forcing many of the animals—those used to a warmer clime—into their winter quarters. At 3:45, fifteen minutes before the zoo closes, she begins her rounds.

The sun is completing its run across the sky, and night has begun to fall, bathing everything in blue that will fade to black—a photographer's backdrop for the Christmas lights that dot the landscape and will soon light up the night sky.

Donna thinks often about the baby growing inside of her. The green, red, and white Christmas lights that outline house awnings and turn pine trees into swirls of light make it impossible to forget the coming holidays, and she wonders what toys she and her husband will buy their baby in the coming years.

She does not know it, but neither she nor her unborn child will live to see Christmas. Her assailant is watching her as she walks through the employee area of the South American exhibit. Hidden in the shadows and waiting to pounce, he watches as she nears the corner. The attack occurs with such speed that she does not have the time to react. Paralyzed with fear, she doesn't scream. She doesn't have time.

A blow to the side of her head knocks Reed to the floor. She flails her arms like a drowning swimmer, thrashing at the air, at her attacker, but these frenetic movements do not help her. On her back on the floor, she feels a tremendous pressure on her neck. Not pain, but pressure—a crushing, enveloping force, like a giant hand encircling her neck and squeezing. Her lips move, but she manages nothing louder than a raspy gasp. She feels the sensation of warmth and of warm fluid running down her neck: blood. And then her vision fades to black . . .

The zookeeper who dropped off Reed at the exhibit returns about forty minutes later at 4:25. The sun has set, and darkness has begun to fall on the zoo, painting the snow an eerie blue color. She walks up the short flight of steps to the outer door of the South American exhibit's employee area. She unlocks the door and is stunned by a sight that freezes her in place: the speckled coat of Naudi—one of the zoo's two resident jaguars—roaming inside the holding area but outside the cages.

The cat first appears in her peripheral vision but stops a few feet away and looks at her; she is now face-to-face with an apex predator. The door leading to the zoo is wide open, and the door behind it, leading out of the zoo, is also open. The cat is essentially a few feet away from freedom. She realizes the tremendous danger represented by the two-hundred-pound cat, which could overcome her at this distance with a single jump and enter the zoo grounds. If he gets past her, he could leave the zoo grounds entirely. She takes a few steps back and slams the door closed. She runs for help. Somewhere, she realizes, on the other side of the door, is Donna Reed.

A few minutes later, two other zookeepers arrive and manage to contain Naudi in an adjacent storage room. When they manage to secure the cat, they find a horrific sight: Donna Reed lying next to a large cage in a pool of her own blood.

Emergency personnel arrive, but they cannot find a pulse . . . Donna Reed and her unborn child have already left the scene.

The zoo's veterinarian arrives shortly after with a tranquilizer gun and shoots the jaguar. The tranquilizers fail to knock out the large animal. Naudi continues to move about the storage area while the emergency personnel remove Reed's body. To prevent another accident, a police officer stands guard with a shotgun . . . just in case.

Naudi and his female mate, Nesha, arrived in 1979 at the John Ball Zoo, where the pair of jaguars became the stars of the South American exhibit.

The jaguar is the only member of the *Panthera* genus native to the New World (the Old World big cats comprise the leopard, lion, and tiger). Their habitat is the jungles and grasslands of Central and South America, but they are occasionally sighted in southwestern America as well. The name *jaguar*, which is of uncertain etymology, may derive from the Guarani word *yaguareté*, meaning "fierce dog"—a suitable epithet. Anyone who comes across a jaguar while hiking through the wilderness may tremble at its terrible beauty, as this big cat is indeed beautiful but very dangerous.

Their coats come in many varieties: a shiny, jet black silk to a gold-and-black spotted camouflage pattern over a yellowish or reddish background and a white underbelly. The number and size of the rosettes forming the cat's camouflage vary in size and shape, as does the general color of the coat.

This apex predator—a juggernaut in its territory—is for the most part a solitary hunter that selects, stalks, and then ambushes its prey. It has some of the strongest jaws in the animal kingdom—a fact that explains its modus operandi, which is unique among the big cats. The jaguar will stalk its prey, then attack it from a blind spot or from behind cover, leaping on the back of larger victims. With smaller victims, it might knock the prey to the ground or even cause a skull fracture with one powerful blow of its paw to the head. The jaguar typically renders its prey immovable by crushing the spinal vertebrae, thus severing the spinal cord, before delivering death by grasping the prey's skull between the ears and subsequently piercing the brain. Some scientists believe that this method of killing comes from a strategy developed from hunting and killing turtles.

In build, the jaguar is the animal kingdom's version of a linebacker: short, stocky, yet large (they can weigh over two hundred pounds), and an excellent athlete. It is a superb climber and swimmer and it typically overpowers animals much larger in size. Its powerful jaws can virtually pulverize the bones of its prey.

With the kill concluded, the jaguar will drag its prey to another spot, where it will begin to devour portions of its victim, beginning with the upper torso. In the wild, the jaguar typically needs on average over three pounds of meat a day, while those in captivity consume four pounds or more a day.

Anyone who encounters a jaguar in the zoo may feel a sense of awe and power and is almost certainly appreciative of the bars, moat, or other barrier keeping the animal in captivity. Anyone who encounters one in the wild feels another sense: terror . . . that is, *if* he sees the jaguar before it attacks. Zoos provide the best of both worlds by allowing visitors to enter the jungle, but one with protective barriers that serve as reminders that their foray into the animal kingdom is mostly fantasy and that also protect them from the animals and vice versa.

That afternoon in December, with the protective barriers removed, the two worlds became one. Although she didn't know it, Donna Reed had entered the jungle, and Naudi had entered the human world. Donna Reed probably didn't see Naudi hiding behind the corner or even when he pounced. And the one-hundred-and-thirty-pound zoo worker didn't have a chance against the nearly two-hundred-pound cat.

It wasn't the first time that tragedy resulted from these two worlds coming into contact, although most such deaths occur when people venture into the animal kingdom, into the realm dominated by apex predators. In 1998, two divers presumably perished (their bodies were never found), most likely killed by bull sharks when a dive boat abandoned them on Australia's Great Barrier Reef—a tragic scenario captured in the film *Open Water*.

In 2003, two men died in parallel incidents half a world apart. A Russian naturalist noted for his work with Russian bears was found in Kronotsky State Reserve, mauled to death by bears. His American parallel, who spent several summers living among bears in Alaska, was killed and partially eaten by bears.

And in 2006, Steve Irwin—the "Crocodile Hunter"—died when a stingray stabbed him in the chest and the spiny barb pierced his heart. A herpetologist with hours of experience in various habitats, Irwin's death underlines the danger inherent when humans enter the animal kingdom.

Like these unfortunate victims, Donna Reed loved animals; she and her husband purchased a farm two years before her death. In fact, her love for animals motivated her to volunteer at the zoo, where eventually she became an employee. Yet unlike the scientists, naturalists, and amateurs who sometimes venture too close to the subjects they study, Donna Reed's death resulted when a predator escaped its enclosure. She loved animals, but her contact with one of them led to her untimely death and subsequent journey to the Kent County Morgue.

Donna Reed arrived at the morgue where the jaguar's modus operandi became apparent in her injuries. Although the jaguar did not chew or feed upon her body after killing her, Reed's body bore the marks of her futile struggle against her powerful assailant. Her hands contained numerous abrasions—defensive wounds that she likely sustained when she attempted to stave off her attacker. Claw marks formed several vertical lines running the length of her back. Several cuts—puncture wounds from the big cat's teeth—appeared where the cat's teeth tore through her face, scalp, and neck. The ferocity of the attack and the force of the jaguar were evident in the gaping wound on the left side of her scalp that shredded much of her left ear.

Reed also sustained two fractured vertebrae, the first and the third cervical vertebrae, located in the neck. She had a fracture at the base of her skull and two puncture wounds to the carotid artery and jugular veins of the neck caused by the jaguar's canine teeth.

The injuries are consistent with the jaguar's preferred method of killing its prey. Naudi attacked Reed from behind, either reaching out and pulling Reed to him, pouncing on Reed, or knocking her to the ground with a swipe of his paw. He outweighed Reed by seventy pounds and likely had little trouble overcoming the zookeeper. Investigators found an interesting item at the scene that provides some perspective about the cat's size: a bloody paw print on the pavement next to a leather glove. The paw was almost as big as the palm of the glove, and Naudi's claws measured over three inches in length!

Once he had wrestled or knocked Reed to the ground, he grasped her neck with his jaws (his upper jaw on the left side of her face and the lower jaw on her right) and bit down, fracturing the cervical vertebrae, piercing the spinal cord and skull, and causing damage to her throat. He held her on the floor while she exsanguinated, or "bled out" from the puncture holes in her left carotid artery and left jugular vein. Donna Reed bled to death, which led to the death of a second victim.

When Donna Reed's heart stopped pumping, the blood and subsequent oxygen supply to her unborn child ceased. Her baby died at about the same time she did, or shortly afterward. Even if emergency personnel had performed a C-section at the scene, they could not have saved the fetus.

An analysis of the death scene provided details that supported the scenario detailed above. The blood spatter that dotted one wall like crimson graffiti marked the spot where the jaguar wrestled Donna Reed to the floor and inflicted the injuries on her neck (the blood pressure causing the arterial spray that painted the wall with her blood). The blood pooled near the drain suggested that the jaguar held Reed at this spot for a time while she bled profusely from her neck wounds. The large amount of blood at the bottom of the drain—at least three to four liters—confirmed this spot as the place where Donna Reed and her unborn child died.

Emergency personnel, however, found her body positioned with her feet toward the drain grate, rotated ninety degrees from the orientation in which she died, suggesting that Naudi moved her body. All of Donna Reed's wounds were inflicted premortem or perimortem. The jaguar moved Donna Reed's body, but apart from the wounds he inflicted during the attack, the cat left the body unmolested.

To provide further confirmation about the details of Reed's injuries and subsequent death, Naudi's jaw was measured (after the zookeepers managed to sedate him). At the Kent County Morgue, pathology personnel made a parallel measurement. A jaguar skull of a similar size was placed on a slightly wary female hospital volunteer to simulate the injuries sustained by Donna Reed. The measurement confirmed that Naudi's jaw and subsequent bite radius was large enough to envelope her entire neck; the jaguar's mouth could open to an astonishing five and a quarter inches, or approximately half the length of a ruler. If you imagine a very large hand squeezing your neck from behind, you can imagine the sensation Donna Reed felt when Naudi applied the deadly choke hold.

After the tragic death, zoo officials scrambled to answer three vital questions: how did the cat get free from its confines, how could they prevent it from happening again, and what should they do with Naudi?

The first question seemed the most important, as the cat's escape had led to Donna Reed's death and could create other potentially dangerous if not fatal situations: *how* did Naudi become free of the holding cage? The zoo and the city launched investigations to answer this question.

In fact, Naudi's escape did not mark the first such incident at John Ball Zoo. Six months earlier, another cat, this time a cougar, got loose and swatted a security guard in the face, causing minor injuries. According to one zoo employee, Naudi was in a belligerent mood the day Donna Reed died; earlier, the cat had lunged at him from behind the holding cage's fencing. Still, the fencing is designed to protect zoo employees and the public from the dangerous felines.

The investigation and the city's subsequent safety report revealed a disturbing answer to the first question. Two zoo workers who came close to a potentially lethal rendezvous with Naudi's one-hundred-and-eighty-pound mate, Nesha, accidentally discovered how Naudi managed to flee his cage. After Donna Reed's fatal encounter with Naudi, the workers helped secure the male jaguar in a storage room of the employee's facility when they noticed an anomaly that likely led to the big cat's escape: a gap between the cyclone fence and the top of a door separating the jaguars' outside cage from inside cage. The gap appeared larger than is typical for such cages.

As the workers examined the door, Nesha appeared at the door entrance and looked through the opening. Her entire head, it appeared, could fit in the opening. If she wanted to, Nesha could have squeezed through the gap and entered the employee area. This is apparently how Naudi escaped. The report concluded that the male jaguar pushed the door open wider and squeezed through the opening between the door and the top of the ramp that led to the holding cages. The opening measured 10 and 3/8 inches wide—more than twice as wide as the initial plan and more than enough to permit the jaguar to squeeze through.

The investigation also focused on the fencing around the zoo complex. The jaguar did come just a few feet away from exiting the building, entering the zoo grounds, and possibly even beyond. If Naudi did escape from the holding facility onto the zoo grounds, the fence to the outside world would represent little obstacle. The powerful cat could simply climb over an eight-foot fence, even one capped with barbed wire. According to some experts, an adult jaguar may even be able to leap over an eight-foot fence. One can imagine the headline and the terror it would create for residents: "Beware: Killer Jaguar on the Loose."

Another concern raised during the investigation involved the availability of firearms to zoo staff should the need arise to shoot an animal. At the time of Donna Reed's death, the zoo facility contained only one firearm capable of stopping an adult jaguar. The zookeepers did have access to a 12-gauge shotgun but only birdshot for ammunition, which would have had little effect in stopping a jaguar on the prowl. While the desired course of action to contain an escaped animal is to tranquilize it with a dart (which is what was used to contain Naudi), a firearm would add a layer of safety for zoo workers, a safety net should the extreme circumstance—like a jaguar running free in the zoo—occur again.

Almost six months after the death of Donna Reed, zoo officials answered the second question—what to do with Naudi and Nesha—by sending the pair of jaguars to a new home: an animal rehabilitation and holding facility north of Los Angeles, California, in the San Fernando Valley. In the early morning hours of May 3, 1986, behind a shroud of secrecy, zoo employees carried the drugged cats on stretchers and loaded them onto a truck to begin their journey west. The move resulted in part from pressure applied by Reed's relatives. The relocation met with mixed reaction from zoo employees: some felt remorse about losing the two beautiful cats, while others felt relief that the animal that caused Reed's death no longer resided in their zoo, where it would have served as a constant reminder of the tragedy.

When such a tragic accident occurs, the finger of blame typically points to something or someone. It's too easy to vilify the animal. One article in the *Grand Rapids Press* referred to Naudi as "the killer cat";[1] another referred to Naudi as "the killer jaguar."[2] Yet one can't blame the cat, because it behaved, one expert noted, as any territorial predator would behave when it feels threatened.[3] No one purposely released the jaguar to initiate a fatal encounter with the pregnant zookeeper. And it would be absurd to blame the victim; Reed didn't free Naudi. In fact, she clearly didn't realize the dangerous situation she stepped into when she entered the holding facility.

The zookeepers could not be blamed, either. The escape did not result from a door carelessly left open. In other words, Donna Reed's death did not result from the negligence of the zookeepers or zoo staff. But shouldn't the zoo officials have known about the design flaw that allowed Naudi to escape?

When the construction on the South American exhibit was completed, the zoo director at the time reviewed the work, as did contractors, but no engineers from the city or any other entity were involved, because, unlike other construction at the zoo, the John Ball Zoological Society coordinated all efforts related to the South American exhibit. Typically, the city hired a consulting engineer to inspect new construction.

The finger of blame would point to the city of Grand Rapids; Owen-Ames-Kimball Company; Scenic-Security Fence Company (the manufacturer of the holding cages); McFadzean, Everly, and Associates; and the John Ball Zoological Society, in a lawsuit initiated by Donna Reed's husband.

The case never made it to trial. Donna Reed's husband, David Reed,* did not intend to bankrupt the city with the suit, and almost a year and a half after the tragic incident, he agreed to a settlement involving a sum much less than he could have won if a civil trial took place: $1.9 million. The defendants shared the fiscal burden of the civil damages, and Reed's family received a lump sum of $400,000 followed by yearly payments until 2007. The city would have lost a much greater sum if a trial did take place.

In the aftermath of Donna Reed's death, zoo officials took steps to improve safety. Some of the holding cages, including the cage of the "killer jaguar," were rewelded. A few months after the tragic accident, in the spring of 1986, the city hired a zoo consulting firm to inspect the John Ball Zoo. Investigators discovered several areas that could prove potentially hazardous to employees and visitors. Among their recommendations: double-bolt locks on the animal cages and a fence around the entire perimeter of the zoo.

Shortly after the death of Donna Reed, the city sold the zoo to the county for the sum of $1.

Today, the John Ball Zoo still sits perched on the side of a hill west of the city. And it now has a fence running around its perimeter, although this provides no real security should another jaguar escape. This shouldn't be a problem. The zoo houses pumas and snow leopards . . . but no jaguars.

## Notes

1. Tom Rademacher and John Sinkevics, "Jaguar Came within 'a Leap' of Freedom," *Grand Rapids Press*, February 12, 1986.

2. Ibid., "Jaguar Exhibit Never Received City Inspection," *Grand Rapids Press*, February 5, 1986.

3. Steven Verburg, "Jaguar That Killed Keeper Finds Home in California," *Grand Rapids Press*, May 4, 1986.

## Klismaphilia

"A" is for the agoraphiliacs, who do it in public . . . or for agonophiliacs, who like it rough . . .
"B" is for blood fetishists, who do it like vampires . . .
"C" is for claustrophiliacs, who like it in tight places (such as cages or coffins) . . . or for coprophiliacs, who (literally) give a shit . . .
"D" is for dacryphiliacs, who do it with tears . . .
"E" is for erotic asphyxiation—the loving chokehold . . .

In the ABCs of sexual fetishism, the letter "K" belongs to klismaphiliacs . . .

If one spends enough time around a morgue, one will see some very bizarre ways in which people have died. Evidence? Consider the strange death of Gary Malchevski.*

Forty-eight-year-old Malchevski worked for an area car dealership as an accounts payable clerk. His supervisor characterized him as an ideal employee, never late for work, never absent. He never took vacation days. He lived alone and kept to himself, eating his lunch in his car instead of in the staff lunchroom. People knew *of* him more than they knew him. He never came to work parties. His desk did not contain the usual photographs of friends and family or the typical clutter. Just a pile of yellow sticky notes stuck to his desk.

"He had this unsettling way of talking with you and not looking into your eyes. He looked off in the distance, at something on a nearby desk, but not directly at you," his supervisor, John Kendrick,* recalls.

The Monday he didn't show up for work, no fewer than fifty-two yellow notes littered his desk—a fact from which investigators deduced that the loner had not intended to leave the world.

That Monday was a typically frigid, sunless January day. Kendrick called his employee three times before making the short trip to Malchevski's small home just before noon. (Malchevski had no emergency contact in his employee file.) The solitary accounts payable clerk didn't answer the door. Kendrick told police that he knocked loud enough "to wake the dead," but no one answered.

He peered through the side window of the detached, one-stall garage, hoping *not* to see Malchevski's Toyota Celica parked inside, hoping that as uncharacteristic as it would be, perhaps Gary Malchevski had visited a local nightclub after work on Friday, met the love of his life, drove to the airport, and caught a red-eye to Las Vegas for a quickie wedding.

Kendrick peeped through the windows of the living room and the kitchen but still saw no signs of life. The venetian blinds in what appeared to be the bedroom were drawn. He tried the back door and, to his surprise, found it unlocked. He opened the door just enough to stick his head inside.

"Hello, Gary," he said in a hushed tone.

No answer.

"Hello." A little louder.

No answer.

"Hello," he shouted.

No answer.

Despite what felt like an invasion of the man's privacy, Kendrick stepped inside the door. He walked up the short flight of steps to the main floor when he noticed a peculiar smell—a sickly-sweet, pungent odor. Although he never smelled it before, Kendrick knew what it represented. He jumped down the steps and out the door and stood in the middle of Malchevski's postage stamp–sized lot. As he dialed the police on his cell phone, he realized his hands were shaking.

Investigators found Gary Malchevski amid a scene the likes of which none of them had ever quite seen before. He had died days before, most likely sometime Friday night (a neighbor reported last seeing him at around six on Friday night), and the lividity indicated that he died in the exact position in which investigators found him.

Malchevski was lying on his left side, his legs apart, with a pair of purple woman's panties slid down to midthigh. He was wearing a T-shirt advertising "Trojan" condoms, and whatever type of sex he was practicing and with whom, he apparently attempted to make it safe sex, as he was wearing a condom. Various pornographic magazines lay open and formed a ring around him. The collage included "nudie" magazines depicting naked models, such as *Playboy* and *Penthouse*, and publications depicting graphic heterosexual and homosexual acts, most of them involving bondage of various types.

Next to the bed stood a coatrack with a hot water bottle dangling from it. A tube from the bottle ran onto the bed and disappeared into Malchevski's rectum. Gary Malchevski had created what appeared to be a homemade enema, but for what purpose?

The scene suggested that Gary Malchevski had engaged in a type of paraphilia called klismaphilia. As defined by *Merriam-Webster's Collegiate Dictionary*, paraphilia consists of "a pattern of recurring sexually arousing mental imagery or behavior that involves unusual and esp. socially unacceptable sexual practices."[1] Paraphilia includes an alphabet soup of varieties. Some of these practices are dangerous and occasionally send their practitioners to the morgue. For example, people who practice sexual asphyxiation experience sexual arousal when their partners choke them (or they asphyxiate themselves—the autoerotic variety). Sometimes, though, a miscalculation can lead to a death.

In the human carnival of sexual fetishism, one of the more unusual practices is klismaphilia—sexual pleasure derived from enemas. Although its name is relatively new (Dr. Joanne Denko coined the term in 1973), the practice itself dates back to antiquity. Several Web sites, chat rooms, and fetish clubs cater to the whims of klismaphiliacs, and either from fellow klismaphiliacs or from his own trial and error, Gary Malchevski figured out a way to rig an apparatus to self-administer enemas.

It appeared that in the midst of sex play, either solo or with a partner, something went wrong and Malchevski died. But how? Perhaps he suffered a massive heart attack and died on the spot.

Gary Malchevski's body traveled to the Kent County Morgue. A complete autopsy on Malchevski revealed no apparent cause of death. No severely narrowed arteries that would have caused a fatal ventricular fibrillation. No skull fractures that would indicate he hit his head (or that someone hit him), thereby sustaining a lethal blunt force head injury.

So how did he die? The question hung over the morgue like a nimbus cloud. The autopsy did reveal a few clues about the decedent's demise. His liver contained fatty change, indicative of a person who consistently consumed large amounts of alcohol. And his colon contained 500 milliliters of a yellow fluid consistent with the contents of the hot water bottle attached to the coatrack and inserted into his rectum.

The contents of the hot water bottle provided another clue: wine. The night he died, Gary Malchevski took at least one wine enema. The toxicology screen would solve the mystery of his death: a sample of his blood taken during the autopsy revealed an ethanol (alcohol) level of 350 milligrams per deciliter (mg/dl). A sample of vitreous humor taken from his eye revealed an even higher concentration, 410 mg/dl.

These ethanol levels indicate that he consumed a lethal dose of wine. A concentration in the vicinity of 400 milligrams per deciliter of ethanol is considered to be lethal. When the blood-alcohol level approaches this level, the alcohol overwhelms the brain stem's ability to control respiration and death results.

Gary Malchevski died from acute ethanol intoxication; he overdosed on alcohol. One single-shot cocktail or beer elevates the blood-alcohol level by about 15 milligrams per deciliter. To reach 410 mg/dl, Gary Malchevski consumed the equivalent of a little over twenty-seven drinks. Instead of drinking himself to death, however, he absorbed the wine from the tube inserted into his rectum. In essence, his body ingested a huge amount of wine at once, like a beer bong with wine, only instead of pouring the booze down his throat . . . you get the picture.

Determining the cause of death in a case involving a paraphilia is the easy part. Determining the manner of death—accident, homicide, suicide—is tricky and represents a potential quagmire for the medical examiner and forensic pathologist. To determine manner of death, the ME must look at the context of the victim's death. Consider a game of Russian roulette in which the player dies. One could argue that the decedent chose an uncommon method of killing himself. One could also argue that the decedent planned on surviving the game and his death resulted from an accident. What did he intend?

Did Malchevski intend to die? If he did, then suicide becomes the manner of death. Some evidence that he planned on dying, such as a suicide note, would help. Yet he left no note, and his coworkers did not characterize him as depressed or despondent. In fact, the sticky notes investigators found in his work cubicle, while far from definitive, suggested that he planned on returning to work the following Monday. Without evidence to the contrary, it seems he settled into bed Friday night to enjoy a dose of his usual elixir and accidentally caused an overdose.

But was he alone the night he died? While various aspects of the scene indicate that he played alone the night he died, sometimes it takes two to tango, and in deaths involving sexual play, if a tango partner participates in the activity that leads to the victim's death, the manner of death becomes homicide (although not necessarily murder). In a case involving erotic asphyxia, one partner chokes or smothers the other partner. A miscalculation can lead to death, and, again, intent becomes a key factor.

Did Gary Malchevski have a tango partner the night he died—a partner who prepared and helped administer the enemas? One can envision a scenario in which the partner, shocked at the victim's unexpected death, flees the scene to avoid the scandal and embarrassment that would result from the article under the front-page headline "Bizarre Death on South Side." Through the unlocked back door and into the night, and anonymity . . .

Some clues suggest that someone else could have been present: the unlocked back door; the condom Malchevski wore when he died, although these do not necessarily indicate the presence of another person. Malchevski could have forgotten to lock the back door, or perhaps he was a trusting sort and didn't typically lock it. And some men use condoms when masturbating.

Besides, police found no concrete evidence that anyone other than Malchevski was ever in the house. No telltale clues of a lover, no dirty garments, lipstick-ringed cigarette butts, champagne flutes with fingerprints . . . nothing. And even if they did find some evidence of a playmate, whom would they question? An exhaustive search uncovered no friends or potential lovers. Just coworkers baffled by the quiet, accounting clerk's dark secret.

While he may have believed his brand of paraphilia to be a safe and enjoyable way to spend a Friday night, Gary Malchevski's death proves that self-sex is not always safe sex. Manner of death: accident.

## Note

1. From *Merriam-Webster's Collegiate Dictionary*.

# 8. things ain't always what they seem

*"Circumstantial evidence is a very tricky thing. It may seem to point very straight to one thing, but if you shift your own point of view a little, you may find it pointing in an equally uncompromising manner to something entirely different."*

—Sherlock Holmes, "The Boscombe Valley Mystery," *The Adventures of Sherlock Holmes* (1891)

In the short story "The Boscombe Valley Mystery," Sherlock Holmes explains the axiom that appearances can be deceptive and the furthest thing from reality. In the same story, Conan Doyle's master detective notes, "There is nothing more deceptive than an obvious fact." In essence, obvious facts can, like the red herrings mystery writers drag across the trail leading to the mystery's solution, mislead investigators and medical examiners. To the medical examiner and investigator, things ain't always what they seem . . .

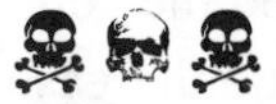

John Bass* loved his wife, Nancy.* They appeared to have an idyllic marriage, their love story set in a small, two-story white house complete with a white picket fence. An accountant by trade, Bass volunteered much of his free time to the local Christian Reformed Church. Everyone in the community reeled when his wife died in a tragic accident. Bass found his wife submerged in a tub of blood-tinged water in the guest bathroom. Apparently knocked unconscious when she struck her head in a fall, she drowned in the bathtub.

The necessary room is a common place for such accidents. Think about it: people visit the bathroom more often than any other room in the house, and it is usually a smaller room with a number of hard edges (countertops, toilet seats, bathtub). During parties, the bathroom becomes complicit in many accidents as teetering revelers relieve themselves, stumbling or passing out and sustaining serious and sometimes lethal head injuries. It is also a place where electricity and water coexist. One ignorant man died while standing in a filled bathtub when he attempted to change a lightbulb.

Because of its reputation, the bathroom has also become the room of choice for murderers attempting to stage accidents . . .

One key element of the Nancy Bass's "accident" made it appear to be no accident: a gash in her scalp incongruous with the blunt edge of the bathtub. She did not sustain this gash when she fell in the bathtub. Officer Rick Neerkin, the first to arrive on the scene, noticed some white particles on the bed that he first thought was spackling from the ceiling, but the ceiling appeared undamaged.[1] Like the laceration on Nancy Bass's head, the white dust was suspicious. John Bass's ruse had fooled no one.

An investigator studying the scene discovered a crack in the toilet tank lid in the master bath, and the contours of the lid fit those of the wound. Together, the crack and the gash led to a conclusion far from what the scene initially suggested: this pious man, a churchgoing man, hit his wife in the head with the heavy toilet tank lid while she slept and staged her drowning in the bathtub.

Things ain't always what they seem . . .

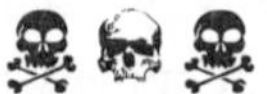

Jane Van Ryn* loved to play board games. Monopoly, Clue, anything (although some said she had a penchant for Scrabble). She passed the long days of her retirement playing with anyone and everyone who would join her: her grandchildren when they visited; other retirees and residents of her retirement community; and her daughter Victoria Van Ryn,* who visited twice each week on Tuesdays and Thursdays. Jane was suffering from lung cancer; the elderly woman's games were numbered.

It was Victoria Van Ryn who discovered her mother lying in a pool of her own blood next to the dining room table. Her well-worn game of Monopoly lay on the table. Piles of Monopoly money were neatly tucked under the board, a few forest-green houses situated on various properties—evidence suggesting that a struggle that led to murder interrupted the game. It appeared that someone had used her love of games as a way to enter her home and murder her as a prelude to or consequence of robbery. While Jane Van Ryn's body traveled to the Kent County Morgue, investigators began the exhaustive task of interviewing everyone who had recently come into contact with her.

The autopsy revealed a shocking twist to the story. The extensive blood at the scene suggested that a violent homicide had occurred, but the cause of death was lung cancer that had eroded a blood vessel. She exsanguinated; she coughed up large amounts of blood caused by the cancer, which explained the extensive amount of blood found at the scene. Jane Van Ryn died at the hand of the fiend known as cancer, not at the hand of a homicidal thief.

Things ain't always what they seem . . .

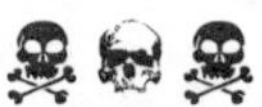

Was it fate, fear, or the fall that killed Lucy Westerhof?*

Lucy Westerhof, an elderly woman visiting a friend, left her friend's apartment to go home. On the way to her car, she met a rogue who snatched her purse. During the theft, Westerhof was knocked to the ground.

Shaken, she retreated back to her friend's apartment to call the police. While giving the story to the police, she collapsed and died. It first appeared that she sustained a lethal head injury when the thief pushed her to the ground.

Instead of Westerhof's death resulting from a linear skull fracture, however, the autopsy revealed that she suffered from a ruptured aneurysm in her brain. The small, delicate blood vessels in the body sometimes contain weak spots, which balloon outward, like thin spots on a bald tire. When the blood bursts through the berrylike out-pouching . . . trouble. While treatable with surgery, most people die from ruptured aneurysms before they reach the hospital.

With the cause of death established, the key question in this case became, what caused the aneurysm to rupture? Conventional medical wisdom maintains that aneurysms rupture without relationship to external events. In other words, when the thief pushed Westerhof to the ground, the impact did not cause the aneurysm to burst. The fall did not kill her. The aneurysm burst because it was time for it to burst. It was fate.

More recent information, however, indicates that stress (associated with increase in blood pressure) could cause an aneurysm to rupture. The bulk of the evidence supports the notion that the stress of being assaulted caused the rupture, and therefore Lucy Westerhof's death was a homicide. The fear of being robbed and assaulted led to her death.

Things ain't always what they seem . . .

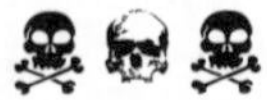

Friends and relatives described Jason Moore* as depressed, despondent. Thirty-five, alone, childless, unemployed, and on the verge of bankruptcy, Moore perhaps felt the weight of life on his shoulders. He loved to gamble and apparently never passed on the opportunity to engage in a game of chance. One friend told investigators an intriguing tale, perhaps hyperbole, that Moore once bet a thousand dollars on which frog would leap from a log first. Most of the time he bet, he lost.

Not surprisingly, over the years the losses accumulated. Moore gambled away his mortgage payments and subsequently lost his house. He lost his Honda Accord on a heartbreaking single hand of cards: a full house bested by a better full house. He became trapped in a vicious cycle like a hamster stuck on an exercise wheel; he gambled, lost, borrowed, and gambled some more.

His suicide, three days before Christmas, surprised no one. However, details of Moore's apparent suicide baffled investigators. He was found dead in bed holding a .22 rifle . . . an odd choice for a suicide.

And in the center of Moore's forehead, investigators found not one but two gunshot wounds. How, they wondered, could he have shot himself in the head twice? Unless his gun misfired, this could not have happened. Moore's suicide appeared to be a homicide. Perhaps underworld creditors came to exact their final payment. A first shot followed by a second—a coup de grâce to ensure the job was done.

The two holes in the skull deceived investigators into believing Moore sustained two gunshot wounds in the head when in fact he sustained just one: a deceptive wound known in forensic circles as a "keyhole defect."

Moore shot himself with the .22 positioned at an oblique, or severe, angle to his skull. The skull is essentially composed of three layers: outer dense, inner dense, and a middle, spongy layer sandwiched in between the two. The bullet fragmented into pieces when it contacted the inner layer of the skull. A portion of the bullet continued into the brain and caused Moore's death. The other portion of the bullet ricocheted off the inner layer of skull, passed back through the forehead, and created an exit wound that at first appeared to be a second entrance wound. This bullet fragment was found embedded in the ceiling. A keyhole defect resulted. The term refers to the appearance of the two holes, one on top of the other, like an antiquated keyhole. Despite the appearance of two entry wounds and thus murder, Moore did inflict the injury, and thus his death resulted from suicide and not homicide.

Things ain't always what they seem . . .

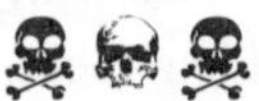

Todd Bayer* had a bit of Jekyll and Hyde in him. When he drank, Mr. Hyde emerged from the usually calm, placid demeanor of the journeyman electrician. One night he came home late after a few rounds at the corner tavern and was greeted by the braying of his three-year-old son Malcolm.*

The next day, Janine Bayer,* who knew enough to stay out of her husband's way after a late night, found her son Malcolm in bed, dead. Janine told the police that her husband had given Malcolm a bath in the wee hours of the morning. She heard loud banging behind the door, but was too afraid to see what was going on.

The cause of death initially appeared to be a result of child abuse. Police took Malcolm's body to the morgue for an autopsy and Todd in handcuffs to jail. Investigators expected to find that Malcolm Bayer died as a result of internal injuries caused by a severe beating.

The autopsy revealed no lacerated organs, no fractured ribs, no skull fractures . . . in short, no injuries indicating that Todd Bayer's evil Mr. Hyde had turned on his own son. The autopsy did uncover several partially digested potassium pills in Malcolm's stomach. Malcolm Bayer had managed to open a container of his grandmother's potassium pills and swallowed some. In high levels, potassium causes the heart to stop. Malcolm died of potassium poisoning.

Every cloud has a silver lining: despite his innocence, Todd Bayer blamed himself for his son's death and rededicated himself to a life without alcohol.

As for his son's death, things ain't always what they seem . . .

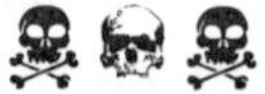

Things ain't always what they seem, even to pathologists, who are not immune from making mistakes based on appearances. A forensic pathologist's mistake, though, can lead to a prison sentence . . .

Eight-month-old Darius Jackson* arrived at the morgue. The pathologist who conducted the autopsy on Darius's body believed that he had been sexually abused—a thesis based on the fact that the infant's anus appeared to be dilated and red. The lining of the rectum was red, and white blood cells were observed microscopically, suggesting a recent injury or infection. Suspicion fell onto Darius's grandfather Bruce,* the child's custodial parent. Bruce Jackson's arrest seemed imminent.

Yet the pathologist who conducted the autopsy lacked specialized forensic training.

The prosecutor, not wanting to make a mistake that could send an innocent man to prison, sent the autopsy report, photographs, and tissue slides to the Kent County medical examiner for review. The pillars of the prosecution's case for child abuse—the "telltale" signs of sexual abuse—began to crumble under scrutiny. The dilated anus, the redness, and the presence of white blood cells—the basis of the case against Bruce Jackson—had a completely innocent explanation. A dilated anus is a well-known and fairly frequent finding in dead infants either related to relaxation of the anal sphincter upon death or upon stool being impacted in the rectum and anus perimortem. The redness observed was simply dilated blood vessels—a nonspecific finding. The white blood cells were sparse and within normal range.

Things ain't always what they seem . . .

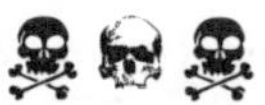

Things ain't always what they seem, but sometimes, the jury convicts anyway . . .

June Devries* discovered her eight-year-old daughter, Therese,* asleep on the couch. It wasn't an uncommon sight. The sleeping angel apparently fell asleep watching television. To her horror, June could not rouse her daughter. Therese had died.

In the autopsy that followed, a blood sample taken from Therese's heart showed an elevated but not lethal (according to a standard toxicology text) level of the prescription antidepressant medication imipramine. June faced a charge for murdering her child by giving her a large dose of the antidepressant medication.

Yet the level of antidepressant in Therese's system was invalid because the sample was taken from the heart, and blood from the heart taken postmortem is well known to falsely show increased quantities of certain drugs, especially antidepressants, because of a condition known as postmortem redistribution. Postmortem redistribution falsely elevates drug concentration by a factor of three, or three times, for imipramine. So to determine the accurate level of the antidepressant in Therese's system, the forensic pathologist who conducted the autopsy needed to divide the level by three. Therefore, the toxicological levels were not high enough to explain her death; Therese did not die from a drug overdose. And the presence of imipramine in Therese's blood was not accidental or homicidal: a physician prescribed the drug as a treatment for bed-wetting.

Both the pathologist and consultant toxicologist for the prosecution did not take redistribution into account when they opined that Therese died of a drug overdose. And, the autopsy also showed an abnormal arrangement of the coronary arteries—a type known to be lethal. Despite abundant medical literature to the contrary, the pathologist dismissed the coronary artery anomaly as trivial. Because of a legal technicality, Dr. Cohle, who testified for the defense, was not allowed to explain with citations from the literature his reason for considering that the heart anomaly was the cause of Therese's death and that the drug level was indeed invalid.

June Devries was found guilty of first-degree murder in the case.

According to the jury, June Devries is guilty of murdering her eight-year-old daughter . . . but things ain't always what they seem.

☠ ☠ ☠

It appeared to be a routine, ordinary case of a driver weaving across the road, perhaps under the influence of a substance or simply exhausted after a long shift at work. It turned into every traffic cop's worst nightmare: a shoot-out that would leave one of the combatants dead.

Officer Jeff Early* had no idea what would transpire when he pulled over the Toyota pickup driven by Jamie Knox.* Unbeknownst to Officer Early, Knox had been diagnosed with paranoid schizophrenia and had sneaked away from home with two of his uncle's handguns, one of which police later found under his car seat and the other which he held as Officer Early approached.

Early noticed nothing out of the ordinary when he approached the driver's side of the Toyota. A loud crack erupted as a bullet ripped through the driver's side window and into Early's forearm. Early, shocked, instinctively began to retreat and, while back-pedaling, fired six shots into the car.

Early's aim appeared to be accurate, and when the smoke and smell of cordite dissipated, Jamie Knox sat slumped over in the driver's seat, dead of a gunshot wound to the head. Jeff Early had returned fire and, in doing so, appeared to have killed a mentally ill man. His return barrage had perforated the car, riddled the side panels and dashboard with holes, and shattered the windows. The shooting, like all police shootings, received intense scrutiny.

It also presented a forensic riddle wrapped in an enigma.

Jamie Knox, whose body traveled to the Kent County Morgue, presented several provocative if not perplexing clues. The only bullet that struck Knox passed through his head, but the bullet entered the skull on the right side, or the side opposite to Officer Early. If Early's story was true, the bullet should have struck Knox on the left or left rear side of his head. In addition, the soot inside the wound indicated that the barrel of the gun used to shoot Knox was pressed against his right temple. This forensic evidence appeared to counter Officer

Early's story, and Jamie Knox's death looked more like an execution, as improbable a scenario as it seemed.

An x-ray of Knox's skull added to the mystery. The bullet that killed Jamie Knox passed through his skull and did not fragment. Police officers typically use hollow-point bullets, which are copper-covered (jacketed) with an exposed lead tip; these bullets expand or "mushroom" soon after impact and remain inside the target instead of passing through and possibly injuring another person. The bullet that killed Jamie Knox was round-nosed and completely encased in copper—a type of bullet that typically passes through a target. In addition, the bullet that killed Knox was a 9-millimeter; Officer Early carried a .40-caliber H & K pistol that afternoon. The bullet that killed Knox did *not* come from Officer Early.

So where did the bullet come from? Not from Knox, it appeared. Investigators found a .38 Smith & Wesson revolver clutched in Knox's right hand. The 9-millimeter projectile, however, is made to be fired from a semiautomatic pistol, not a revolver. A close examination of Knox's handgun solved this puzzle; investigators found a spent 9-millimeter cartridge in Knox's .38 Smith & Wesson.

Fitted together, the puzzle pieces—the gunpowder indicating a tight-contact wound, the 9-millimeter bullet that killed Knox, the spent 9-millimeter shell in Knox's .38—formed a picture of what occurred the afternoon of the "shoot-out." While it appeared that Jamie Knox had opened fire on Officer Early, in fact, he had shot himself in the head. The bullet passed through his head, through the driver's side window, and into Officer Early's forearm, where it remained for over two weeks until it shifted and a physician removed it. Early returned fire, but none of the six bullets struck Knox. A ballistics test on the bullet taken from Early's arm confirmed that it indeed came from the .38 found in Jamie Knox's right hand.

Things ain't always what they seem.

## Note

1. Rick Neerken, city of Grandville police officer, interview with Tobin T. Buhk, March 20, 2007.

# "double trouble"

## A Conclusion to the Case Discussed in the Introduction: "Moonlighting"

What happened to Bryan McBride, who crashed his snowmobile into a pine tree on a Friday night in mid-December? The question dangled in the air of the Kent County Morgue like the foul odor of decomposition.

Bryan McBride did a little moonlight snowmobile riding with his brother, Andrew. When they became separated, Andrew packed up and left. A little while later, other snowmobile riders discovered a body lying on the ground in a heap next to the smashed remains of a snowmobile; Bryan McBride, it appeared, had died in a tragic accident. Or had he? The fact that Andrew and Bryan McBride were identical twins led to speculation that one twin killed the other and assumed his identity.

After the autopsy, the seed Dr. Cohle planted with his speculation about the twins began to grow. A *Law & Order* fanatic, I began to spin convoluted webs of conspiracies—like a spider on amphetamines—to explain Bryan McBride's death.

For parents, twins complicate matters. Multiple births mean multiple diapers, clothes, toys, presents at Christmas . . . if they cross the law, twins complicate matters for authorities as well.

The DNA card, which consists of four bright red blotches of blood on a piece of cardboard the size of an index card, can provide no help in establishing the identity of a victim if he or she is a twin. The DNA of identical twins is identical. Therefore, a twin enjoys a genetic reasonable doubt in cases where authorities cannot tell which twin committed a crime. Consider a hypothetical scenario: a serial rapist is on the loose, and police have obtained DNA samples from semen and skin fragments retrieved from his previous victims. Police manage to identity a suspect, a victim picks him out of a lineup, and a DNA sample is taken. They have a match. They have identified and caught the serial rapist.

Except he's a twin, and he quickly blames the rapes on his identical twin, who under questioning throws the blame, like a hot potato, back at his twin. The twins are playing a game of Monkey in the Middle, and the police, well, they are the monkeys caught in the middle. Who do they charge? If they have no evidence to differentiate one twin from another, they cannot proceed. Even if they did make it to a trial, each twin would testify against the other and thus construct a reasonable doubt for the jurors. What can the police do? Throw both twins in prison? That would lead to one innocent person incarcerated . . . unless they both committed the rapes.

The McBride brothers committed no rapes or murders, but the fact that they are twins complicates matters. In a typical accident, authorities must ascertain cause of death, but in this case, they must also establish the victim's identity (also true with accidents in which the victim's face is obliterated).

Bryan McBride, I had convinced myself, was in fact Andrew McBride. Bryan, whose criminal history included convictions and subsequent prison stints for assault and rape, became enraptured with his twin brother's girlfriend, Denise. In high school, the two brothers would play practical jokes on their girlfriends by switching. They enjoyed duping others but never took the joke too far. Neither brother married or had children, nor, one could argue, had they grown up. They lived together, thirty-eight-year-old daredevils, living a hedonistic lifestyle. Their jobs—one a tool and die maker and the other an auto mechanic—provided enough cash flow to support the real love of their lives: speed. Their pole barn contained their toys: a pair of motorcycles, a pair of quads, a pair of Jet Skis, and a pair of snowmobiles.

The twins seemed inseparable. Then came Denise, a striking brunette in her late twenties with crystal blue eyes. She fell for Andrew McBride, often spending the night in his room where Bryan could easily overhear the sounds of their passion. Bryan became intoxicated with Denise and even suggested to Andrew that they switch places so he could enjoy her. Unlike his high school relationships, however, Andrew had fallen in love, and the notion of sharing his love with anyone, even his twin brother, felt like lying on a bed of needles.

Night after night, Bryan McBride thought about Denise, how she would feel lying next to him, whispering into his ear, her thigh caressing his. Her image forced away all other thoughts, like a malignant tumor growing larger each day. He began to avoid going home, instead stopping at a local bar, spending a portion of his paycheck on cocktails. One day, he came across an old high school friend. A conversation began with a voice across the bar, "Hey, Andrew McBride."

For an hour, he conversed with a high school chum as his brother, then he realized that he could pass for his brother . . .

This, however, is merely a figment of an overactive imagination. A fiction . . .

On Monday, following the Saturday autopsy of Bryan/Andrew McBride, police matched the fingerprints taken at the Kent County Morgue with those on file and concluded that the man killed last Friday night was none other than Bryan McBride. Also on Monday, Dr. Cohle received the toxicology report.

The toxicology report removed any question marks about the cause of death. According to the surviving twin, he and his brother visited a tavern and downed a few glasses of liquid insulation before venturing out into the cold night. Blood, however, does not lie, and the blood sample indicated that Bryan McBride consumed more than a few drinks.

The blood-alcohol level is measured in a ratio of milligrams to deciliters, expressed as mg/dl. In Michigan, the legal limit for operating an automobile is 80 milligrams per deciliter, or 0.08 percent. A person of average body weight (70 kilograms or 154 pounds) would reach this limit after consuming about five to six single-shot cocktails or beers. As a point of reference, one cocktail or beer raises the blood-alcohol level by 15 milligrams per deciliter.

At the time he died, Bryan McBride's blood-alcohol level was 0.22 percent, or almost three times the legal limit to operate a motor vehicle. This means that at two hundred and fifty pounds—almost a hundred pounds more than the average adult male—he probably consumed at least fifteen to twenty drinks. During his moonlight ride, Bryan McBride felt no pain, indeed, but as much alcohol as he consumed prior to and/or during his moonlight ride, he didn't consume enough to kill him. The forensic rule of thumb for an overdose of alcohol, called an ethanol overdose, is 400 milligrams per deciliter. When the blood-alcohol level transcends this level, the alcohol overwhelms the brain stem, stopping breathing.

Consuming twenty drinks and then operating a snowmobile at high speed in a dark forest—foolish, absolutely, but deadly only in conjunction with an injury, like the concussion he likely sustained when he struck the tree. No subdural hemorrhage was discovered during the autopsy, but this does not eliminate the possibility that he suffered a concussion. Instead, the combination of the concussion he sustained when he struck the tree coupled with the alcohol overwhelmed his ability to breathe and caused his death.

He was not the victim of a malignant twin bent on a devious plan to trade identities, but he could have been; the skeletons in the ME's closet illustrate that appearances can drastically conflict with the reality underneath; that the clothes a victim wears sometimes hide the naked truth.

Bryan McBride died as a result of a tragic accident. He traveled from the morgue to a funeral home that would prepare him for the final stage in his earthly existence. Case closed. The Kent County medical examiner had solved another forensic mystery . . .

. . . and the Kent County Morgue has acquired another skeleton in the closet.

# sources

Ackerman-Haywood, Jennifer. "Wife Dies, and Now the Charge Is Murder." *Grand Rapids Press*, September 4, 1999.

"Additional Information regarding the Investigation into Scott Woodring." Michigan State Police press release, July 14, 2003. http://www.michigan.gov/msp/0,1607,7-123-1586_1710-71845—,00.html (accessed April 3, 2007).

Agar, John. "Standoff Suspect Called Dangerous." *Grand Rapids Press*, July 9, 2003.

"Aide Denied Case Review in 5 Deaths." *Grand Rapids Press*, May 5, 1993.

Antiquities Wellington Inn. http://www.wellingtoninn.com/index.php (accessed March 30, 2006).

Autopsy Report for Barbara Ann Biehn (amended), March 26, 2004, May 25, 2005 (amendments), Office of the Kent County Medical Examiner.

Autopsy Report for Chris Schoenborn, December 10, 1982, Office of the Kent County Medical Examiner.

Autopsy Report for David Crawford, May 1, 1996, Office of the Kent County Medical Examiner.

Autopsy Report for Dennis Alt, December 10, 1982, Office of the Kent County Medical Examiner.

Autopsy Report for Dennis Finch, May 14, 1998, Office of the Kent County Medical Examiner.

Autopsy Report for Dorothy Perkins, March 11, 1987, Office of the Kent County Medical Examiner.

Autopsy Report for Edith Cook, December 3, 1988, Office of the Kent County Medical Examiner.

Autopsy Report for Grover Crosslin, September 4, 2001, Office of the Kent County Medical Examiner.

Autopsy Report for Kevin Marshall, July 8, 2003, Office of the Kent County Medical Examiner.

Autopsy Report for Linda Teeter, March 18, 2003, Office of the Kent County Medical Examiner.

Autopsy Report for Manual Longoria, May 18, 2004, Office of the Kent County Medical Examiner.

Autopsy Report for Marguerite Chambers, November 30, 1988, Office of the Kent County Medical Examiner.

Autopsy Report for Mary Louise Moynahan, March 11, 1987, Office of the Kent County Medical Examiner.

Autopsy Report for Onunwa Iwuagwu, April 5, 1985, Office of the Kent County Medical Examiner.

Autopsy Report for Raul Ramirez, May 18, 2004, Office of the Kent County Medical Examiner.

Autopsy Report for Rolland Rohm, September 5, 2001, Office of the Kent County Medical Examiner.

Autopsy Report for Scott Woodring, July 14, 2003, Office of the Kent County Medical Examiner.

Bagwell, Jennifer. "Barred from View: How Michigan Keeps the Lid on Allegations of Widespread Sexual Abuse against Female Inmates." *Metro Times*. http://www.metrotimes.com/19/25/Features/newBarred.htm (accessed October 17, 2006).

Barber, Barrie. "Finch Tried to Get Clark Committed." *Traverse City Record-Eagle*. May 22, 1998. http://www.record-eagle.com/news/clark/22gun.htm (accessed March 30, 2006).

Barnes, John. "Suspect's Note May Bolster Evidence in Slaying." *Grand Rapids Press*, April 17, 1985.

———. "Murder Suspect Bout Blames Murder on Girlfriend." *Grand Rapids Press*, August 6, 1985.

———. "Bout Jury Hears Witnesses Tell Conflicting Stories about Killing." *Grand Rapids Press*, August 7, 1985.

———. "Girlfriend Says She Feared Alleged Killer." *Grand Rapids Press*, August 8, 1985.

———. "Murder Defendant Bout Alleges Cover-up by Lawyer, Girlfriend." *Grand Rapids Press*, August 9, 1985.

———. "Bout Admitted Guilt in Murder; Lawyer Testifies." *Grand Rapids Press*, August 13, 1985.

———. "Bout Jury Weighs Evidence." *Grand Rapids Press*, August 14, 1985.

———. "Girlfriend of Murderer Bout Gets Year in Jail, Judge's Warning." *Grand Rapids Press*, October 1, 1985.

———. "'I'm Not a Murderer.'" *Grand Rapids Press*, May 24, 1987.

———. "Bout Is Denied New Trial as Top Witness Clams Up." *Grand Rapids Press*, May 30, 1987.

Barnes, John, and Doug Guthrie. "Bout Convicted; Victim's Widow Wishes Penalty Were Harsher." *Grand Rapids Press*, August 15, 1985.

Barnes, John, and Tom Rademacher. "Warrants Tell of Plot to Murder Nigerian." *Grand Rapids Press*, April 8, 1985.

Barnes, John, Arn Shackelford, Elizabeth Slowik, and Tom Rademacher. "Police Hint Slaying, Phony Bills Linked." *Grand Rapids Press*, April 6, 1985.

"Beheading Suspect Called Incompetent." *Grand Rapids Press*, August 17, 1996.

Blakely, Dave. Telephone interview with Tobin T. Buhk, December 3, 2007.

*The Book of Common Prayer and Administration of the Sacraments and Other Rites and Ceremonies of the Church according to the Use of the Protestant Episcopal Church in the United States of America*. New York: James Pott and Company, 1892.

Buhk, Kerry, PhD. Personal interview with Tobin T. Buhk, October 17, 2006.

Campbell, Alan. "Defense: Killing Was Self-Defense." *Leelanau Enterprise*, March 3, 2005. http://www.leelanaunews.com/editorial.php?id=1344 (accessed November 12, 2006).

———. "Expert Doubts O'Non Self-Defense Claim." *Leelanau Enterprise*, March 10, 2005. http://www.leelanaunews.com/editorial.php?id=1363 (accessed November 12, 2006).

———. "Juror: No Doubt of O'Non's Guilt." *Leelanau Enterprise*, March 24, 2005. http://www.leelanaunews.com/editorial.php?id=1390 (accessed November 12, 2006).

———. "Robyn O'Non Jury Seated." *Leelanau Enterprise*, August 3, 2006. http://www.leelanaunews.com/editorial.php?id=2373 (accessed November 12, 2006).

———. "3 to 15 Years for Robyn O'Non." *Leelanau Enterprise*, September 7, 2006. http://www.leelanaunews.com/editorial.php?id=2442 (accessed November 12, 2006).

Carlson, Peter. "Was Rainbow Farm Another Waco?" *Washington Post*, January 27, 2002.

Carr, Tom. "Slade Gets Life for Beating Girlfriend." *Traverse City Record-Eagle*, November 21, 2001. http://www.record-eagle.com/2001/nov/21slade.htm (accessed April 3, 2007).

Cauffiel, Lowell. *Forever and Five Days*. New York: Kensington Books, 1992.

Cohle, Stephen D., Charles W. Harlan, and Gretel Harlan, "Fatal Big Cat Attacks." *American Journal of Forensic Medicine and Pathology* 11, no. 3 (1990): 208–12.

Collins, Susan. "Woman Ordered to Stand Trial for Murder." *Grand Rapids Press*, June 16, 1988.

Collins, Susan, and Ken Kolker. "Suspect Relates Bizarre Tale of Killing." *Grand Rapids Press*, December 6, 1988.

"Confession of Mom Accused in Deaths of 3 Children Ruled Admissible in Trial." *Grand Rapids Press*, November 1, 1991.

Court Documents, *State of Indiana, Kosciusko County, v. Jason M. Fisher*, Cause No.: 43C01-0101-CF-0090.

Court Documents, *State of Indiana, Kosciusko County, v. Ralph "Fred" Fisher*, Cause No.: 43C01-0201-MR-1.

———. Information for probable cause affidavit, filed January 2, 2002.

———. Defense attorney Thomas Leatherman's letter to prosecution, dated January 28, 2002.

———. Defense attorney Thomas Leatherman's memorandum in support of motion to dismiss, filed January 28, 2002.

———. Defense attorney Thomas Leatherman's motion to discharge, filed January 28, 2002.

———. Defense attorney Thomas Leatherman's motion to dismiss, filed January 28, 2002.

———. Defense attorney Thomas Leatherman's motion of alibi, filed March 1, 2002.

———. State's reply to defendant's alibi notice, filed March 8, 2002.

Cox, Michael. "Grieving Widow Denies Slain Nigerian Was Involved in Counterfeiting Plot." *Grand Rapids Press*, April 9, 1985.

Deep, Said. "Victim's Kin Find Guilt, Anger in Trial Verdict." *Grand Rapids Press*, September 21, 1989.

———. "Monitor Is Key to First Volley in Spencer Trial." *Grand Rapids Press*, January 28, 1992.

———. "Mother Admitted Killing Baby, Two Officers Testify." *Grand Rapids Press*, January 29, 1992.

———. "Panel Was '100 Percent Sure' Mother Killed Her Son, Juror Says." *Grand Rapids Press*, January 31, 1992.

———. "Spencer Blames Lawyer and Juror in Bid for New Trial." *Grand Rapids Press*, March 14, 1992.

Deiters, Barton. "'Worst Fears' Lead to Slaying of Officer." *Grand Rapids Press*, July 8, 2003.

———. "Suburban Detroit Police Investigate Body Found in Ottawa County." *Grand Rapids Press*, March 27, 2004.

Deiters, Barton, and John Agar. "Convicted Killer's Story Sways Dutch, but Judge Is Unmoved." *Grand Rapids Press*, June 22, 2004.

Donker, Robert. Personal interview with Tobin T. Buhk, August 17, 2007.

Durbin, Dee-Ann. "'We Like Them. They Were Good People.'" *Grand Rapids Press*, September 5, 2001.

Echlin, Bill. "Defense Suggests 'Friendly Fire' in Clark Case." *Traverse City Record-Eagle*. June 25, 1998. http://www.record-eagle.com/news/clark/25clark.htm (accessed March 30, 2006).

Eddy, David. Telephone interview with Tobin T. Buhk, August 23, 2006.

Emrick, Corky. "Murder Trial to Begin Tuesday." *Sturgis Journal*, March 15, 2004. http://www.sturgisjournal.com/print.asp?ArticleID=15803&Section ID=2&SubSectionID=65 (accessed May 11, 2006).

———. "Murder Trial Begins." *Sturgis Journal*, March 17, 2004. http://www.sturgisjournal.com/print.asp?ArticleID=15838&SectionID=2&SubSectionID=65 (accessed May 11, 2006).

———. "Victim's Friends Testify." *Sturgis Journal*, March 18, 2004. http://www.sturgisjournal.com/print.asp?ArticleID=15844&SectionID=2&SubSectionID=65 (accessed May 11, 2006).

———. "Outburst Lands Victim's Brother in Jail; Jury Hears Taped Confession." *Sturgis Journal*, March 19, 2004. http://www.sturgisjournal.com/print.asp?ArticleID=15857&SectionID=2&SubSectionID=65 (accessed May 11, 2006).

———. "Murder Trial Nears End." *Sturgis Journal*, March 24, 2004. http://www.sturgisjournal.com/print.asp?ArticleID=15883&SectionID=2&SubSectionID=65 (accessed May 11, 2006).

———. "Jury Deliberation Begins." *Sturgis Journal*, March 25, 2004. http://www.sturgisjournal.com/print.asp?ArticleID=15891&SectionID=2&SubSectionID=65 (accessed May 11, 2006).

———. "Guilty on All Counts." *Sturgis Journal*, March 26, 2004. http://www.sturgisjournal.com/print.asp?ArticleID=15898&SectionID=2&SubSectionID=65 (accessed May 11, 2006).

———. "Authorities Say Getting Help Could Have Saved Teeter." *Sturgis Journal*, March 27, 2004. http://www.sturgisjournal.com/print.asp?ArticleID=15906&SectionID=2&SubSectionID=65 (accessed May 11, 2006).

Erbaugh, Roger, DDS. Personal interview with Tobin T. Buhk, July 14, 2006.

"Examiners Disagree over Cause of Death." *Traverse City Record-Eagle*, June 2, 2006. http://www.record-eagle.com/2006/jun/02unger.htm (accessed April 3, 2007).

Finger, Christine. "Killer's Parents Charged." *Traverse City Record-Eagle*, January 11, 2006. http://www.archives.record-eagle.com/2006/jan/11onon.htm (accessed December 5, 2007).

Fitrakis, Bob. "Siege at Rainbow Farm Leaves Two Dead." *Free Press*, October 1, 2001. http://www.freepress.org/journal.php?strFunc=display&strID=96&strJournal=14 (accessed July 20, 2007).

Flesher, John. "Attorneys Clash over Key Testimony in Slaying Case." *Daily Oakland Press*, July 8, 2004. http://theoaklandpress/com/stories/070804/loc_20040708031.shtml (accessed April 3, 2007).

———. "Experts Differ on Cause of Death." *Grand Rapids Press*, September 9, 2004.

———. "Prosecutors, Defense Offer Contrasting Portrayals." *Traverse City Record-Eagle*, May 4, 2006. http://www.record-eagle.com/2006/may/04unger.htm (accessed April 3, 2007).

———. "Unger Found Guilty." *Traverse City Record-Eagle*, June 22, 2006. http://www.record-eagle.com/2006/jun/22unger.htm (accessed April 3, 2007).

"Free Harry Bout." http://www.geocities.com/freeharrybout (accessed May 31, 2006).

"Friends of Florence Unger Testify." *Traverse City Record-Eagle*, May 19, 2006. http://www.record-eagle.com/2006/may/19unger.htm (accessed April 3, 2007).

"Friend: Wife's Death Was Imagined." *Traverse City Record-Eagle*, May 20, 2006. http://www.record-eagle.com/2006/may/20unger.htm (accessed April 3, 2007).

Gmiter, Tanda. "Husband on Trial in Wife's Brutal Slaying." *Grand Rapids Press*, January 26, 2000.

———. "Husband Found Guilty of Beating Wife to Death." *Grand Rapids Press*, January 28, 2000.

Guthrie, Doug. "Judge Orders Infant's Body Exhumed." *Grand Rapids Press*, December 28, 1990.

———. "Book Sheds New Light on Alpine Murders." *Grand Rapids Press*, March 5, 1992.

———. "New Details Revealed in Book Reliving Alpine Manor Deaths." *Grand Rapids Press*, March 15, 1992.

———. "Pal Regrets Inability to Help Victim: The Young Man Who Befriended David Crawford in Class Later Gave Him a Ride to the Sparta Area." *Grand Rapids Press*, May 3, 1996.

———. "Teen Suspect in Beheading Case Fit for Trial, Report Says." *Grand Rapids Press*, January 18, 1997.

———. "Husband Found Guilty of Beating Wife to Death." *Grand Rapids Press*, January 28, 2000.

———. "Man Gets at Least 14 Years for Beating Wife to Death." *Grand Rapids Press*, March 14, 2000.

———. "Mistake Shortens Murderer's Sentence." *Grand Rapids Press*, August 22, 2000.

———. "'My Life Is Over,' Shooting Victim's Message Says; Jurors Hear Sandra Duyst's Voice Mail Message, Telling Her Husband to 'Enjoy Your Life.'" *Grand Rapids Press*, March 9, 2001.

Guthrie, Doug, and Theresa D. McClellan. "Mom's Concern Aided Police: Dental Records Provide Identity in Beheading Case." *Grand Rapids Press*, May 2, 1996.

"Gunman Kills TC Officer." *Traverse City Record-Eagle*, May 13, 1998. http://www.record-eagle.com/news/clark/13shoot.htm (accessed March 30, 2006).

Harger, John, and Joe Snapper. "Neighbors Reluctant to Condemn Suspect; They Share Fear of Government, but Want Him Punished If Proven Guilty." *Grand Rapids Press*, July 10, 2003.

"The Harry Bout Story." *Injustice Line*. http://www.injusticeline.com (accessed January 8, 2006).

Hogan, John. "6 Years After Slayings, Family Still Fighting the Pain." *Grand Rapids Press*, December 5, 1988.

———. "Mother of Four Is Dead Following Alleged Argument." *Grand Rapids Press*, December 22, 1988.

———. "History of Abuse Preceded Killing; Husband Sought." *Grand Rapids Press*, December 23, 1988.

———. "'Tragic Coincidence' May Have Been Three Murders." *Grand Rapids Press*, December 12, 1990.

———. "Second Child of Wayland Woman Killed, Officials Say." *Grand Rapids Press*, February 19, 1991.

———. "Report OKs Trial of Mom Accused of Killing Son." *Grand Rapids Press*, July 17, 1991.

———. "Don't Know What Happened, Suspect Claims in Son's Death." *Grand Rapids Press*, July 18, 1991.

———. "Woman Facing Trial in Son's Suffocation Is Charged in Death of 2 Other Children." *Grand Rapids Press*, January 25, 1992.

———. "Didn't Take Her Son's Life, Spencer Tells Allegan Jury." *Grand Rapids Press*, January 30, 1992.

———. "Family Gets $50,000 in Nursing Home Death." *Grand Rapids Press*, October 31, 1992.

Hogan, John, and Theresa D. McClellan. "Authorities Look Again at Deaths of Mother's Two Girls." *Grand Rapids Press*, December 13, 1990.

*Jack in the Box* (documentary film). Directed by David Schock, PhD. PenULTIMATE, Ltd.

Kohlmeier, R. E., C. A. McMahan, and V. J. M. DiMaio. "Suicide by Firearms." *American Journal of Forensic Medical Pathology* 22 (2001): 337–40.

Kolker, Ken. "Two Arrested in Nursing Home Deaths." *Grand Rapids Press*, December 5, 1988.

———. "Friends Remember Murder Victim as Open, Giving." *Grand Rapids Press*, May 5, 1996.

Kolker, Ken, and Susan Collins. "Autopsy Done in Nursing Home Death." *Grand Rapids Press*, December 1, 1988.

———. "Friends, Co-Workers Describe 2 Aides." *Grand Rapids Press*, December 6, 1988.

Kuipers, Dean. "Siege at Rainbow Farm." *Playboy*, October 2003.

Lawrence, James Sterling. Telephone interview with Tobin T. Buhk, August 7, 2007.

Lee, Amy. "Cause of Death Debated in Unger Case." *Detroit News*, September 9, 2004. http://detnews.com/metro/ungertrial/b01-268329.htm (accessed April 3, 2007).

Leith, Scott. "Beheading Suspect, 17, Injured in Two-Story Fall at Jail." *Grand Rapids Press*, February 1, 1997.

Lipka, Ruth Anne. "Police Seek Information on Missing Milford Woman." *Times-Union* (Warsaw, IN), January 24, 2001.

———. "Milford Woman Feared Murdered." *Times-Union* (Warsaw, IN), January 25, 2001.

———. "Milford Woman's Body Found." *Times-Union* (Warsaw, IN), January 26, 2001.

———. "Charges Brought against Murder Suspect." *Times-Union* (Warsaw, IN), January 27, 2001.

———. "Suspect Posts Bond, Details Emerge in Murder. *Times-Union* (Warsaw, IN), January 29, 2001.

———. "Autopsy Shows Vroman Suffered Head Wounds." *Times-Union* (Warsaw, IN), January 30, 2001.

———. "Sixth Arrest Likely, Vehicle Recovered in Vroman Case." *Times-Union* (Warsaw, IN), February 8, 2001.

———. "Fisher Trial to Stay Here." *Times-Union* (Warsaw, IN), April 12, 2001.

———. "Fisher Faces More Charges in Murder of Milford Woman." *Times-Union* (Warsaw, IN), December 14, 2001.

———. "Murder Charges Brought against Ralph Fisher." *Times-Union* (Warsaw, IN), January 7, 2002.

———. "Son Says Dad Killed Kathy Vroman." *Times-Union* (Warsaw, IN), January 9, 2002.

———. "Conspiracy Charge Dropped in Ralph Fisher's Case." *Times-Union* (Warsaw, IN), January 17, 2002.

———. "Attorney Seeks to Have Fred Fisher Released." *Times-Union* (Warsaw, IN), January 30, 2002.

———. "Defense Attorney Says Ralph Fisher Has Alibi." *Times-Union* (Warsaw, IN), March 19, 2002.

———. "Jason Fisher Testifies against His Father." *Times-Union* (Warsaw, IN), March 20, 2002.

———. "Victim's Husband Testifies That Witness Is Lying." *Times-Union* (Warsaw, IN), March 21, 2002.

———. "Defense Rests in Ralph Fisher Murder Trial." *Times-Union* (Warsaw, IN), March 22, 2002.

———. "Ralph Fisher a Free Man." *Times-Union* (Warsaw, IN), March 23, 2002.

———. "Fisher Murder Charge Dropped." *Times-Union* (Warsaw, IN), April 9, 2002.

———. "Fisher Sentenced for Theft, Burglary." *Times-Union* (Warsaw, IN), October 10, 2002.

———. "Aldrich Granted Modification of His Jail Sentence." *Times-Union* (Warsaw, IN), November 9, 2002.

Martindale, Mike. "MI Husband Behaved Oddly at Wife's Drowning Scene." *Detroit News*, May 5, 2006.

Martinez, Fernando. Personal interview with Tobin T. Buhk, October 25, 2006.

McClellan, Theresa D. "Charges Dropped in Deaths of 2 Children." *Grand Rapids Press*, June 30, 1993.

———. "'Nothing We Could Do with Him.'" *Grand Rapids Press*, May 14, 1996.

———. "Trooper Is Remembered for Courage." *Grand Rapids Press*, July 9, 2003.

McClellan, Theresa D., and Daniel J. Eizans. "Answers Elude Investigators So Far." *Grand Rapids Press*.

McClellan, Theresa D., and Doug Guthrie. "Cops Recount Gruesome Discovery." *Grand Rapids Press*, May 1, 1996.

McClellan, Theresa, and Jim Mencarelli. "Jaguar Gets Loose at Zoo, Kills Keeper." *Grand Rapids Press*, December 9, 1985.

McClellan, Theresa D., and Kelley Root. "Mom's Troubled Life Was a Treadmill of Drugs, Birth, Death." *Grand Rapids Press*, December 12, 1990.

McDougal, Dennis. *Angel of Darkness: The True Story of Randy Kraft and the Most Heinous Murder Spree*. Grand Central Publishing, 1992.

"Medical Examiner Says Farm Pair Were Strangled." *Grand Rapids Press*, December 28, 1982.

Mencarelli, Jim, and Thomas D. Smith. "Search Intensifies around Hastings for Missing Sisters; No Leads Yet." *Grand Rapids Press*, March 4, 1987.

———. "Slain Sister Began Lending Money to Builder in 1982." *Grand Rapids Press*, March 12, 1987.

Mencarelli, Jim, Thomas D. Smith, and Ken Kolker. "Bankrupt Builder Held in Sister Killings." *Grand Rapids Press*, March 11, 1987.

Miller, Daniel T. Personal interview with Tobin T. Buhk, May 2, 2007.

Miller, Jennie. "Hairdresser Perceived Mark Unger as Habitual Liar." *Woodward Talk*, June 7, 2006. http://nl.newsbank.com/nlsearch/we/Archives?p_action=doc&p_docid=115DC52C34F6A3B8 (accessed August 6, 2007).

———. Wayland City Police Department supplementary incident report, September 28, 1990.

Morlock, Jerry. "Mystery Still Clouds Deaths of Two Men." *Grand Rapids Press*, December 12, 1982.

Morlock, Jerry, and Arn Shackelford. "Why and How Young Rural Men Met Death Baffles Investigators." *Grand Rapids Press*, December 10, 1982.

Neerken, Rick. Personal interview with Tobin T. Buhk, March 20, 2007.

Neil, Ron. Michigan Department of State Police supplemental incident report, December 13, 1990.

———. Personal interview with Tobin T. Buhk, August 16, 2006.

"News Copter Hit by Bullets in Standoff." Associated Press. *Grand Rapids Press*, September 2, 2001.

Newton, Michael. "All about Randy Kraft: Changeling." Court TV Crime Library. http://www.crimelibrary.com/serial_killers/predators/kraft/2.html (accessed October 23, 2006).

———. "All about Randy Kraft: Death Row." Court TV Crime Library. http://www.crimelibrary.com/serial_killers/predators/kraft/10.html (accessed October 23, 2006).

———. "All about Randy Kraft: Death Trip." Court TV Crime Library. http://www.crimelibrary.com/serial_killers/predators/kraft/4.html (accessed October 23, 2006).

———. "All about Randy Kraft: Hedonist." Court TV Crime Library. http://www.crimelibrary.com/serial_killers/predators/kraft/3.html (accessed October 23, 2006).

———. "All about Randy Kraft: Scorecard." Court TV Crime Library. http://www.crimelibrary.com/serial_killers/predators/kraft/8.html (accessed October 23, 2006).

———. "All about Randy Kraft: Task Force." Court TV Crime Library. http://www.crimelibrary.com/serial_killers/predators/kraft/5.html (accessed October 23, 2006).

O'Brien, Bill. "Clark Seeks Venue Change for Trial." *Traverse City Record-Eagle*. August 29, 1998. http://www.record-eagle.com/1999/clark/29venue.htm (accessed March 30, 2006).

———. "Clark House May Change into an Inn." *Traverse City Record-Eagle*. August 4, 1999. http://www.record-eagle.com/1999/aug/04clrkbb.htm.

Perlman, Lisa. "Woman's Talk of Killing Babies 'Naturally Flowed,' Sergeant Recalls." *Grand Rapids Press*, July 1, 1993.

*People v. Bauder*, 269 Mich. App. 174 (2005).

*People v. Datema*, 448 Mich. 585; 533 N.W. 2d 272 (1995).

*People v. Kraft*, in the Supreme Court of California, S013187, Super. Ct. No. C52776. http://www.lawrepository.com (accessed May 25, 2006).

*People v. Lange*, 251 Mich. App. 247; 650 N.W. 2d 691 (2002).

*People v. McSwain*, 259 Mich. App. 654 (2003).

*People v. Slade*, Mich. App. 238129 (2003), unpublished opinion. http://courtofappeals.mijud.net (accessed April 3, 2007).

*People v. Spencer* trial transcripts, volume III of IV; File No.: 91-8787-FH.

Pritchard, James. "Father Expected Standoff to End Badly." *Grand Rapids Press*, September 4, 2001.

———. "Police Gunfire Kills Second Man in Vandalia Standoff." *Grand Rapids Press*, September 4, 2001.

———. "Investigators Sift through Rubble, Backers Keep Up Protests at Farm." *Grand Rapids Press*, September 6, 2001.

Rademacher, Tom. "'I Would Have Been Next,' Says Estranged Wife of Death Suspect." *Grand Rapids Press*, April 14, 1985.

Rademacher, Tom, and John Sinkevics. "Jaguar Exhibit Never Received City Inspection." *Grand Rapids Press*, February 5, 1986.

——— . "Jaguar Came within 'a Leap' of Freedom." *Grand Rapids Press*, February 12, 1986.

Rademacher, Tom, and Elizabeth Slowik. "Body Found Buried in Concrete; 3 Held." *Grand Rapids Press*, April 5, 1985.

Raymer, Marjory. "Court Hearing for Clark Delayed." *Traverse City Record-Eagle*. May 27, 1998. http://www.record-eagle.com/news/clark/27nohear.htm (accessed March 30, 2006).

"Report Says Police, FBI Acted in Self-Defense in Fatal Farm Standoff." Associated Press. *Grand Rapids Press*, January 8, 2002.

Repper, Venus. Personal interview with Tobin T. Buhk, August 17, 2007.

Revere, C. T. "Mutilation Victim's Mom Says Son Wanted to Be Animator." *Grand Rapids Press*, May 4, 1996.

Rochester, Mark. "Hooker Is Found Guilty of Murdering 'John.'" *Grand Rapids Press*, October 29, 1988.

Roelofs, Ted. "Horror of Bizarre Killing Weighs Heavily on Residents." *Grand Rapids Press*, May 1, 1996.

———. "Suspect Suffers Hallucinations, Court Told." *Grand Rapids Press*, August 20, 1996.

———. "Locked Up 17 Years, Killer Seeks New Trial." *Grand Rapids Press*, May 23, 2002.

Rowe, Rod. "Son Says Father Is Murderer." *Goshen News*, March 20, 2002. http://www2.goshennews.com/news/files/2002/3/3-20-2002/news3.html (accessed August 1, 2007).

———. "Defense Offering Alibi to Murder." *Goshen News*, March 21, 2002. http://www2.goshennews.com/news/files/2002/3/3-21-2002/news1.html (accessed August 1, 2007).

———. "Jury Verdict Expected Today." *Goshen News*, March 22, 2002. http://www2.goshennews.com/news/files/2002/3/3-22-2002/news2.html (accessed August 1, 2007).

———. "Jury Finds Ralph 'Fred' Fisher Not Guilty of Murder." *Goshen News*, March 23, 2002. http://www2.goshennews.com/news/files/2002/3/3-23-2002/news1.html (accessed August 1, 2007).

Sauer, Norm, PhD. Biological profile for John Doe, June 10, 2002.

———. Personal interview with Tobin T. Buhk, September 27, 2006.

"Silent Witness Is Sentenced for Contempt." *Grand Rapids Press*, June 2, 1987.

Sloane, David. "Suspect Brought Back to Indiana." *Times Union* (Warsaw, IN), February 10, 2001.

———. "Vroman Receives 4-Year Sentence." *Times Union*, (Warsaw, IN), June 6, 2001.

Smith, Stacey. "Prosecutor Says Slade Partied until Arrest." *Traverse City Record-Eagle*, September 14, 2001. http://www.record-eagle.com/2001/sep/14slade.htm (accessed April 3, 2007).

———. "Witness: Barth Intended to End Ties with Slade." *Traverse City*

*Record-Eagle*, September 15, 2001. http://www.record-eagle.com/2001/sep/15sladet.htm (accessed April 3, 2007).

———. "Slade Tried to Revive Barth." *Traverse City Record-Eagle*, September 19, 2001. http://www.record-eagle.com/2001/sep/19slade.htm (accessed April 3, 2007).

———. "Slade's Home Familiar to Police." *Traverse City Record-Eagle*, September 20, 2001. http://www.record-eagle.com/2001/sep/20slade.htm (accessed April 3, 2007).

———. "Jurors Deliberate Slade Verdict." *Traverse City Record-Eagle*, September 21, 2001. http://www.record-eagle.com/2001/sep/21slade.htm (accessed April 3, 2007).

Smith, Stacey, and Cari Noga. "Wanted Man Arrested in Kingsley Store." *Traverse City Record-Eagle*, September 22, 2000. http://www.record-eagle.com/2000/sep/22kill.htm (accessed April 3, 2007).

"Sovereign Citizens Movement." Anti-Defamation League. http://www.adl.org/learn/Ext_US/SCM.asp?xpicked=4&item=20 (accessed July 20, 2006).

"Standoff Supporters Sue over Autopsy Files." Associated Press. *Grand Rapids Press*, January 22, 2002.

Storey, Ian. "Clark Declines Insanity Defense." *Traverse City Record-Eagle*, July 25, 1998. http://www.record-eagle.com/1999/clark/25clrk.htm (accessed March 30, 2006).

———. "Clark Attorney Wants Evidence Thrown Out." *Traverse City Record-Eagle*, September 6, 1998. http://www.record-eagle.com/news/clark/6thrown.htm (accessed March 30, 2006).

———. "Clark Trial." *Traverse City Record-Eagle*, September 17, 1998. http://www.record-eagle.com/news/clark/17clark.htm (accessed March 30, 2006).

———. "Clark's Arsenal Pricey, but Legal." *Traverse City Record-Eagle*, October 18, 1998. http://www.record-eagle.com/news/clark/18guns.htm (accessed March 30, 2006).

———. "Home of Accused Murderer up for Sale." *Traverse City Record-Eagle*, November 6, 1998. http://www.record-eagle.com/news/clark/6clarkj.htm (accessed March 30, 2006).

———. "Jury in John Clark's December Murder Trial Will Likely Be Sequestered, a First in Traverse City." *Traverse City Record-Eagle*,

November 6, 1998. http://www.record-eagle.com/news/clark/6clarkj.htm (accessed March 30, 2006).

———. "Clark: Shooting Was in Self-Defense: Prosecutor Argues Slaying of Police Sergeant Was Premeditated." *Grand Traverse Herald*, December 2, 1998. http://www.gtherald.com/news/clark/2clarktr.htm (accessed March 30, 2006).

———. "Clark Trial: Jury Gets a Look at Weapon's Cache." *Traverse City Record-Eagle*, December 6, 1998. http://www.record-eagle.com/news/clark/06clark.htm (accessed March 30, 2006).

———. "Jury Weighs Murder Case against Clark." *Traverse City Record-Eagle*, December 9, 1998. http://www.record-eagle.com/news/clark/9clarktr.htm (accessed March 30, 2006).

———. "Clark Faces Life Behind Bars." *Traverse City Record-Eagle*, December 10, 1998. http://www.record-eagle.com/news/clark/10clarkt.htm (accessed March 30, 2006).

———. "'I Hope You Rot in Prison.'" *Traverse City Record-Eagle*, January 16, 1999. http://www.record-eagle.com/news/clark/16clark.htm (accessed March 30, 2006).

———. "Slade Has Long History of Run-Ins with Law." *Traverse City Record-Eagle*, September 22, 2000. http://www.record-eagle.com/2000/sep/22sus.htm (accessed April 3, 2007).

———. "Slade to Face Open Murder." *Traverse City Record-Eagle*, April 13, 2001. http://www.record-eagle.com/2001/apr/13slade.htm (accessed April 3, 2007).

———. "How Events Unfolded in May of 1998." *Traverse City Record-Eagle*, May 11, 2003. http://www.record-eagle.com/2003/may/11finch2.htm (accessed March 22, 2006).

———. "Examiners Don't Agree." *Traverse City Record-Eagle*, February 1, 2004. http://www.record-eagle.com/2004/feb/01unger.htm (accessed April 3, 2007).

———. "Two Sought in Connection with Deaths." *Traverse City Record-Eagle*, May 20, 2004. http://www.record-eagle.com/2004/may/20slay.htm (accessed November 12, 2006).

———. "Police Believe Suspect Left State." *Traverse City Record-Eagle*, June 26, 2004. http://www.record-eagle.com/2004/jun/26onon.htm (accessed November 12, 2006).

———. "Suspicious Death: Preliminary Hearing for Mark Unger Begins."

*Traverse City Record-Eagle*, July 7, 2004. http://www.record-eagle.com/2004/jul/07unger.htm (accessed April 3, 2007).

———. "Defense Attorneys Challenge Expert Witness Appearance." *Traverse City Record-Eagle*, July 8, 2004. http://www.record-eagle.com/2004/jul/08unger.htm (accessed April 3, 2007).

———. "O'Non: I Was Just Defending Myself." *Traverse City Record-Eagle*, November 21, 2004. http://www.record-eagle .com/2004/nov/21onon.htm (accessed November 12, 2006).

———. "Alleged O'Non Helper Sought." *Traverse City Record-Eagle*, February 14, 2005. http://www.record-eagle.com/2005/feb/14onon.htm (accessed November 12, 2006).

———. "O'Non Trial Slated to Start Today." *Traverse City Record-Eagle*, March 1, 2005. http://www.record-eagle.com/2005/mar/01onon.htm (accessed November 12, 2006).

———. "Doctor Testifies about Victims' Injuries. *Traverse City Record-Eagle*, March 9, 2005. http://www.record-eagle.com/2005/mar/09onon.htm (accessed November 12, 2006).

———. "3 More Refuse to Testify in O'Non Trial." *Traverse City Record-Eagle*, March 10, 2005. http://www.record-eagle.com/2005/mar/10onon.htm (accessed November 12, 2006).

———. "O'Non Takes Stand: 'I Was Shot at First.'" *Traverse City Record-Eagle*, March 11, 2005. http://www.record-eagle.com/2005/mar/11onon.htm (accessed November 12, 2006).

———. "Former Girlfriend Testifies to Plans." *Traverse City Record-Eagle*, March 16, 2005. http://www.record-eagle.com/2005/mar/16onon.htm (accessed November 12, 2006).

———. "O'Non Guilty of Murder." *Traverse City Record-Eagle*, March 17, 2005. http://www.record-eagle.com/2005/mar/17onon.htm (accessed November 12, 2006).

———. "O'Non Sentenced to Life in Prison." *Traverse City Record-Eagle*, April 26, 2005. http://www.record-eagle.com/2005/apr/26onon.htm (accessed November 12, 2006).

———. "Divorce Papers Preceded Death." *Traverse City Record-Eagle*, May 6, 2006. http://www.record-eagle.com/2006/may/06unger.htm (accessed April 3, 2007).

———. "Witnesses Recount Unger's Financial Woes." *Traverse City*

*Record-Eagle*, May 11, 2006. http://www.record-eagle.com/2006/may/11unger.htm (accessed April 3, 2007).

———. "Jurors See Photos of Death Scene." *Traverse City Record-Eagle*, May 12, 2006. http://www.record-eagle.com/2006/may/12unger.htm (accessed April 3, 2007).

———. "Medical Examiner Defends Homicide Ruling." *Traverse City Record-Eagle*, May 13, 2006. http://www.record-eagle.com/2006/may/13unger.htm (accessed April 3, 2007).

———. "Woman Testifies of Finding Body at Resort." *Traverse City Record-Eagle*, May 18, 2006. http://www.record-eagle.com/2006/may/18unger.htm (accessed April 3, 2007).

———. "Man Gets Jail for Tampering: Killer's Dad Admitted Trying to Sway Case." *Traverse City Record-Eagle*, July 5, 2006. http://www.archives.record-eagle.com/2006/jul/06onon.htm (accessed December 5, 2007).

Sullivan, Patrick. "Doctor: Death No Accident." *Traverse City Record-Eagle*, September 9, 2004. http://www.record-eagle.com/2004/sept/09unger.htm (accessed April 3, 2007).

Sypert, Tracy L. "Settlement in Death of Zoo Employee Totals $1.9 Million." *Grand Rapids Press*, March 5, 1987.

———. "Fate of Graham in Deaths of Elderly." *Grand Rapids Press*, September 20, 1989.

———. "Killing Story Too Real to Be False: Jurors." *Grand Rapids Press*, September 21, 1989.

"Target 8 Investigation Uncovers New Information about Deadly Standoff in Fremont." *Wood TV*. http://www.woodtv.com/global/story.asp?s=1892048&ClientType=Printable (accessed June 6, 2006).

"Testimony Focuses on Paint Chips." *Traverse City Record-Eagle*, May 26, 2006. http://www.record-eagle.com/2006/may/26unger.htm (accessed April 3, 2007).

Thyng, Michael. Telephone interview with Tobin T. Buhk, August 25, 2007.

Tunison, John. "A Lonely End." *Grand Rapids Press*, September 21, 2002.

———. "Body Not That of Missing Macomb Woman; Mystery Remains." *Grand Rapids Press*, April 1, 2004.

———. "Conference Helped Police Solve Mystery: Experts Confirmed Theory Body Floated from Wisconsin to Pigeon Lake." *Grand Rapids Press*, October 26, 2004.

———. "Unsolved Mystery: Police Still Trying to Identify Body Found in Lake Nine Months Ago." *Grand Rapids Press*, December 29, 2004.

Verburg, Steven. "Jaguar That Killed Keeper Finds Home in California." *Grand Rapids Press*, May 4, 1986.

"Vroman Charged in New York." *Times-Union* (Warsaw, IN), February 2, 2001.

Wertz, Rich. "Man Charged with Open Murder in Shooting of Police Officer." *Traverse City Record-Eagle*, May 14, 1998. http://www.record-eagle.com/news/clark/14seige.htm (accessed March 30, 2006).

———. "Investigators Find Explosives in House: Bomb-Sniffing Dogs Missed Explosives Earlier Because of Clutter in John Clark's Home." *Traverse City Record-Eagle*, May 16, 1998. http://www.record-eagle.com/news/clark/16evac.htm (accessed March 30, 2006).

Wertz, Rich, and Bill O'Brien. "Gunman Kills TC Officer." *Traverse City Record-Eagle*, May 13, 1998. http://www.record-eagle.com/news/clark/13shoot.htm (accessed March 30, 2006).

West, Peg. "Cruz Bound Over for Trial in Murder, Beheading Case." *Grand Rapids Press*, May 14, 1996.

———. "Slaying Victim Remembered for His Life." *Grand Rapids Press*, December 7, 1997.

———. "Prosecutor Warns of Grisly Video." *Grand Rapids Press*, December 9, 1997.

———. "Witness Tells Jurors He Viewed Severed Head." *Grand Rapids Press*, December 10, 1997.

———. "Head Was Severed as Trophy, Cop Says." *Grand Rapids Press*, December 11, 1997.

———. "Beheading Trial Turns to Suspect's Sanity." *Grand Rapids Press*, December 15, 1997.

———. "Demons Controlled Beheading Suspect, Court Told." *Grand Rapids Press*, December 16, 1997.

———. "Prosecution May Play Audio Portion of Gruesome Beheading Tape." *Grand Rapids Press*, December 17, 1997.

———. "Prosecutors Play Tape to Counter Cruz Defense." *Grand Rapids Press*, December 18, 1997.

———. "Victim's Mother Finds No Forgiveness for Cruz." *Grand Rapids Press*, December 19, 1997.

———. "Teen Guilty in Beheading Gets Life Term." *Grand Rapids Press*, December 29, 1997.

———. "Slaying Victim's Mom Knows Son Is with God." *Grand Rapids Press*, December 31, 1997.

Wilkins, Korie. "Man Charged in Death of His Estranged Wife." *Daily Oakland Press*, May 20, 2004. http://theoaklandpress.com/stories/052004/pol_20040520073.shtml (accessed April 3, 2007).

Wishnia, Steven. "End of the Rainbow." http://user.aol.com/station019/farmend.htm (accessed April 3, 2007).

Witsil, Frank. "Unger Jury to Visit Site of Death Today." *Detroit Free Press*, May 3, 2006.

# acknowledgments

For their help in the creation of this work, the authors wish to thank the following:

Members of the Kent County medical examiner's staff for their assistance in providing information about the cases discussed in the text, case files, autopsy reports, and photographs: administrative assistants Sue Atwood and Jodi Patton; autopsy assistants and death scene investigators Paul Davison, Jason Chatman, Joel Talsma, and, in particular for her help in processing images and taking the author photograph that appears on the back cover, morgue assistant Lindsey Bonner. Since autopsies provide the focal point of the cases discussed, the Kent County medical examiner's office provided vital assistance to which this work owes its life.

For lending their expertise to this work, the authors also wish to thank the following: for information about forensic odontology and its application to various cases, Roger Erbaugh, DDS; for information about DID and Munchausen by proxy syndrome, Kerry C. Buhk, PhD; for an inside look at a forensics anthropology laboratory and the application of anthropology to criminal cases, professor of physical anthropology at Michigan State University and forensic anthropologist Norm Sauer, PhD.

For sharing their experiences and knowledge, the authors wish to thank members of various law enforcement agencies, including local, state, and federal law enforcement; for information about the Keith Prong and Diane Spencer investigations, Michigan state police detective sergeant (retired) Ron Neil; for information about the Diane Spencer investigation, including providing access to key evidence and court records, Wayland police chief Dan Miller; for information about the Barbara Biehn investigation, Michigan state police cold case detective Dave Eddy and Ottawa County detective Dave Blakely; for demonstrating the use of forensic art, Michigan state police trooper Fernando Martinez; for information about the John Doe and Barbara Biehn cases, Ottawa County detectives Venus Repper and Robert Donker. For information about the Nancy Bass* murder, City of Grandville police officer Rick Neerken. For crime scene photographs from the John Doe case, the Ottawa County sheriff's department. For information about the Kathy Vroman case, Michigan state trooper Michael Thyng.

For the use of the photograph of the jaguar skull on the hospital volunteer's neck, Wolters Kluwer. The photograph originally appeared in the following publication: Stephen D. Cohle, MD, Charles W. Harlan, MD, and Gretel Harlan, MD, "Fatal Big Cat Attacks," *American Journal of Forensic Medicine and Pathology* 11, no. 3 (1990): 208–12.

At Prometheus Books, we'd like to thank Grace M. Conti-Zilsberger, Steven L. Mitchell, and Joe Gramlich.

For navigating the sometimes turbulent waters of the world of publishing, our literary agent Mike Hamilburg, of the Mitchell J. Hamilburg Agency in Los Angeles, California, and his assistant Joanie Kern.

And last but not least, the authors would like to thank their families for their loving support.

# index

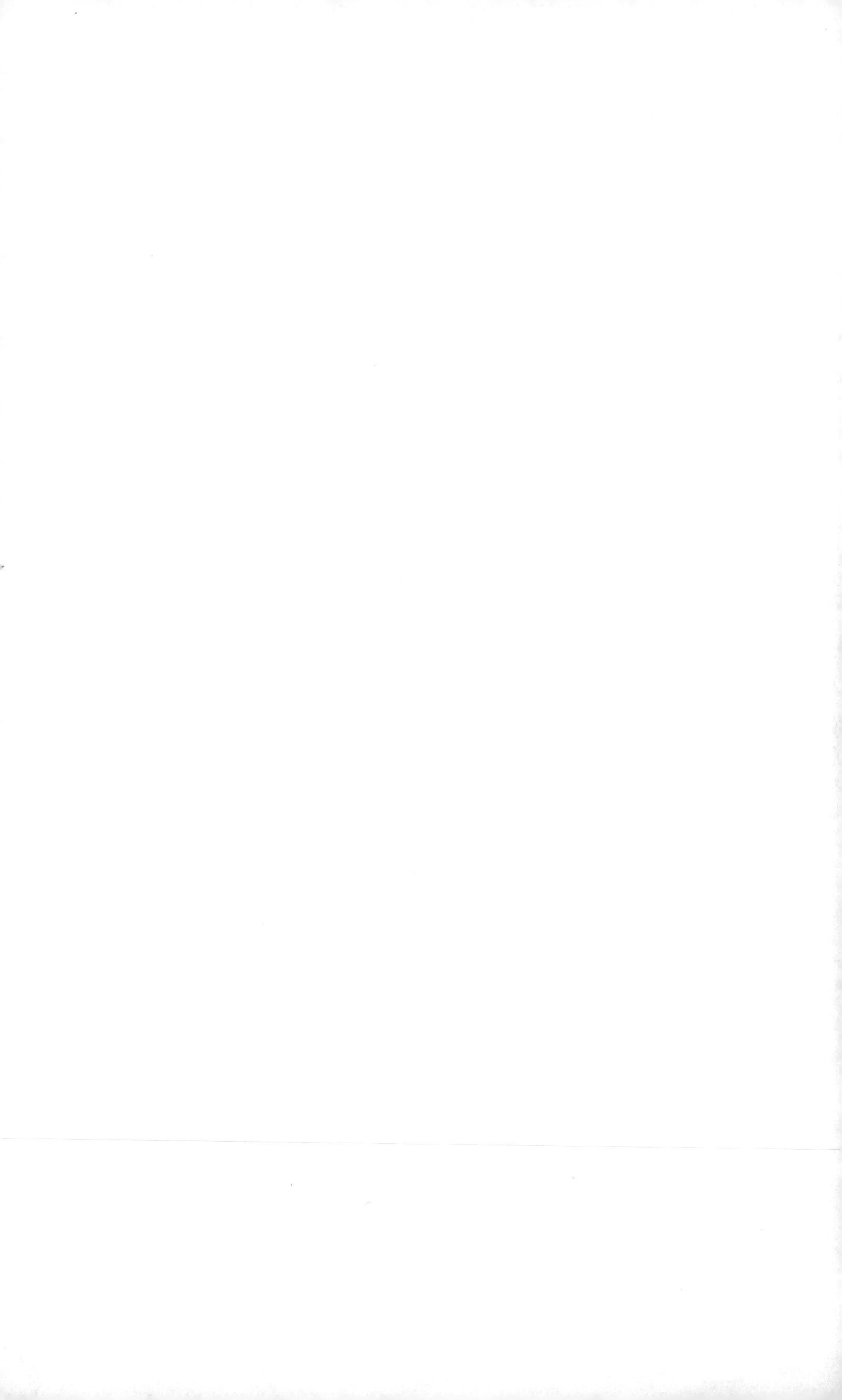